HEALTH SERVICE GOVERNANCE

ICSA STUDY TEXT

HEALTH SERVICE GOVERNANCE

CLAIRE LEA

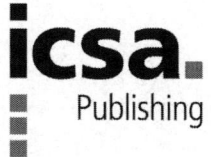

First published 2012

Published by ICSA Information & Training Ltd
16 Park Crescent
London W1B 1AH

© ICSA Information & Training Ltd, 2012

The author and publisher would like to acknowledge and thank Brian Coyle, author of the ICSA study text, *Corporate Governance*, extracts from which are included in this text.

All rights reserved. No part of this publication may be reproduced, stored in a retrieval system, or transmitted, in any form, or by any means, electronic, mechanical, photocopying, recording or otherwise, without prior permission, in writing, from the publisher.

Designed and typeset by
Florence Production Ltd, Stoodleigh, Devon
Printed by
Hobbs the Printers Ltd, Totten Hampshire

British Cataloguing in Publication Data
A catalogue record for this book is available from the British Library.

ISBN 978 1 860 725036

Contents

How to use this study text viii
Health Service Governance syllabus xi
Acronyms and abbreviations xvii
Acknowledgements xix

PART ONE: The governance landscape 1

Chapter 1 Definitions and issues in governance 3
  1 Defining the NHS 3
  2 Defining governance 4
  3 Principles of good corporate governance 8
  4 Key issues in governance 10
  5 A brief history of corporate governance 15
  6 Governance in the public sector 18
  7 Arguments for and against governance regimes 21
  8 Governance and the voluntary sector 22

Chapter 2 The NHS landscape 26
  1 History and context 26
  2 Principles and values of the NHS 27
  3 Rights and pledges provided by the constitution 28
  4 Statement of NHS accountability 31
  5 Other NHS bodies 34
  6 Relationships with stakeholders and local accountability 35
  7 Health and Social Care (HSC) Act 2012 36

Chapter 3 Governance, the law and the company secretary 41
  1 Governance and the law 41
  2 UK healthcare law 42
  3 Company law and other legislation 49
  4 Compulsory regulation and voluntary best practice 51
  5 The role of the company secretary 53

PART TWO: General principles of health service governance 63

Chapter 4 Issues in health service governance 67
  1 Defining health service governance 67
  2 Consequences of poor health service governance 67
  3 Consequences of poor corporate governance 69
  4 Common themes in poor governance 70
  5 Theoretical frameworks 71
  6 Stakeholders 76
  7 Approaches to governance 79

Contents

Chapter 5   The regulatory framework   83
    1   Voluntary frameworks for governance   83
    2   Codes for health service governance   85
    3   *UK Corporate Governance Code*   92
    4   Other codes   93
    5   Ethics and governance   94
    6   The reality of health service governance   97

Chapter 6   Governance of foundation trusts   99
    1   Foundation trusts overview   99
    2   Regulation   101
    3   Governance structures   103
    4   Membership   105
    5   Council of governors   106
    6   Elections   111
    7   Foundation Trust Network   112
    8   The future for foundation trusts   113
    9   The governance challenge   114

PART THREE: Health service governance in practice   121

Chapter 7   The board of directors   123
    1   Governance responsibilities of the board   123
    2   Board structures   126
    3   The powers of directors   128
    4   The duties of directors to their organisation   129
    5   The statutory duties of directors   133
    6   Liability of directors   136
    7   *NHS Code of Conduct and Accountability*   138
    8   Matters reserved for the board   139
    9   The roles of chairman and chief executive officer (CEO)   140
    10   Size and composition of the board   145
    11   Non-executive directors (NEDs)   147
    12   Senior independent directors (SIDs)   152
    13   Board committees and non-executive directors (NEDs)   153
    14   Effectiveness of non-executive directors (NEDs)   153

Chapter 8   Governance and boardroom practice   157
    1   Good boardroom practice   157
    2   Board behaviour   159
    3   Appointments to the board   162
    4   Nomination committees   165
    5   Succession planning   170
    6   Refreshing board membership   171
    7   Induction and training of directors   172
    8   Performance evaluation of the board   175
    9   Conflicts of interest   180
    10   Hospitality policy and registers   182

Chapter 9   Remuneration issues   187
    1   Remuneration as a governance issue   187

2 Principles of senior executive remuneration 193
3 Elements of remuneration for executive directors and other senior executives 195
4 The design of performance-related remuneration 196
5 The remuneration committee 198
6 The remuneration of non-executive directors (NEDs) 200
7 Compensation for loss of office 202
8 Disclosure of directors' remuneration details 203
9 Further guidance 205

Chapter 10 Reporting and the role of audit 209
1 Reporting and health service governance 209
2 Directors' duties and responsibilities for financial reporting 218
3 Relationship between internal and external audit 220
4 The role and responsibilities of external audit 223
5 The audit committee 231
6 Disclosure of governance arrangements 238
7 The business review 238

PART FOUR: Risk management and internal control 241

Chapter 11 Identifying operational and strategic risks 243
1 Risk management and governance 243
2 The nature of risk 245
3 Business risks and internal control risks 246
4 Responsibilities for risk management 247
5 Risk committees and risk managers 248
6 Risk management policies, systems and procedures 249

Chapter 12 Internal control systems 253
1 Elements of an internal control system 253
2 The UK corporate governance framework for internal control 259
3 The *Turnbull Guidance* on internal control 260
4 The Annual Governance Statement (AGS) (previously the SIC) 262
5 Internal audit 265
6 Emergency preparedness and business continuity 267
7 Whistleblowing procedures 269

Appendix 1 The UK Corporate Governance Code 275
Appendix 2 NHS Foundation Trust Code of Governance 292
Appendix 3 The Healthy NHS Board: principles for good governance 309
Appendix 4 FRC Guidance on Board Effectiveness 341
Appendix 5 FRC Guidance on Audit Committees 348
Appendix 6 Guidance on internal control (The Turnbull Guidance) 361

Glossary 368
Directory 377
Index 379

How to use this study text

ICSA study texts developed to support ICSA's Chartered Secretaries Qualifying Scheme (CSQS) follow a standard format and include a range of navigational, self-testing and illustrative features to help you get the most out of the support materials.

Each text is divided into three main sections:

- introductory material
- the text itself, divided into Parts and Chapters
- additional reference information

The sections below show you how to find your way around the text and make the most of its features.

Introductory material

The introductory section of each text includes a full contents list and the module syllabus, which reiterates the module aims, learning outcomes and syllabus content for the module in question.

Where relevant, the introductory section will also include a list of acronyms and abbreviations or a list of legal cases for reference.

The text itself

Each **part** opens with a list of the chapters to follow, an overview of what will be covered and learning outcomes for the part. Part openings also include a case study, which introduces a real-world scenario related to the topics covered in that part. Questions based on this case and designed to test the application of theory into practice appear in the chapters and at part endings (see below).

Every **chapter** opens with a list of the topics covered and an introduction specific to that chapter. Chapters are structured to allow students to break the content down into manageable sections for study. Each chapter ends with a summary of key content to reinforce understanding.

Part opening
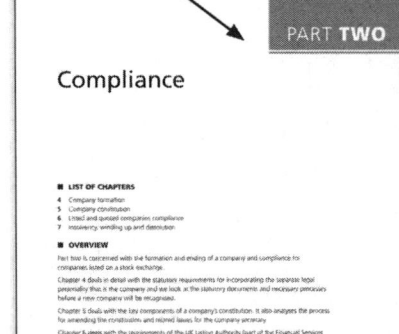

Chapter opening
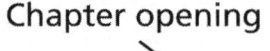
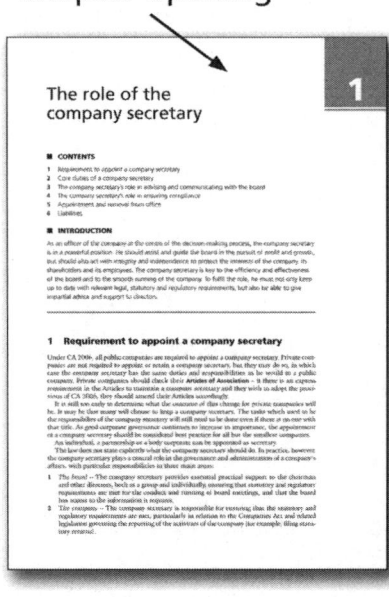

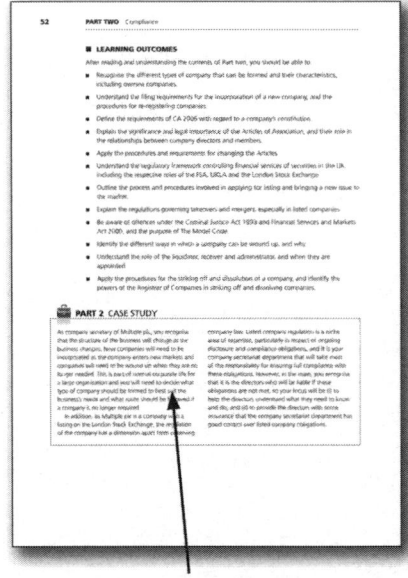
Part case study

Features

The text is enhanced by a range of illustrative and self-testing features to assist understanding and to help you prepare for the examination. Each feature is presented in a standard format, so that you will become familiar with how to use them in your study.

The texts also include tables, figures and checklists and, where relevant, sample documents and forms.

Case Examples

Case examples present short, illustrative case studies which look at how concepts are applied in practice.

Checklist

Sample wording

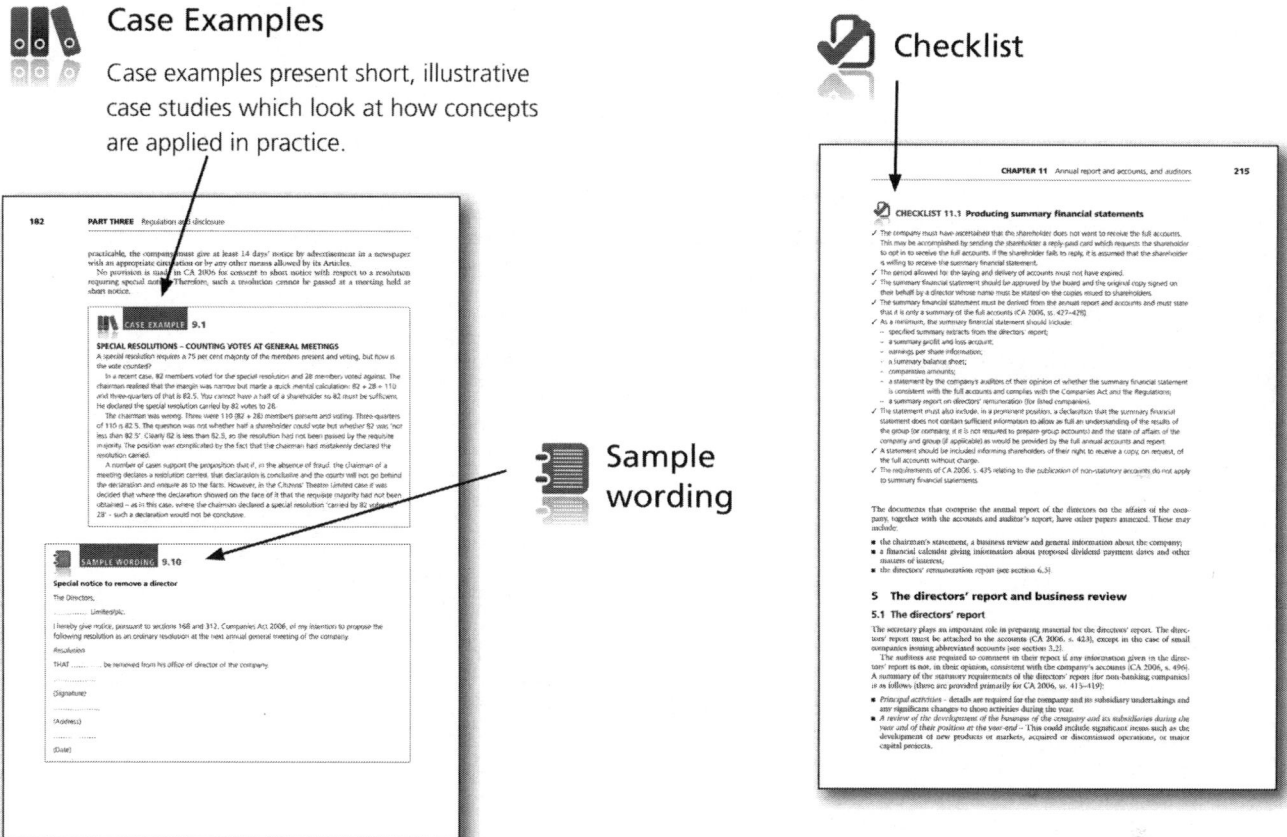

Case Law

Case law summaries provide overviews of significant legal cases.

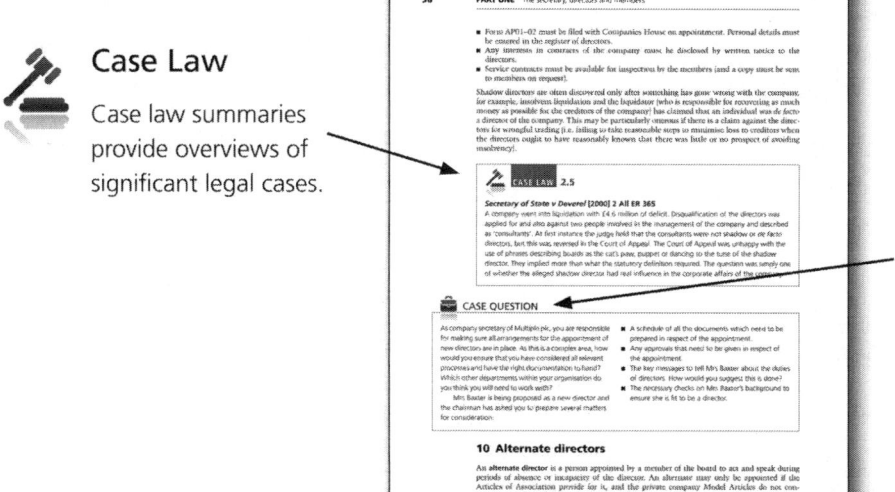

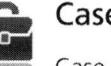

Case Questions

Case questions relate to the part opening case study, encouraging you to apply the theory you're learning to a real-world business scenario.

How to use this study text

Definitions
Key terms are highlighted in bold on first use and defined in the end of book glossary.

Stop and Think
Stop and think boxes encourage you to reflect on how your own experiences or common business scenarios relate to the topic under discussion.

Test your Knowledge
Short, revision-style questions to help you re-cap on key information and core concepts.

Part case questions

Glossary

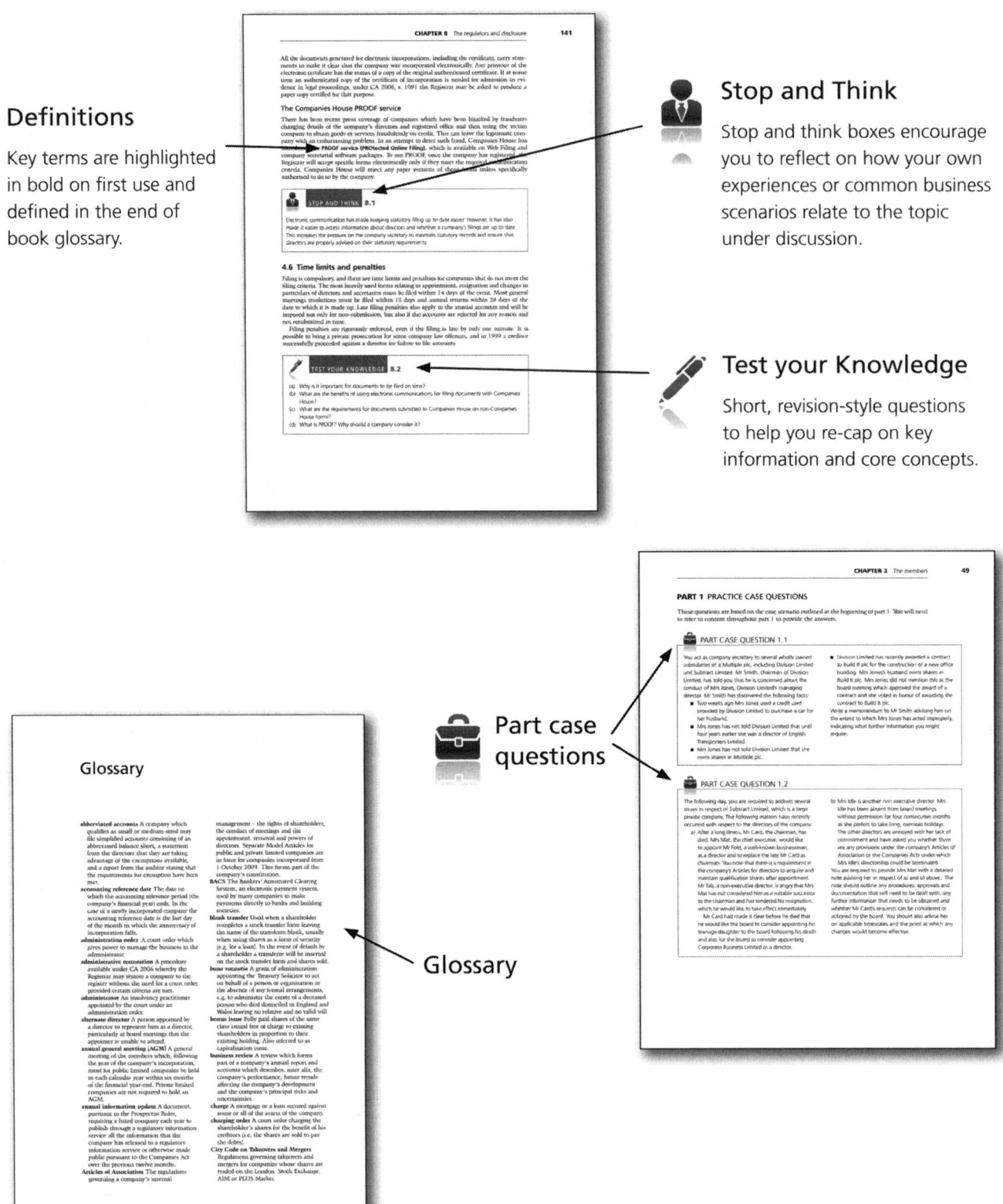

Reference material

The text ends with a range of additional guidance and reference material. Most texts will include Appendices, which comprise additional reference material specific to that module.

Other reference material includes a glossary of key terms, a directory of further reading and web resources and a comprehensive index.

Health Service Governance syllabus

Module outline and aims

The aim of the Health Service Governance module is to equip the company secretary with the knowledge and key skills necessary to act as adviser to governing bodies across the NHS in England. The advice of the company secretary will include all aspects of the governance obligations of NHS organisations in England, covering not only legal duties, but also applicable and recommended standards of best practice.

The module enables the development of a sound understanding of health service governance principles and practices in the NHS in England. It will also enable you to support the development of good governance and stakeholder dialogue throughout the organisation, being aware of legal obligations and best practice.

Learning outcomes

On successful completion of this module, you will be able to:

- Appraise the frameworks underlying governance law and practice as they apply to the NHS in England.
- Distinguish between and compare the legal obligations for governance and recommended best practice.
- Advise on governance issues across all principal types of NHS organisation, ensuring that the pursuit of strategic objectives is in line with regulatory developments and developments in best practice.
- Analyse and evaluate situations in which governance problems arise and provide recommendations for solutions.
- Demonstrate how general concepts of governance apply in a given situation or given circumstances.
- From the perspective of a company secretary, provide authoritative and professional advice on matters of health service governance.
- Assess the relationship between governance and performance within organisations.
- Apply the principles of risk management and appraise the significance of risk management for good governance.
- Compare the responsibilities of NHS organisations to different stakeholder groups, and advise on issues of ethical conduct and the application of principles of corporate responsibility or corporate citizenship.

Syllabus content

History and development of governance – weighting 15%

General overview of the NHS and its reporting lines.

Timeline for key Corporate Governance developments and general overview of their impact on the NHS

Overview of latest developments

General principles of health service governance – weighting 20%

Candidates are expected to demonstrate an awareness of all areas of health service governance, and to be able to review common themes. They will be able to understand the scope of health service governance, the various issues with which such governance is concerned, and how these issues relate to each other. While emphasis will be placed on the application of health service governance in the NHS in England, due regard will also be given to areas of corporate governance and their relevance to the NHS in England.

Meaning of health service governance

- Difference between governance and management
- Purpose of good governance

Key theories and models of governance

- Agency theory, transaction cost theory
- Stakeholder value approach, enlightened stakeholder approach, stakeholder approach

Governance, risk and financial stability

- The balancing of conflicting objectives

Potential consequences of poor governance

- Business failure and the contribution of poor governance

Governance and ethics, corporate ethics, corporate codes of ethics, professional ethics as applied in the NHS in England

Key issues in governance

- Role and composition of the board, remuneration of directors and senior executives, accounting and audit, relations with stakeholders

Applying best practice in governance: voluntary and regulatory approaches, rules or principles, concept of 'comply or explain'

Governance problems for group structures

Governance issues in the public sector

- Nolan Principles

Governance issues in the voluntary sector (charities)

Specific guidance and requirements for NHS charities, including Financial Reporting.

Overview of other relevant governance issues, including quality, finances and PFI scheme.

Legal and regulatory aspects of governance

This section focuses on the legal and regulatory measures on governance in the NHS in England.

Governance aspects of relevant Acts and regulations, especially Health Acts and the Companies Act 2006

- Statutory duties of directors, and the concepts of duty of care and skill and fiduciary duty on which these statutory duties are based
- An awareness of the requirements for reporting on directors' remuneration is required, but not the detailed regulations

EU Green Paper and competition law

Law relating to insolvency and regulations relating to assessment of going concern status.

Codes of corporate and health service governance practice and reports on governance

Candidates will be expected to demonstrate an awareness of the prominent codes or reports on governance and to be aware of current developments, such as when these codes or reports are being reviewed or re-drafted.

- UK Corporate Governance Code
- Monitor Code of Governance for NHS foundation trusts
- The Healthy NHS board
- For future reference: other Clinical Commissioning Group publications on consortia.

Role of the company secretary

Role of the company secretary in the identification of governance issues, and the application of governance rules and principles in practice.

Comparison of the governance role of the company secretary and the role of the legal team, whether legal services are available 'in-house' or externally procured.

The application of governance rules and principles – weighting 45%

Candidates will be required to discuss in detail statutory rules and the principles or provisions of governance codes, and apply them to specific situations or case studies. Candidates will also be expected to understand the role of the company secretary in providing support and advice regarding the application of best governance practice in the NHS in England.

The broad areas that will be examined are as follows:

The board of directors or governing council

Role of the board and the role of the Council of Governors and their respective governance responsibilities.

Unitary and two-tier boards

- Boards of directors
- NHS foundation trust boards of governance

Matters reserved for the board

- Department of Health guidelines
- For future reference: other ICSA guidance

Roles of the chairman, chief executive officer and accountable officer

Size, structure and composition of the board: board balance, independence

Independent non-executive directors

- Functions of the independent NED

Good boardroom practice

- Responsibilities of the chairman and company secretary

Appointments to the board: nominations committee, council of governors

- Contribution of the nominations committee to good governance
- Higgs Guidance on duties of the nomination committee
- Tyson Report

Information and professional development for board members

- Induction and ongoing training
- Role of the company secretary in the efficient provision of information
- Directors and external professional advice
- For future reference: Governor advisory panel

Effectiveness of the board, its committees and individual board members. Performance evaluation of the board

- Monitor Code of Governance for NHS foundation trusts
- Annual performance evaluation of the board, its committees and individual directors

- Higgs Guidance on performance evaluation
- FRC *Guidance on Board Effectiveness*

Re-election of board members and Council of Governors

- Retirement by rotation

Boardroom ethics

- Link to statutory duties of directors and Council of Governors

Conflicts and declarations of interest

Liability of directors: directors' and officers' liability insurance

- The reasons for and nature of directors' liability

Personal interests of directors in transactions of their company or subsidiary companies

Independent and non-independent non-executive directors: their role and effectiveness

- Good practice suggestions from the Higgs Report
- Senior independent director: role
- Criticisms of the ineffectiveness of NEDs.

Remuneration of directors and senior executives

Principles of remuneration structure: elements of remuneration.

Remuneration policy

The design of performance-related remuneration

- Elements of a remuneration package
- Theories of performance-related pay and accountability
- Deciding a remuneration package for senior executives
- *For future reference: NHS Commissioning Board guidance on pay*

Role of the remuneration committee

- Higgs Guidance on role of the remuneration committee
- Code of Governance for NHS Foundation Trusts

Compensation for loss of office

Disclosures of directors' remuneration

- Candidates will be expected to show an awareness of issues relating to the disclosure of directors' remuneration in the annual report and accounts, but not the detail (e.g. not the detail of the directors' remuneration report).

Reporting to stakeholders and external audit

Financial reporting, going concern status (review of future solvency): responsibilities of the board, executive management and the external auditors.

- The need for reliable financial reporting: true and fair view
- The nature of the going concern statement and its relevance for governance
- Directors' responsibility for the financial statements
- Responsibility of the external auditors
- Responsibility for the discovery of fraud

Role of the audit committee: the audit committee and the external auditors

- Composition of the committee and skills of committee members
- Department of Health and Monitor guidance
- *For future reference: NHS Commissioning Board guidance*

Independence of the external auditors

- The significance of auditor independence: threats to auditor independence
- Auditors and non-audit work

Principles of reporting requirements for good governance: accountability, transparency

- The meaning of accountability
- The meaning of transparency
- Balancing statutory and mandatory reporting requirements with meaningful engagement with stakeholders

Disclosures of governance arrangements

Reporting non-financial information: business review or operating and financial review

- The significance of narrative reporting for better governance.

Relations with stakeholders

The equitable treatment of stakeholders.

- The meaning of equitable treatment: examples of inequitable treatment

Rights and powers of stakeholders

Dialogue and communications with major stakeholders – achieving meaningful engagement

Constructive use of the annual general meeting

Risk management and internal control – weighting 20%

Candidates will be able to discuss aspects of risk facing an organisation, and to comment and advise on the systems in place for the identification and assessment of risks, the management of risk and monitoring the effectiveness of risk management and internal control systems.

The nature of risks facing NHS organisations in England: categories of risk

- The difference between 'business risk' and 'governance risk' (internal control risk); strategic risk and operational risk; and clinical risk and non-clinical risk

Risk tolerance levels: risk and return, risk appetite

Responsibilities for risk management and internal control: board of directors, executive management, audit committee, internal and external auditors

- Risk management committees in NHS organisations (with reference to Department of Health guidance on controls assurance, 1999)

Risk management policies, systems and procedures

Risks in the business environment

- The implications of business risk and strategy selection for governance: a general understanding only is required

Internal control risks: financial, operational and compliance risks

Elements of an internal control system

- The Turnbull Guidance and subsequent reviews of this guidance
- The Department of Health guidance on controls assurance in the NHS in England

Function, scope and status of internal audit and internal auditors: independence of the internal auditors: the need for internal audit

- Role of internal audit within an internal control system
- Standards for internal audit in the NHS in England

Identifying key risk areas: key performance indicators

Disaster recovery and business continuity plans

Whistle-blowing policy and procedures
- ICSA best practice on whistle-blowing procedures
- *For future reference: NHS constitution and supporting guidance*

Reviewing and reporting on the effectiveness of the risk management system

Reviewing and reporting on the effectiveness of the internal control system
- UK Corporate Governance Code requirements, Turnbull guidelines and subsequent reviews of this guidance
- Monitor Governance Code for NHS foundation trusts requirements.

Acronyms and abbreviations

ABI	Association of British Insurers
ACCA	Association of Chartered Certified Accountants
AGM	annual general meeting
AGS	annual governance statement
AHAs	area health authorities
BAF	Board Assurance Framework
CACG	Commonwealth Association for Corporate Governance
CBC	Community Based Care organisation
CCA	Civil Contingencies Act 2004
CEO	Chief executive officer
CCGs	Clinical Commissioning Groups
CFO	chief financial officer
CFSMS	Counter Fraud and Security Management Service – now called NHS Protect
CHAI	Commission for Healthcare Audit and Inspection
CHI	Commission for Health Improvement
CIPFA	Chartered Institute of Public Finance and Accountancy
COSO	Committee of Sponsoring Organizations
CQC	Care Quality Commission
CQUINs	Commissioning for Quality Improvement
CRO	chief risk officer
CSR	corporate social responsibility
DH	Department of Health
DHAs	District health authorities
DTR	Disclosure Rules and Transparency Rules
EPLO	Emergency Planning Liaison Officer
EU	European Union
FOIA	Freedom of Information Act
FPCs	family practitioner committees
FRAB	Financial Reporting Advisory Board
FRC	Financial Reporting Council
FReM	*Financial Reporting Manual*
FSA	Financial Services Authority
FT	foundation trust
FTN	Foundation Trust Network
HPA	Health Protection Agency
HSC	Health and Social Care
IBE	Institute of Business Ethics
ICAEW	Institute of Chartered Accountants in England and Wales
ICGN	International Corporate Governance Network
IFAC	International Federation of Accountants
LINks	Local Involvement Networks
LLA	liability limitation agreement
NAO	National Audit Office
NAPF	National Association of Pension Funds
NCVO	National Council of Voluntary Organisations
NDPBs	non-departmental public bodies
NEDs	non-executive directors
NHS	National Health Service
NHSCB	NHS Commissioning Board
NHS FT ARM	*NHS Foundation Trust Annual Reporting Manual*

NICE	National Institute of Clinical Excellence
NSFs	National Service Frameworks
NYSE	New York Stock Exchange
OECD	Organisation for Economic Co-operation and Development
OF	Operating Framework
OPM	Office for Public Management
OSC	Overview and Scrutiny Committee
PCT	primary care trust
PFI	Private Finance Initiative
PPI	Patient and Public Involvement
PROMs	patient reported outcome measures
RHA	Regional Health Authority
SEC	Securities and Exchange Commission
SHAs	strategic health authorities
SIC	Statement on Internal Control
SID	senior independent director
Solace	Society of Local Authority Chief Executives and Senior Managers
SOX	Sarbanes-Oxley Act
TITO	time in/time out sessions
TSR	total shareholder return
VFM	Value for money
VSM	Very Senior Managers

Acknowledgements

The publishers would like to thank the following organisations for permission to reproduce the following material:

Appendix 2 and Figure 10.1

The NHS Foundation Trust Code and Figure 10.1, Annual Planning and Monitoring Cycle are reproduced with kind permission of Monitor © Monitor, 2010.

Appendix 1 and Appendices 4–6

The UK Corporate Governance Code, The FRC Guidance on Board Effectiveness, The FRC Guidance on Audit Committees and The Guidance on Internal Control are © FRC and adapted and reproduced with the kind permission of the Financial Reporting Council. All rights reserved. For further information see www.frc.org.uk or call +44 (0)20 7492 2300.

Every effort has been made to locate and acknowledge sources and holders of copyright material in this study text. In the event that any have been inadvertently overlooked, please contact the publisher.

PART **ONE**

The governance landscape

■ LIST OF CHAPTERS

1   Definitions and issues in governance
2   The NHS landscape
3   Governance, the law and the company secretary

■ OVERVIEW

The term 'governance' is commonly used, but it is often hard to define exactly what it means and what its objectives should be. To ensure clarity throughout this text certain terms need to be understood to have a defined meaning. These definitions may be somewhat false in a general sense and outside of this text may well be used interchangeably. Adhering to these definitions within the purposes of this study text will, however, enable the reader to distinguish between different landscapes in which governance needs to be understood.

The defined meanings are as follows.

- **Corporate governance:** the governance applied to the corporate commercial business world, including public and private companies.
- **Health service governance:** the governance applied to NHS organisations.
- **Public sector governance:** the governance applied across the wider public sector including the NHS.
- **Governance:** this term will be used to refer to the concepts of governance, which are generally applicable regardless of landscape.

This text focuses on the aspects of health service governance that are concerned with the practices and procedures for ensuring that the individual parts of the National Health Service (NHS) are run in such a way that they achieve their objectives and are in line with public sector values such as value for money (VFM) and providing universal and free healthcare benefits to all those in need. Health service governance can be defined as a process for monitoring and control to ensure that management runs the organisation in the interests of those stakeholders, which, quite rightly will also include the Department of Health (DH) as well as patients and employees. This is an interesting contrast to the objectives of a company in the private sector that may decide to maximise the wealth of its owners (the shareholders), subject to various guidelines and constraints and with regard to other groups or individuals with an interest in what the company does.

Health service governance operates on two levels: first, the manner in which the government department (DH) is held to account by the electorate for the way in which it manages the provision of healthcare; and second, the way in which individual parts of the NHS are governed and to what purpose. This text focuses on the aspects of health service governance that are concerned with the practices and procedures for ensuring that the individual parts of the NHS are run in such a way that they achieve their objectives and are in line with public sector values such as VFM and providing universal and free healthcare benefits to all those in need.

The first part of this study text introduces the NHS, outlines the concepts of governance and their significance for the health service and for the wider corporate business world. It also highlights the particular nuances within the NHS and makes a direct contrast with the approaches taken by corporate governance. It explores the role of the NHS Constitution in establishing health service governance and the implications of the Health and Social Care (HSC) Act 2012. It will also consider the legal aspects to governance and how the role of the company secretary is a vital part of the governance toolkit, helping to ensure that best practice and the law are followed.

Chapter 1 explains the nature and scope of the NHS and health service governance, the principles of good governance, and the voluntary and regulatory approaches that are used to apply best practice (i.e. the generally accepted best way of doing something) in corporate governance. A comparison of governance in the NHS, the wider public sector, the voluntary sector and the corporate commercial world will be made and the various codes of best practice that have developed will be explored.

Chapter 2 explains the nature and scope of the NHS Constitution, the principles and values that it codifies, and the rights and pledges that are made to patients and staff. The system of responsibility and accountability for making decisions in the NHS is explored and an outline of the changes under the HSC Act 2012 is given.

Chapter 3 considers the extent to which best practice in both health service governance and corporate governance is imposed on organisations by the law or other regulations. There are two different approaches to establishing a system of best practice in governance. One approach is to establish voluntary principles and guidelines, and invite (or expect) organisations to comply with them. A second approach is to establish laws and other regulations for governance that organisations must obey. In practice, many countries combine legal and regulatory requirements with voluntary principles and codes of conduct. The chapter concludes with an explanation of the role of the company secretary in applying best practice in governance, including complying with governance principles and provisions.

■ LEARNING OUTCOMES

Part One should enable you to:

- understand the specific dynamics that apply to health service governance within the NHS
- discuss the underlying differences between governance in the NHS and the wider corporate commercial world
- describe the key aspects of the NHS Constitution and their relevance to health service governance
- distinguish between and compare the legal obligations for governance and recommended best practice
- understand the changes being implemented by the HSC Act 2012
- discuss the role of the company secretary in providing authoritative, credible and professional advice on governance both within the NHS and the corporate commercial world.

Definitions and issues in governance

■ CONTENTS

1 Defining the NHS
2 Defining governance
3 Principles of good corporate governance
4 Key issues in governance
5 A brief history of corporate governance
6 Governance in the public sector
7 Arguments for and against governance regimes
8 Governance and the voluntary sector

■ INTRODUCTION

This chapter explains the nature and scope of the NHS and health service governance, the principles of good governance, and the voluntary and regulatory approaches that are used to apply best practice (i.e. the generally accepted best way of doing something) in governance. The chapter also compares governance in the NHS, the wider public sector, the voluntary sector and the corporate commercial world and explores the various codes of best practice that have developed.

1 Defining the NHS

The NHS is the shared name of three of the four publicly funded healthcare systems in the United Kingdom. They provide a comprehensive range of health services, the vast majority of which are free at the point of use to residents of the United Kingdom.

The NHS in England was created by the NHS Act 1948, which actually created a NHS for both England and Wales. Responsibility for the NHS in Wales was passed to the Secretary of State for Wales in 1969, leaving the Secretary of State for Social Services responsible for the NHS in England alone. Only the English NHS is officially called the NHS, the others being NHS Scotland and NHS Wales. In Northern Ireland it is called Health and Social Care (HSC) rather than the NHS. Each system operates independently, and is politically accountable to the relevant government: the Scottish Government, Welsh Government, the Northern Ireland Executive or the UK Government (for the English NHS). While this study text specifically focuses on the NHS in England, any areas of significant difference for the other three UK healthcare systems will be highlighted.

Despite their separate funding and administration, there is no discrimination when a resident of one country of the United Kingdom requires treatment in another, although a patient will often be returned to their home area when they are fit to be moved. The financial and administrative consequences are dealt with by the organisations involved and no personal involvement by the patient is required.

The NHS in England has agreed a formal constitution which, in one document, lays down the objectives of the NHS, the rights and responsibilities of the various parties involved in healthcare in England (patients, staff, trust boards) and the guiding principles that govern the service. It was first published on 21 January 2009 as part of a ten-year plan to provide the highest quality of care and service for patients in England. Previously these rights and responsibilities had evolved in common law or through UK or European Union (EU) law, or were policy pledges by the NHS and government. These have now been written into the constitution.

In summary, the guiding principles of the NHS are as follows:

- The NHS provides a comprehensive service, available to all irrespective of age, gender, disability, race, sexual orientation, religion or belief, respecting their human rights.
- Access to NHS services is based on clinical need, not an individual's ability to pay (except in exceptional circumstances sanctioned by Parliament).
- The NHS aspires to the highest standards of excellence and professionalism to provide high quality care that is safe, effective and focused on the patient experience.
- NHS services must reflect the needs and preferences of patients, their families and their carers.
- The NHS works across organisational boundaries and in partnership with other organisations in the interest of patients, local communities and the wider population. The NHS is an integrated system of organisations and services bound together by the principles and values reflected in the constitution.

The DH is the government department responsible for policy in health and social care matters. It is also responsible for the NHS in England along with a few elements of the same matters that are not otherwise devolved to the Scottish, Welsh or Northern Irish governments. The DH then delegates powers to the various authorities and Boards that it has established to oversee and scrutinise the provision of healthcare. This structure will be altered radically in 2012/2013 by the HSC Act 2012. The impact of this legislation and the revised structure for the NHS is set out in Chapter 2.

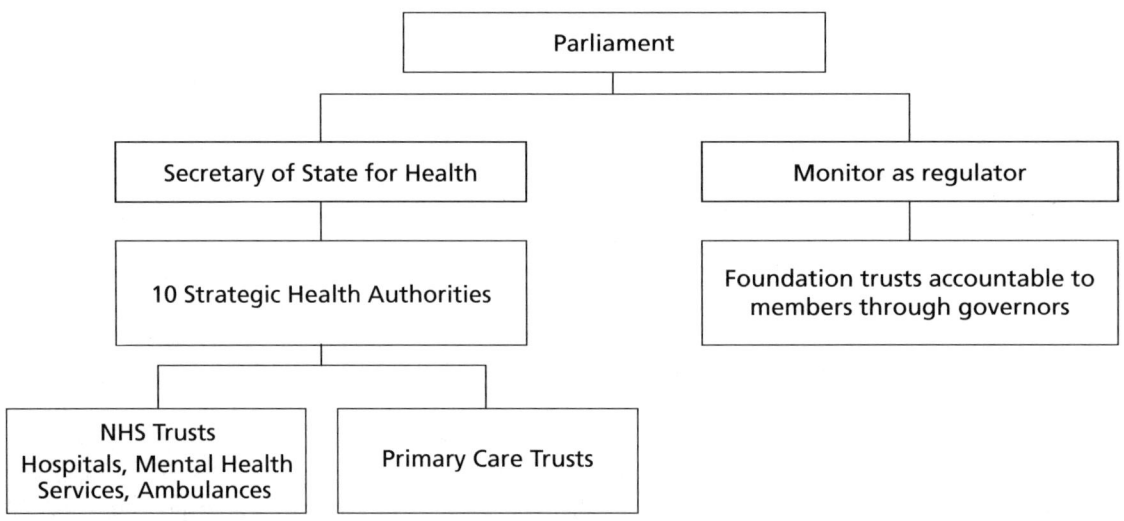

FIGURE 1.1 Structure of the NHS before the Health and Social Care Act 2012
(Source: www.nhshistory.net)

2 Defining governance

'Governance' refers to the way in which something is governed and to the function of governing. The governance of a country, for example, refers to the powers and actions of the legislative assembly, the executive government and the judiciary.

Health service governance operates on two levels: first, the manner in which the government department (DH) is held to account by the electorate for the way it manages the provision of healthcare; and second, the way in which individual parts of the NHS are governed and to what purpose. This study text is concerned with the latter of these two aspects of governance. It is concerned with the practices and procedures for trying to ensure that the individual parts of the NHS are run in such a way that they achieve their objectives and are in line with public sector values such as VFM and providing universal and free healthcare benefits to all those in need.

This provides an interesting contrast to the objectives of a company in the private sector, which may decide to maximise the wealth of its owners (the shareholders), subject to various guidelines and constraints and with regard to other groups or individuals with an interest in what the company does.

The study of governance within the NHS is complicated by the overuse of the term 'governance'. As the introduction has established, this text is concerned purely with health service governance, namely the practices and procedures for ensuring that the individual parts of the NHS are run in such a way that they achieve their objectives and are in line with public sector values such as VFM and providing universal and free healthcare benefits to all those in need. However, the role of the NHS company secretary is made more complex (and therefore potentially more interesting) by the way in which the term 'governance' is used so widely.

In the NHS there is quality governance, information governance, governance risk ratings for foundation trusts and board governance to name just a few. Health service governance as set out by this text is defined as the practices and procedures by which power is shared and exercised by the board of directors (and the council of governors in foundation trusts), and how the holders of power in the organisation should be held accountable for what they do. At times the text will refer to these other areas of governance to ensure that the breadth of the role of the NHS company secretary can be fully considered. Such references will specifically highlight the type of governance that is being referred to, e.g. quality governance.

Guidelines and constraints in both the public and private sector include behaving in an ethical way and in compliance with laws and regulations. Other groups with an interest in how an organisation acts include employees, customers, suppliers, the communities in which the organisation operates and the general public. Individuals, organisations or groups with an interest in how an organisation operates are called **stakeholders**. Health service governance can be defined as a process for monitoring and control to ensure that management runs the organisation in the interests of those stakeholders, which, quite rightly will also include the DH as well as patients and employees. The numerous stakeholders and the variety of their roles will be explored in Chapter 4.

By comparison companies in the private sector are mostly governed in accordance with the interests of the shareholders but it can be argued that they should also be governed in the interests of all its major stakeholders, not just its owners. This argument is particularly relevant to large companies whose activities have a big impact on the economy and society.

The work of Lord Hutton and the Commission on Ownership Report, *Plurality, Stewardship and Engagement*, published in March 2012, raises interesting questions about the responsibilities of companies to consider the interests of a wider group of stakeholders. The Commission was established following the recent banking crisis and the expenses scandal in government where the balancing interests has proven to be a key factor. Another recent example was that of the successful takeover of Cadbury by Kraft.

 CASE EXAMPLE 1.1

Kraft, the world's second-largest food maker with annual revenues of $42 billion, appealed directly to Cadbury's shareholders after the Cadbury's board rejected its proposal. Kraft stressed it was committed to working towards a recommended transaction and to maintaining a constructive dialogue. Cadbury put out a statement, confirming it had received an 'unsolicited' proposal from Kraft that was conditional on financing and due diligence. 'The board of Cadbury reviewed the proposal with its advisers and rejected it,' it said. 'The board is confident in Cadbury's standalone strategy and growth prospects as a result of its strong brands, unique category and geographic scope and the continued successful delivery of its Vision into Action plan. The board believes that the proposal fundamentally undervalues the group and its prospects.' However, the final offer proved to be too attractive for the shareholders and the board was required to act in their best interests even though the board did not believe the takeover was in the interests of a wider group of stakeholders.

Governance is not an easy concept to understand. In the case of governing a country, it would be concerned with who has the power to rule and what the governors of the country should be trying to achieve. The government of a democratic country presumably sets itself the objective of protecting its people and acting in their best interests, whatever these might be. Powers are shared between the legislative, executive and judiciary, but it is a matter of debate how these powers should be shared and exercised. In the UK, for example, there is healthy political debate about the respective powers of Parliament, the Prime Minister and the Cabinet, the UK law courts, and the powers of the government bodies and courts of the EU.

In the NHS, similar issues of governance arise. While corporate governance is concerned with how powers are shared and exercised by different groups, to ensure that the objectives of the organisation are achieved, health service governance is concerned with the rights to health provision for the general public, the political direction being given by the DH, and other interest groups such as employees, suppliers and the local community.

Corporate governance includes how powers are shared and exercised by the directors, and how the holders of power in the organisation should be held accountable for what they do. Both companies and NHS organisations are legal entities or 'legal persons' established according to statutory obligations such as the Companies Act or Health and Social Care Act legislation. As a person, they are able to enter into contracts and make business transactions. They can own assets and owe money to others, and they can sue and be sued in law. However, although it is a legal person, decisions about what the company or organisation should do are taken by individuals in the company or organisation's name.

- Just as a country has citizens, a company has members. The members of a company are its owners, the 'equity' shareholders. The membership of large companies changes constantly, as investors buy and sell the company's shares.
- The citizens of a country, even in a democracy, have relatively few powers. Power is in the hands of the legislative (Parliament) and the executive (the government). Similarly, shareholders have relatively few powers, and these are restricted mainly to certain voting rights. Power is in the hands of the board of directors, or perhaps just one or two individual directors on the board.
- For large companies, the main issue with corporate governance is the relationship between the board of directors and the shareholders, and the way in which the board exercises its powers. The relationship between the shareholders and the board can be described as a 'principal–agent' relationship. In some companies other stakeholders may have significant influence.

Principles of corporate governance are based on the view that a company should be governed in the interests of the shareholders, and possibly also in the interests of other stakeholder groups. The board ought to use its powers in an appropriate and responsible way, and should be accountable in some ways to the shareholders (and other stakeholders, perhaps).

In health service governance, this idea of membership is more complex. In foundation trusts there is a clear membership structure but the members are not strictly speaking the owners of the trust, they are the recipients of the health services provided and might be seen as 'proxy shareholders' on behalf of the general public. Further complications arise as the foundation trust (FT) is still required to consider the views of the community it serves regardless of whether they are members or not and is also required to consider the views of its other stakeholders such as local authorities, primary care trusts (PCTs), **strategic health authorities (SHAs), clinical commissioning groups (CCGs)**. For non-FT organisations there is no established membership structure and there is an equivalent variety of stakeholders. It is this variety of stakeholders and the different levels of influence that they are able to exercise within the NHS that makes the idea of health service governance an interesting and challenging subject.

The significant distinction between corporate governance and health service governance is the relationship between the board of directors and its variety of stakeholders, and the way in which the board exercises its powers. Principles of health service governance are based on the view that the organisation should be governed in such a way that balances the requirements of a wide variety of stakeholders. The board is required to use its powers in an appropriate and responsible way, and is accountable in different ways to each of the stakeholders.

2.1 Why is governance important?

Regardless of sector, governance is a key issue as it regulates the power and decision making of a small group of people who have been given a large responsibility for the stewardship of the assets of a third party. In the context of the NHS, this stewardship involves both public assets and healthcare services. It really can be a matter of life and death as well as a matter of severe financial loss. As a result NHS organisations have clear aims that have been set out in the NHS constitution and they should be governed in such a way that they move towards the achievement of these aims.

Although NHS organisations and companies exist as a legal person, in reality each organisation is the organised, collective effort of many different individuals. They are controlled by boards of directors in the interests of their stakeholders. The interests of the board and the stakeholders ought to coincide, but in practice they may be in conflict with each other. The challenge of good health service governance is to find a way in which the interests of a wide variety of stakeholders and the directors can all be sufficiently satisfied.

For companies the challenge still remains but it rests largely on balancing the interests of the board of directors and the shareholders.

2.2 Governance and management

It is important to recognise the difference between the governance of any organisation and its management.

Powers to manage the affairs of an NHS organisation, or a company, are given to the board of directors, but most of these powers are delegated to a **chief executive officer** (CEO) or managing director, and are delegated further to **executive directors** and executive managers. The board of directors should retain some powers and responsibilities, and certain matters should be reserved for board decision-making rather than delegated to the management team (see Chapter 8).

The board of directors should also be responsible for monitoring the performance of the management team. However, the board of directors itself is not responsible for day-to-day management. It is responsible for governing the organisation. Responsibilities for governance go beyond management, and governance should not be confused with management. Even so, it is probably true to say that when a senior executive manager is 'promoted' to the board, he or she may consider the position of an executive director to be a recognition of his senior executive position. However, the promotion of an executive manager to the board creates new responsibilities for governance that are not related to management. The executive director ought to think as a member of the board, rather than as a senior executive, in performing his duties as a director.

This concept is known as the **unitary board** where there is an effective single board that is collectively responsible for controlling the organisation or company, with no one individual having unfettered powers of decision making. When an executive director becomes a board member, they are part of that collective responsibility for ensuring the achievement of corporate aims and objectives and must not solely contribute to discussions and decisions in the light of their particular executive function.

TEST YOUR KNOWLEDGE 1.1

a Why is health service governance challenging for NHS organisations?
b What is the difference between governance and management?

3 Principles of good corporate governance

Several concepts apply to sound corporate governance in all countries where international investors invest their money. Many of these are ethical in nature and the King Code (see Chapter 3) describes them as the 'overarching corporate governance principles':

- fairness
- accountability
- responsibility
- transparency.

These principles are directly applicable to an understanding of health service governance and are set out here with examples from both corporate and health service governance.

3.1 Fairness

Fairness refers to the principle that all shareholders should receive equal consideration. **Minority shareholders**, for example (see Chapter 3), should be treated in the same way as majority shareholders. This concept might seem fairly straightforward in the UK, where the rights of minority shareholders are protected to a large extent by company law. In some countries, however, minority shareholder rights are often disregarded by the larger shareholders and the board of directors. There should also be fairness in the treatment of stakeholders other than shareholders.

The NHS Constitution sets out a number of rights and pledges that underpin the principle of fairness, e.g. the right to access, right to drugs, right to complain, staff rights.

3.2 Accountability

Decision-makers who act on behalf of an organisation should be accountable for the decisions they make and the actions they take. In a company, the board of directors should be accountable to the shareholders, the company's owners. Shareholders should be able to assess the actions of their board of directors and the committees of the board, and have the opportunity to query them and challenge them. In an NHS organisation a variety of stakeholders will provide that level of accountability. A problem with accountability is deciding how the directors should be accountable, and in particular over what period of time.

According to the financial theory for companies, if the objective of a company is to maximise the wealth of its shareholders, this will be achieved by maximising the financial returns to shareholders through increases in profits, dividends, prospects for profit growth and a rising share price. It might therefore follow that directors should be held accountable to shareholders on the basis of the returns on shareholder capital that the company has achieved. However, there is no consensus about the period over which returns to shareholders and increases in share value should be measured. Performance can be measured over a short term of one year at a time, or over a long term of (say) five or ten years – or even longer. In practice, it is usual to measure returns over the short term and assess performance in terms of profitability over a 12-month period. In the short term, however, a company's share price may be affected by influences unrelated to the company's underlying performance, such as excessive optimism or pessimism in the stock markets generally. In the short term, it is also easier to soothe investors with promises for the future, even though current performance is not good. It is only when a company fails consistently to deliver on its promises that investor confidence ebbs away.

If company performance were to be judged by the return to shareholders over a 12-month period, the directors would focus on short-term results and short-term movements in the stock market price. Short-termism is easy to criticise, but difficult to disregard in practice if performance targets ignore the long term. They should really be looking after the underlying business of the company and its profitability over the longer term.

Writing in the *Financial Times* (29 January 2002), John Kay, reflecting on the reasons given by the former finance director of Marconi for the company's financial collapse in 2000, commented:

'[A director's] job is to run a business that adds value by means of the services it provides to customers. If he succeeds, it will generate returns to investors in the long term. And this is the only mechanism that can generate returns to investors. The problem is that the equivalence between value added in operations and stock market returns holds in the long run but not the short. Share prices may, for a time, become divorced from the fundamental value of a business. This has been true of most share prices in recent years. In these conditions, attention to **total shareholder returns** distracts executives from their real function of managing businesses.'

The problem of accountability remains, however. Even if it is accepted that company performance should not be judged by short-term financial results and share price movements, how can the board be made accountable for its contribution to longer-term success?

By way of contrast, accountability for an NHS organisation can be measured in a number of ways:

- **Regulators:** Care Quality Commission (CQC), Monitor.
- **Commissioners:** National Commissioning Board, Clinical Commissioning Groups, GPs.
- **Political scrutiny:** DH, overview and scrutiny committees, health and wellbeing boards, Healthwatch.
- **Public opinion:** patient surveys, Patient Choice agenda, national staff surveys.

However, the issue of short-termism remains as changes in government policy often drives the form of accountability that is practiced by the regulators, commissioners and political scrutineers. The views expressed by public opinion can also focus on very local issues that need to be balanced against wider healthcare changes for the public benefit.

The NHS Constitution sets out that the NHS is accountable to the public, communities and patients that it serves. The government ensures that there is always a clear and up-to-date statement of NHS accountability for this purpose (see Chapter 3).

3.3 Responsibility

The board of directors is given authority to act on behalf of the company, and a further principle of corporate governance is that it should accept full **responsibility** for the powers that it is given and the authority that it exercises. A board of directors should understand what its responsibilities are, and should carry them out to the best of its abilities.

Accountability goes hand in hand with responsibility. The board of directors should be made accountable to the shareholders for the way in which it has carried out its responsibilities. Similarly, executive management should be responsible for the exercise of powers delegated to them by the board of directors, and should be made accountable to the board for their achievements and performance.

3.4 Transparency

Transparency means **openness**. In the context of corporate governance, this is a willingness by the company to provide clear information to shareholders and other stakeholders about what the company has done and hopes to achieve, without giving away commercially sensitive information. It might be useful to think of openness in terms of its opposite, which is to be a 'closed book' and refuse to divulge any information whatsoever.

Transparency should not be confused with 'understandability'. Information should be communicated in a way that is understandable, but transparency is concerned more with the content of the information that is communicated.

A principle of good governance is that stakeholders should be informed about what an organisation is doing and plans to do in the future, and about the risks involved in its business strategies.

Transparency in NHS organisations is set out by the requirements of the Freedom of Information Act (FOIA) 2000 and the requirements of openness set out in the Nolan Standards in Public Life (see Section 6.1). The NHS Constitution requires that the system of responsibility and accountability for making decisions in the NHS should be transparent and clear to the public, patients and staff.

> **TEST YOUR KNOWLEDGE 1.2**
>
> a What are the 'overarching corporate governance principles'?
> b How does the NHS Constitution underpin these principles?
> c How can accountability for an NHS organisation be measured?

4 Key issues in governance

Good governance should promote the best long-term interests of the organisation. It requires an effective board of directors, with an appropriate balance of skills and experience, and well-motivated individuals as directors. The composition of the board, its functions and responsibilities, and its effectiveness, are therefore core issues in governance.

At the heart of the debate about corporate governance lie the conflicts of interest, or potential conflicts of interest, between shareholders, the board of directors as a whole and individual board members, and possibly also a number of other stakeholder groups. The directors may be tempted to take risks and make decisions aimed at boosting short-term performance. Many shareholders are more concerned about the longer term, the continuing survival of their company and the value of their investment. If a company gets into financial difficulties, professional managers can move on to another company to start again, whereas shareholders suffer a financial loss.

Issues in corporate governance where a conflict of interests might be apparent are:

- financial reporting and auditing
- directors' remuneration
- company–stakeholder relations
- risk-taking and the management of risk
- effective communication between the directors and shareholders
- ethical conduct and corporate social responsibility (CSR).

Similar issues arise in health service governance. One stakeholder group may have a particular focus on an area of service delivery while the directors have to manage the wider provision of healthcare services. The directors often have to manage the competing interests of patient groups and the financial decisions contained within government policy. The directors have to consider their own careers within the NHS, managing the performance requirements of the regulators and any consideration of a longer term strategy for the particular body for whom they are responsible. These issues will be considered in more detail in the chapters that follow.

4.1 Financial reporting and auditing

The directors may try to disguise the true financial performance of their company by 'dressing up' the published accounts and giving less than honest statements. '**Window-dressed**' accounts make it difficult for stakeholders to reach a reasoned judgement about the financial position of the company. In NHS organisations misleading published accounts make it difficult for stakeholders to assess whether public funding is being correctly managed and expended on the key areas of service delivery that is required.

Concerns about misleading published accounts in the corporate commercial world provided an early impetus in the 1980s and early 1990s to the movement for better corporate governance in the UK. Accounting irregularities in a number of companies led to a tightening of accounting standards, although the problems of window dressing are unlikely ever to disappear completely. Concerns about financial reporting in the USA emerged with the collapse of Enron in 2001 (see Case example 1.2), which filed for bankruptcy after 'adjusting' its accounts. This was followed by similar problems at other US companies, such as telecommunications group WorldCom (which admitted to fraud in its accounting), Global Crossing and Rank Xerox. Problems then emerged in some European companies, most notably the Italian group Parmalat at the end of 2003. It was also suggested that incomprehensible or misleading accounts contributed to the global banking crisis in 2007–2009, with banks such as Lehman Brothers (which collapsed in 2008) possibly using questionable accounting practices to disguise the true state of their financial position. A corporate governance issue is the question of the extent to which the directors were aware in each case of the impending collapse of their company, and if they knew the problems why shareholders were not informed much sooner. It is now widely accepted that the directors of a company should be responsible for giving an assurance to their shareholders that they consider their company to be a going concern that will not collapse within the next 12 months.

When the annual financial statements of a company prove to have been misleading, questions are inevitably raised about the effectiveness of the external auditors. There are two main issues relating to the external audit of a company:

- whether it should be the job of the auditors to discover financial fraud and material errors
- the problem of the relationship between a client company and its auditors, and the extent to which the auditors are independent and free from the influence of the company's management.

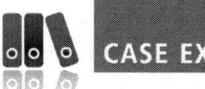

CASE EXAMPLE 1.2

Enron was founded in 1985 with the merger of two US natural gas pipelines. In the 1990s it diversified into selling electricity and other activities; by 2000 it was one of the world's largest companies when measured by reported annual revenue. It appeared to have a highly competent board of directors and **audit committee**. However, although investors and regulators were not aware of it at the time, the rapid growth in the reported assets and profits of Enron was attributable largely to misleading accounting practices. It inflated the value of its reported assets (sometimes recording expenses as assets) and it kept liabilities off its balance sheet by means of establishing 'special purpose entities'. It also anticipated profits by becoming the first non-financial services company to adopt 'mark to market' accounting techniques. This enabled it to earn profits on long-term contracts 'up front' as soon as the contract started. In one case it claimed a large profit on a 20-year contract agreed with Blockbuster Video in 2000, and continued to claim the profit even after the project failed to work successfully and Blockbuster pulled out of the deal.

Senior management were rewarded on the basis of annual earnings and were highly motivated to continue reporting large increases in profits, regardless of the longer-term consequences. Investors began to have doubts about the reliability of Enron's reported profits in 2001. A **'whistleblower'** (see Chapter 12) reported her concerns to the chief executive officer, but her allegations of dubious accounting practices were ignored. However, in October 2001 Enron was eventually forced to announce that it would be re-stating its accounts for 1997–2000 to correct accounting violations. The Securities and Exchange Commission (SEC) announced an investigation into the company, and the stock price collapsed. There were also doubts about whether Enron had sufficient liquidity (cash) to remain in business for long. Its debt was downgraded to junk bond status and in December 2001 the company filed for bankruptcy.

The company's auditors were Arthur Andersen, one of the 'big five' global accounting firms. The firm – in particular its Houston office – took extraordinary measures to protect its client. When the SEC investigation was announced in 2001, Andersen staff attempted to cover up evidence of negligence in its audit work by destroying several tons of documents, and many e-mails and computer files. The firm, especially the Houston office, was accused of losing its independence to Enron and over-reliance on income from the non-audit work that it did for the company. Arthur Andersen was charged with obstructing the course of justice by shredding the documents and destroying the files. Although a guilty verdict was subsequently overturned by the Supreme Court, this was too late to save the firm from the loss of its major clients, and collapse.

Several Enron employees were brought to trial for a number of financial crimes. Andrew Fastow, a former chief financial officer (CFO) of Enron, was found guilty of crimes including fraud, money laundering, insider trading and conspiracy. Two former chief executive officers, Kenneth Lay and Jeffrey Skilling, were charged with a range of financial crimes and brought to trial in 2006. Both were found guilty: Skilling was imprisoned and Lay died before sentence was passed.

If auditors are subject to influence, they might be persuaded to agree with a controversial method of accounting for particular transactions, which shows the company's performance or financial position in a better light. Arthur Andersen, which collapsed in 2002, appears to have lacked independence from its major client Enron (see Case example 1.2).

Financial reporting is also vital for NHS organisations and it is subject to a great level of scrutiny. It must be remembered that the financial position of an NHS organisation is closely linked to its performance targets and the level of activity it is involved in. While there is some guidance on how targets should be measured in order that the correct financial data can be collated, the pressure to reach performance targets can lead to irregularities in the measurement of target data.

CASE EXAMPLE 1.3

An NHS finance director took a leading teaching hospital to an employment tribunal over claims he was sacked for '**whistleblowing**' over fiddled statistics for cancelled operations. The director queried why a senior executive had instructed a junior member of staff to record the number of weekly cancelled operations as zero, instead of the recorded number, in a form sent to the DH to help determine the hospital's performance rating. It then emerged that the figure zero had been entered for a number of weeks, during which time a number of operations were believed to have been cancelled on the day of the operation for non-clinical reasons – though no such cancellations were ever recorded. The hospital had been under pressure because of its poor record on cancelled operations, and evidence of improvement would have gained it a greater share of a large performance fund made available by the DH.

CASE EXAMPLE 1.4

Over a three-month period a trust's financial position deteriorated significantly so that instead of a modest surplus the trust was forecasting a significant deficit. When the deterioration became apparent, the trust failed to raise the matter promptly or notify Monitor, the regulator, of risks associated with its recovery plan. The *Compliance Framework* requires trusts to report any material, actual or prospective changes that may affect their ability to comply with any aspect of their authorisation.

The trust submitted a re-forecast plan to Monitor, setting out a recovery in the following quarter. This largely relied on a significant reduction in staff costs. However given the record of the trust in consistently overspending on pay, Monitor was not convinced that the recovery plan would be delivered. Furthermore the re-forecast showed a significant liquidity risk in the medium term that the board had taken no steps to mitigate or put in place contingencies. Overspend on pay had been reported to every board meeting over a protracted period, but plans to deal with the overspend were not due to take effect until the following financial year and the trust failed to identify that the situation would not be remedied in the short term.

There was no evidence that the level of challenge in the boardroom on financial issues was sufficient in the light of the level of financial deterioration. Despite the urgent need to improve the financial situation Monitor noted that evidence suggested that the board was not sufficiently engaged in holding the executive to account for delivery of improvements and had tolerated slippage in delivery and extended timelines. The trust remained under enhanced monitoring arrangements until it was deemed to no longer be in breach of its terms of authorisation.

4.2 Directors' remuneration

In the corporate commercial world directors may reward themselves with huge salaries and other rewards, such as bonuses, a generous pension scheme, **share options** (see Chapter 11) and other benefits. Institutional shareholders do not object to high remuneration for directors. However, they maintain that rewards should depend largely on the performance of the company and the benefits obtained for the shareholders. The main complaint about 'fat cat' directors' remuneration is that when the company does well, the directors are rewarded well, which is fair enough, but when the company does badly, the directors continue to be paid just as generously.

Interest in arguments about directors' pay has varied between different countries. In the UK, concerns led to the establishment of the Greenbury Committee in the 1990s and the production of the **Greenbury Report**. Directors' remuneration has remained a contentious issue ever since. In 2002 company law was changed by the Directors' Remuneration Report Regulations, requiring listed companies to produce a directors' remuneration report annually and to invite shareholders to vote on the report at the company's annual general meeting (AGM).

Within NHS organisations there is, to a certain extent, a greater level of regulation. All NHS organisations (except NHS foundation trusts) are required to follow either the Very Senior Managers (VSM) Pay Framework or Agenda for Change. The VSM Pay Framework is published by DH. VSM means chief executives, executive directors and others with board-level responsibility who report directly to the CEO. At present the VSM Framework applies to senior staff in PCTs, ambulance trusts, SHAs and special health authorities. The government has declared a pay freeze for 2011/12 and 2012/2013.

The Agenda for Change system allocates posts to set payscales using a job evaluation scheme. Directors within acute and mental health trusts have their pay set within this system unless they are a foundation trusts. All foundation trusts have the freedom to use local terms and conditions when setting pay for all employees, however, in practice all but one (Southend University Hospital NHS Foundation Trust) has continued to be guided by VSM and to operate Agenda for Change for their staff. This may change as the pressure to find cost improvement efficiencies increases.

4.3 Company–stakeholder relations

Most decision-making powers in an organisation are held by the board of directors. The governance debate has been about the extent to which professional managers, acting as board directors, exercise those powers in the interests of their principal stakeholder (e.g. shareholders) and other stakeholders in the organisation, and whether the powers of directors should be restricted. This aspect of governance is about:

- the structure of the board of directors and the role of independent **non-executive directors (NEDs)**
- the responsibilities of the board of directors
- the duties of directors.

And particularly in corporate governance:

- the powers of shareholders under company law and whether these should be extended by corporate law reform, e.g. by giving shareholders the right to approve the company's remuneration policy or its remuneration packages for board members (see Chapter 9)
- whether shareholders actually make full use of the powers they already have, for example by voting not to re-elect directors.

And particularly in health service governance:

- the rights granted under the NHS Constitution to the public and staff
- the decisions about service delivery and manner in which services are delivered.

4.4 Corporate governance and risk management

In the corporate commercial world and as a general rule, investors expect higher rewards to compensate them for taking higher **business risks** (see Chapter 11). If a company makes decisions that increase the scale of the risks it faces, profits and dividends should be expected to go up. Another issue in corporate governance is that the directors might take decisions intended to increase profits without giving due regard to the risks. In some cases, companies may continue to operate without regard to the changing risk profile of their existing businesses. When investors buy shares in a company, they have an idea of the type of company they are buying into, the nature of its business, the probable returns it will provide for shareholders and the nature of its business and **financial risks** (see Chapter 11). To shareholders, investment risk is important, as well as high returns. Directors, on the other hand, are rewarded on the basis of the returns the company achieves, linked to profits or dividend growth, and their remuneration is not linked in any direct way to the risk aspects of their business. Some companies are also guilty of poor procedures and systems, so that the risk of breakdowns, errors and fraud can be high. In addition to controlling 'business risk', companies should also have effective internal controls for managing **operational risks** (see Chapter 11). Risk management is now recognised as an ingredient of sound corporate governance.

In health service governance **risk management** is equally as crucial; not only does it set out to protect public assets and the use of the taxpayers' money, it also protects the quality of the healthcare services being delivered. Risk is managed at two levels: first, at a strategic/management level; and second, at a day-to-day operational level. The focus of that risk management has to be on the management of business risks associated with running an NHS organisation, which will include the financial, IT and ethical risks while at the same time managing the clinical risks involved in the delivery of healthcare services. Risk management in healthcare is governed by a mixture of legislature-, regulatory- and standards-based guidance. The same is true, however, for NHS organisations, as for companies, that operational issues that may lead to a significant risk of poor care or fraud should be brought to the board's attention.

When referring to 'risk management' in health service governance, the issues have to be mainly 'internal control' and quality performance. Public sector organisations in general have had a long history of wasteful spending, inefficiency, errors and fraud. NHS organisations, along with other local government bodies, are now required by law to publish an annual governance statement (AGS) each year.

4.5 Information and communication

Another issue in corporate governance is communication between the board of directors and the company's shareholders. Shareholders, particularly those with a large financial investment in the company, should be able to voice their concerns to the directors and expect to have their opinions heard. Small shareholders should at least be informed about the company, its financial position and its plans for the future, even if their opinions carry comparatively little weight.

The responsibility for improving communications rests with the companies themselves and their main institutional shareholders. Companies can make better use of the annual report and accounts to report to shareholders on a range of issues and the policies of the company for dealing with them. The annual report and accounts should not be simply a brief **directors' report** (see also Chapter 10) and a set of financial statements. The company should explain its operations and financial position in a business review and report on a range of governance issues, such as directors' remuneration, internal controls and risk management and policies on health, safety and the environment. Many companies now use their website to report on such matters. A company can also try to encourage greater shareholder attendance and participation at AGMs as a method of improving communications and dialogue. Electronic communications, including electronic voting, should also be considered. For their part, institutional investors should develop voting policies and apply these in general meetings. Where necessary, they can vote against the board to alert the directors to the strength of their views.

In health service governance it is an explicit aspect of government policy that stakeholders are to be involved in the design and delivery of their own healthcare, therefore, public information from NHS organisations about their services and future plans is vital. Providing opportunities for the views and opinions of stakeholders to be heard is a key driver within health service governance. Better informed boards of directors will make better healthcare decisions and the increased focus on patient choice results from research in the UK and overseas that treatments are more effective if patients choose, understand and control their own care. Patient choices now include the right to choose a GP, which hospital to go to and the right to be involved in decisions about their own healthcare.

This right to choose, combined with the introduction of 'internal' or 'quasi' market policies, has led to a greater degree of information about the performance of individual consultants and hospitals. This has introduced the commercial concepts of marketing and market share, and a much greater awareness of costs, efficiency and accountability.

Further, the introduction of the FOIA 2000 provided a clear procedure for all public bodies to respond to requests for information about their organisations (see Chapter 3).

Added to this the requirements to make NHS annual accounts, reports from regulators (e.g. Monitor, CQC), national NHS surveys (staff survey, patients survey) and the introduction of Quality Accounts for all providers of healthcare services, all serve to ensure a greater transparency in the relationships with NHS stakeholders.

4.6 Ethical conduct and corporate social responsibility

The relevance of ethical conduct to governance has already been described. There is also a growing recognition that organisations need to consider social and environmental issues, for commercial reasons and governance reasons, as well as ethical reasons. Many stakeholders and many customers expect organisations to have regard to social issues and environmental issues; furthermore, the financial risks from government regulation to protect the environment continue to grow. Social and environmental issues can therefore affect reputation, sales, profits and the share price.

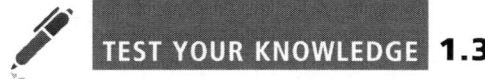

TEST YOUR KNOWLEDGE 1.3

List six key issues in health service governance.

5 A brief history of corporate governance

5.1 Corporate governance in the UK

Concerns about corporate governance have grown over time. The main impetus for better practices in corporate governance began in the UK in the late 1980s and early 1990s. The Report of the Committee on the Financial Aspects of Corporate Governance (the 'Cadbury Report') was published in 1992, and was later described as 'a landmark in thinking on corporate governance'. The report included a Code of Best Practice (the **Cadbury Code**), and UK listed companies came under pressure from City institutions to comply with the requirements of the code.

In 1995, a working group was set up to look into the relationship between companies and institutional investors. It was chaired by Paul Myners, who was then chairman of Gartmore plc, and produced the **Myners Report**, which made a number of recommendations about how the relationship between institutional investors and company management should be conducted. The Report included suggestions for improving the communications between companies and institutional investors and for the conduct of AGMs. The significance of the Myners Report is that it urged institutional investors to reassess their role as shareholders, their responsibilities for ensuring good corporate governance and the success of the companies in which they invest. When a company is performing badly, institutional investors should try to do something to put matters right, instead of selling their shares and washing their hands of the company.

Myners went on to argue that unless institutional investors voluntarily became more active in the governance of companies and exercised their rights more forcibly, they should be compelled to do so by legislation. Representative bodies of the **institutional investor** organisations, such as the Association of British Insurers (ABI) and the National Association of Pension Funds (NAPF), responded by issuing guidelines for their members on corporate governance issues and principles of corporate governance.

On the recommendation of the Cadbury Committee, another committee was set up to review progress on corporate governance in UK listed companies. This committee issued the **Greenbury Report** in 1995, which focused mainly on directors' remuneration. At the time, the UK press was condemning 'fat cat' directors, particularly those in newly privatised companies. The Greenbury Report issued a Code of Best Practice on establishing remuneration committees, for disclosures of much more information about the remuneration of directors and remuneration policy, and for more control over notice periods in directors' service contracts and compensation payments in the event of early termination of contracts.

A Committee on Corporate Governance, chaired by Sir Ronald Hampel, was set up in 1995 to review the recommendations of the Cadbury and Greenbury Committees. The final report of the **Hampel Committee** was published in 1998. This covered a number of governance issues, such as the composition of the board and role of directors, directors' remuneration, the role of shareholders (particularly institutional shareholders), communications between the company and its shareholders, and financial reporting, auditing and internal controls. The Hampel Report also suggested that its recommendations should be combined with those of the Cadbury and Greenbury Committees into a single code of corporate governance. This suggestion led to the publication of the original 1998 **Combined Code** on Corporate Governance (Combined Code), which applied to all UK listed companies.

Corporate governance issues remained in the spotlight in the UK, and two influential reports were produced in January 2003. The **Higgs Report**, commissioned by the government, considered the role and effectiveness of NEDs. The **Smith Report**, commissioned by the Financial Reporting Council (FRC), provided guidance for audit committees. The responsibility for the Combined Code was transferred to the FRC and in 2003 a revised Combined Code was issued, incorporating many of the Higgs and Smith recommendations.

Although the Combined Code has been voluntary, the UK Listing Rules included an obligation on listed companies to disclose the extent of their compliance with it. Listed companies were required to state that they have complied in full with the provisions of the code, or must explain any non-compliance. This **'comply or explain' rule** for listed companies applies to all provisions of the Code.

The *UK Code* and related guidelines are now the responsibility of the FRC. The FRC has reviewed and amended the Combined Code regularly, and in June 2010 issued a revised version of the code, under the new name of the **UK Corporate Governance Code**.

The global financial markets and world economy were badly damaged by the banking crisis that emerged in 2007 and 2008. In the USA, Lehman Brothers collapsed and other banks and brokerage firms were taken over to prevent their collapse. In the UK, Northern Rock bank collapsed in 2007 and in 2008 Royal Bank of Scotland was virtually nationalised. At the same time, the government acquired a major stake in Lloyds TSB Bank after Lloyds had agreed to take over another ailing bank, HBOS. Recognition of governance problems in UK banks led to a review by Sir David Walker and the **Walker Report** (2009). Some recommendations of the Walker Report have been included by the FRC in the 2010 UK Corporate Governance Code.

In May 2011, the FRC began consulting on possible amendments to the code that would require companies to publish their policy on boardroom diversity and report against it annually, as recommended by Lord Davies in his **'Women on Boards' report** published in February 2011, and to consider the board's diversity among other factors, when assessing its effectiveness. In October 2011 the FRC announced that these changes would be implemented in a revised version of the code to be issued in 2012 and apply to financial years beginning on or after 1 October 2012. In September 2011, the FRC announced that it intended to consult on proposed further changes to the code in relation to audit committees and audit retendering. This consultation will begin in early 2012, and should any changes be agreed as a result they would also be incorporated into the revised code that will apply from 1 October 2012.

Some aspects of corporate governance have been brought into UK law, with much of the initiative coming from the EU and **EU Directives**. New regulations in 2002 were introduced for greater disclosures of directors' remuneration by listed companies, replacing similar regulations that had been included in the Listing Rules. The Companies Act 2006 introduced **statutory duties** of directors (similar to the duties that existed previously in common law and equity), and contains a requirement for quoted companies to be more accountable to shareholders by publishing a business review in narrative form each year. Amendments to the Fourth and Seventh EU Company Law Directives approved in 2006 included a requirement for quoted companies to include a corporate governance statement in their annual reports, and amendments to the Eighth Company Law Directive in 2008 requires 'public interest entities' (which include listed companies) to have an audit committee consisting of independent NEDs and to publish an annual corporate governance statement.

A largely separate, although interconnected, development has been a growing awareness on the part of large companies of the potential risks to their reputation and long-term success from failures to comply with laws and regulations or to act ethically. Many companies have also claimed to recognise the potential long-term benefits from acting in a socially responsible manner.

TEST YOUR KNOWLEDGE 1.4

What is the 'comply or explain rule' in corporate governance for listed companies?

5.2 Corporate governance in other countries

Although the UK is seen as a leading country in the development of a corporate governance framework, there have been similar developments in many other countries. For many countries, particularly developing countries, good corporate governance is seen as an essential basic requirement for attracting foreign investment capital. In South Africa, a code of corporate governance was developed by the King Committee. This was revised and strengthened in 2002 and again in 2009 (King III, see chapter 4). On an international basis, recommended principles on corporate governance have been published by the Organisation for Economic Co-operation and Development (OECD).

The USA appeared to show little concern for better corporate governance throughout the 1990s, although there were some activist institutional shareholders such as CalPERS. The situation changed dramatically with the collapse of Enron in 2001 and some other major companies. The major auditing and accountancy firm Arthur Andersen, caught up in the Enron scandal and prosecuted for obstructing the course of justice, collapsed and was broken up in 2002 (see Case example 1.2). Recommendations for change were proposed by the New York Stock Exchange (NYSE), and statutory provisions on corporate governance were introduced in 2002 with the Sarbanes-Oxley Act (SOX). However, the adequacy of corporate governance provisions in the USA (and the UK) has been questioned following the banking crisis in 2007–2009.

Many other countries now have corporate governance codes and legislation covering aspects of corporate governance practice. The regulations and guidelines vary between countries. A summary of the laws and guidelines in each country can be found on the website of the European Corporate Governance Institute.

STOP AND THINK 1.1

From what you have read or heard in news reports, identify a recent example of pressures for better corporate governance that is bringing about changes in a company's management, policies or practices.

What challenges or opportunities might such improvements bring to an NHS organisation?

5.3 National variations in corporate governance

As stated earlier, the need for good corporate governance is a matter of international concern. However, it is important to be aware that although corporate governance has become a matter of some interest in many countries, the pace of change and the nature of corporate governance vary substantially between countries.

Much of the pressure for change has come from institutional investors, particularly in the USA, who have invested fairly heavily in companies in other countries. As shareholders in foreign companies, US investors expect to be allowed to exercise their right to vote and to be treated on an equal footing with other equity shareholders. In countries where minority shareholder rights are not always well respected, US investor influence has probably been influential in the corporate governance changes that have been introduced. The **International Corporate Governance Network (ICGN)** is a voluntary organisation established to promote good governance practice worldwide; this has issued a corporate governance code, based largely on the UK model. Its objective is to raise standards of corporate governance globally, to meet the requirements and expectations of global investors.

In many developing countries, there have been substantial investments in recent years by multinational companies. It might be expected that US and UK multinationals would establish a system of corporate governance within their subsidiaries along similar lines to the parent company, e.g. with NEDs on the board representing interest groups in the local country. Many multinationals are aware of their reputation in overseas markets, and alert to the demands of pressure groups as well as governments in the countries where they have operating subsidiaries.

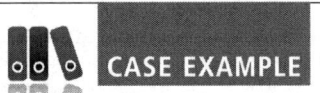 **CASE EXAMPLE 1.5**

RiskMetrics is a US shareholder advisory group that advises shareholders holding up to 20% of some leading German companies. It criticised the decision of Infineon (a German company that manufactures electronic chips) to appoint an individual as chairman-designate that it considered unsuitable, and advised its clients to support a rival candidate for the chairmanship at the company's AGM in 2010. Its view was supported by Hermes, the UK investment fund and a major German institutional investor.

In January 2010, as a result of the pressure, the chairman-designate promised to step down early, saying he would serve only one year instead of five if elected as chairman. The opposing shareholders were pleased with the offer, but insisted that an acceptable compromise had to include the appointment of their candidate to the supervisory board. (In Germany, shareholders can appoint board members, but the supervisory board members elect the chairman.)

6 Governance in the public sector

6.1 Nolan's seven principles of public life

A key development for the governance of the UK public sector was the Nolan Committee on Standards in Public Life. The Committee was set up in 1995 in response to concerns that the conduct of some politicians was unethical and, in particular, allegations of MPs taking cash for putting parliamentary questions. While the Committee focused on MPs, its terms of reference also covered government departments and non-departmental public bodies (**NDPBs**). The Principles, set out in the following text, were originally intended as guidelines for individuals who were involved in public affairs and public bodies, whether as paid employees or as non-paid members of governing bodies. They are now considered to have much wider relevance and have formed the basis in the UK for developing governance guidelines for both the public sector and the voluntary sector.

- **Selflessness**. Holders of public office should take decisions solely in terms of the public interest. They should not do so to gain financial or other material benefits for themselves, their family or their friends.

- **Integrity**. Holders of public office should not place themselves under any financial or other obligation to outside individuals or organisations that might influence them in the performance of their duties.
- **Objectivity**. In carrying out public business, including making public appointments, awarding contracts or recommending individuals for rewards and benefits, holders of public office should make choices on merit.
- **Accountability**. Holders of public office are accountable for their decisions and actions to the public and must submit themselves to whatever scrutiny is appropriate to their office.
- **Openness**. Holders of public office should be as open as possible about the decisions and actions that they take. They should give reasons for their decisions and restrict information only when the wider public interest clearly demands.
- **Honesty**. Holders of public office have a duty to declare any private interests relating to their public duties and to take steps to resolve any conflicts arising in a way that protects the public interest.
- **Leadership**. Holders of public office should promote and support these principles by leadership and example.

The public sector includes central government, state government (in some countries) and local government, state-run health and education services and many other regulatory and advisory bodies. While many of the principles of good corporate governance can be applied to the governing bodies of the public sector, there are also significant differences as have been set out before. For example, public bodies are not profit-making and are not accountable to shareholders.

The public sector has therefore adapted principles of good governance to its own specific circumstances, and to some extent the definition of 'governance' for the public sector differs in some ways from 'governance' of companies. In the UK, the Chartered Institute of Public Finance and Accountancy (CIPFA) and Solace (the Society of Local Authority Chief Executives and Senior Managers) published a governance framework aimed at local government bodies called 'Delivering Good Governance in Local Government: framework' (2007). This sets out principles of governance that local government bodies are encouraged to adopt and apply to their own particular circumstances. This Framework defines governance as:

> '[H]ow local government bodies ensure that they are doing the right things, in the right way, for the right people, in a timely, inclusive, open, honest and accountable manner. It comprises systems and processes, and cultures and values, by which local government bodies are directed and controlled and through which they account to, and engage with, and, where appropriate, lead their communities.'

6.2 Good Governance Standard for Public Services

The Independent Commission for Good Governance in Public Service was established by the Office for Public Management (OPM) and the CIPFA, in partnership with the Joseph Rowntree Foundation. The role of the Commission was to develop a common code and set of principles for good governance across all public services in the UK.

In 2004 it published *Good Governance Standard for Public Services*. This is a guide for everyone concerned with governance in the public services, and applies to all organisations that work for the public using public money. Its application therefore extends from public sector bodies to all private sector organisations that use public money to work for the public.

In justifying the need for the application of good governance principles and practice in the public service sector, the Commission has commented that:

- good governance encourages public trust and participation, whereas
- bad governance fosters low morale and adversarial relationships.

The Commission's Good Governance Standard, which builds on Nolan's Principles, consists of six main principles, each with supporting principles, together with guidelines on how these might be applied in practice. It is useful to look at these and compare them with the principles (described earlier) that apply to good governance in the commercial (profit-making) sector. There are many similarities between these principles and those that should apply in corporate governance to companies.

The six main principles and their supporting principles are as follows:

1. Focusing on the organisation's purpose and on its outcome for citizens and users of the organisation's services.

    - Being clear about the purpose of the organisation and its intended outcomes for citizens and service users. It is suggested that the concept of 'public value' may be useful in helping organisations to identify their purpose and intended outcomes.
    - Making sure that users receive a high-quality service.
    - Making sure that taxpayers get VFM.

2. Performing effectively in clearly defined functions and roles.

    - Being clear about the functions of the organisation's governing body. It is recommended that the governing body should describe in a published document its approach to achieving each of its stated functions. This document can then be used as a basis for measuring actual performance and achievements by the governing body. Functions could include, for example, 'scrutinising the activities and performance of the executive management' and 'making sure that the voice of the public is heard in discussions and decision-making'.
    - Being clear about the responsibilities of the non-executive and the executive governors; these will differ. Many governing bodies consist of both executives and non-executive members (who may be unpaid for their services). However, they should have equal status in discussions on policy and strategy. The Framework recommends that the roles of CEO and chairman of the governing body should not be held by the same individual.
    - Making sure that these responsibilities are properly carried out.
    - Being clear about the relationship between the governors and the public, so that both sides in this relationship know what to expect from the other.

3. Promoting values for the whole organisation and demonstrating good governance through behaviour.

    - Putting the values of the organisation into practice. The governing body should take the lead in doing this.
    - Individual governors behaving in ways that uphold and exemplify effective governance.

4. Taking informed and transparent decisions and managing risk.

    - Being rigorous and transparent about how decisions are taken by the governing body. There should be clearly defined levels of delegation within the organisation. The governing body should not be concerned with matters that are more properly delegated to management. It should also be clear about what the objectives of its own decisions are.
    - Using good quality information, advice and support.
    - Making sure that an effective risk management system is in operation.

5. Developing the capacity and capability of the governing body to be effective.

    - Making sure that the governors have the skills, knowledge and experience to perform well.
    - Developing the capabilities of individuals with governance responsibilities.
    - Striking a balance in the membership of the governing body between continuity and renewal.
    - The creation and refreshing of a governing body is similar in many respects to similar guidelines in corporate governance, although in the public sector, some governors may be elected representatives.

6. Engaging stakeholders and making accountability real.

    - Understanding formal and informal accountability relationships.
    - Taking an active and planned approach to dialogue with and accountability to the public.
    - Taking an effective and planned approach to accountability to staff.
    - Engaging effectively with institutional stakeholders. Institutional stakeholders in the public sector are very different from institutional shareholders in the corporate world. In local government, for example, institutional stakeholders include bodies representing local people. Engagement with stakeholders should help to improve the accountability of the public sector body to the public.

These are general principles, and individual public sector bodies can develop their own codes of governance that are consistent with and based on these principles.

6.3 State-owned industries in emerging countries

The Commonwealth Association for Corporate Governance (CACG) issued a set of guidelines in 1999, which makes particular reference to state-owned industries in the emerging countries of the Commonwealth. In emerging countries:

- most of the largest and economically significant industries are state-owned, and the private sector is often very small
- many directors are not independent, and are often political appointments
- there is a severe shortage of individuals with the necessary skills to act as directors.

The CACG argued that although state-owned industries differ from public companies, the directors of these industries have a duty to taxpayers and the community:

> 'While the conventional fiduciary relationships between shareholders and the board (as found in the private sector) do not necessarily apply, directors of state enterprises nevertheless owe a fiduciary responsibility to account to a country's taxpayers and the communities which such enterprises serve for the efficient utilisation of state-owned assets.'

They owe a duty to taxpayers for the proper use of the money raised in taxes. They also owe a duty to the communities for the efficient delivery of services (electricity, water and so on). CACG also suggested that sound corporate governance in state-owned industries is extremely important in developing economies because they provide a role model for companies in the growing private sector. If state-owned industries govern themselves well, private companies can be persuaded to do the same. If state-owned industries are badly governed, it will be difficult to persuade the private sector to do anything better.

7 Arguments for and against governance regimes

There are differences of opinion about the benefits of governance, and whether these justify the costs of compliance with governance regulations.

It is therefore useful to consider just what the benefits of good governance might be, and what the arguments are against having laws or codes of governance practice. The main arguments in favour of having a strong governance regime are as follows:

- Good governance will eliminate the risk of misleading or false financial reporting, and will prevent organisations from being dominated by self-seeking CEOs or chairmen.
- By reducing the risks of scandals, and promoting fairness, accountability, responsibility and transparency in organisations, stakeholders (particularly shareholders) will be better protected. In the corporate commercial world this should add generally to confidence in the capital markets, and help to sustain share prices.
- It has been argued that organisations that comply with best practice in governance are also more likely to achieve success. Good governance and good leadership and management often go hand in hand. Badly governed organisations may be very successful, and well-governed organisations may fail; however, the probability is greater that badly governed organisations will be less successful and more likely to fail than well-governed ones.
- Well-governed organisations will often develop a strong reputation and so will be less exposed to **reputation risk** (see Chapter 11) than organisations that are not so well governed. Reputation risk can have an adverse impact on stakeholders such as investors, customers and suppliers.
- Good corporate governance encourages investors to hold shares in companies for the longer term, instead of treating shares as short-term investments to be sold for a quick profit. Companies benefit from having shareholders who have an interest in their longer-term prospects.

The main arguments against having a strong governance regime for organisations focus on costs, benefits and value and are as follows:

- It is argued that, for many organisations, compliance with a code of governance is a **box-ticking exercise** as they adopt the required procedures and systems without considering what the potential benefits might be. The only requirement is to comply with the 'rules' and put a tick in a box when this is done. Governance requirements therefore create a time-and-resource-consuming bureaucracy, with compliance officers, and divert the attention of the board of directors from more important matters.
- Good governance is likely to reduce the risk of scandals and unexpected organisational failures. However, it could be argued that the current regulations or best practice guidelines are far too extensive and burdensome.
- When regulations and recommended practice become burdensome, there is an inevitable cost, in terms of both time and money, in achieving compliance. It could be argued that less regulation is better regulation. However there has not yet been an authoritative assessment of the costs of governance compliance with the benefits of better governance systems.

Organisations that are obliged to comply with governance regulations or best practice are at a competitive disadvantage to rival organisations from countries or regimes where governance regulation is weaker. This is one of the criticisms of widening the number of providers of healthcare beyond that of NHS organisations. If they are not subject to the same level of scrutiny and regulation then the playing field is not level.

Within corporate governance this argument is weaker than it used to be as governance regimes have extended to more countries. There is no evidence, for example, that UK companies have lost competitiveness because of the relatively strong governance regime in the UK.

The connection between good governance and good financial results (due to good leadership and management) has not yet been proven or demonstrated.

TEST YOUR KNOWLEDGE 1.5

a What are the arguments in favour of and against the application of governance codes of practice?
b What are the aims of the ICGN?

8 Governance and the voluntary sector

The voluntary sector includes a wide range of organisations, including charities and mutual self-help groups. Many UK charities are established as a trust, which is governed by a board of trustees. Large charities employ full-time managers and employees, whereas others rely entirely on voluntary and unpaid help.

Governance in the voluntary sector has been defined as:

> '[T]he way that trustees work with chief executives and staff (where appointed), volunteers, service users, members and other stakeholders to ensure their organisation is effectively and properly run, and meets the needs for which the organisation was set up.'
>
> 'Good Governance: a code for the voluntary and community sector', 2005

The development of codes and rules for corporate governance and public sector governance has also influenced the voluntary sector. For example, the National Council of Voluntary Organisations (NCVO) adapted Nolan's seven principles of public life into a code of conduct for charity trustees; and the Charity Commission's Statement of Recommended Practice requires larger charities to include a statement on risks in their annual report.

Awareness of the need for good governance has also developed in the voluntary sector response to sector-specific issues, including:

- the increase in size and importance of the voluntary sector, particularly as a result of the contracting out of public service to voluntary organisations

- a perception of a decline in public confidence in charities – charities and other bodies have tried to improve their standards of governance as a way of retaining public confidence in what they are doing
- greater competition for funding – charities with better standards of governance may succeed better in attracting funds from government and the public
- a lack of clarity about the duties of voluntary board members, and in particular concerns about the liabilities of charity trustees – these concerns are similar to those in corporate governance, about the responsibilities of the board, the duties of directors and the potential liability of directors
- a growing demand for accountability to users and beneficiaries of the services provided by charities
- demands for greater transparency on how charities spend their donated income, and in particular the proportion spent ('wasted') on administration.

8.1 'Good Governance: a code for the voluntary and community sector'

Guidance called 'Good Governance: a code for the voluntary and community sector' was published in October 2010 as a second edition of the Code, which was originally published in 2005.

The code sets out best practice for governing a voluntary or community organisation. It is not mandatory but organisations that comply with the code are invited to state this in their Annual Report and other relevant published material, and pledge their support for the code by signing up to the online charter. The code focuses on six key principles that trustees and board members should follow and provides clear information about what those principles imply in practice.

It states that 'effective boards will provide good governance and leadership' as follows:

1. Members of the board will understand their role and responsibilities collectively and individually in relation to:

    - their legal duties
    - their stewardship of assets
    - the provisions of the governing document
    - the external environment
    - the total structure of the organisation

    and in terms of

    - setting and safeguarding the vision, values and reputation of the organisation
    - overseeing the work of the organisation
    - managing and supporting staff and volunteers, where applicable.

2. The board will ensure that the organisation delivers its stated purposes or aims by:

    - ensuring organisational purposes remain relevant and valid
    - developing and agreeing a long term strategy
    - agreeing operational plans and budgets
    - monitoring progress and spending against plan and budget
    - evaluating results, assessing outcomes and impact
    - reviewing and/or amending the plan and budget as appropriate.

3. The board will have a range of appropriate policies and procedures, knowledge, attitudes and behaviours to enable both individuals and the board to work effectively. These will include:

    - finding and recruiting new board members to meet the organisation's changing needs in relation to skills, experience and diversity
    - providing suitable induction for new board members
    - providing all board members with opportunities for training and development according to their needs
    - periodically reviewing their performance both as individuals and as a team.

4 As the accountable body, the board will ensure that:

- the organisation understands and complies with all legal and regulatory requirements that apply to it
- the organisation continues to have good internal financial and management controls
- it regularly identifies and reviews the major risks to which the organisation is exposed and has systems to manage those risks
- delegation to committees, staff and volunteers (as applicable) works effectively and the use of delegated authority is properly supervised.

5 The board will behave with integrity by:

- safeguarding and promoting the organisation's reputation
- acting according to high ethical standards
- identifying, understanding and managing conflicts of interest and loyalty
- maintaining independence of decision making
- delivering impact that best meets the needs of beneficiaries.

6 The board will lead the organisation in being open and accountable, both internally and externally. This will include:

- open communications, informing people about the organisation and its work
- appropriate consultation on significant changes to the organisation's services or policies
- listening and responding to the views of supporters, funders, beneficiaries, service users and others with an interest in the organisation's work
- handling complaints constructively, impartially and effectively
- considering the organisation's responsibilities to the wider community, e.g. its environmental impact.

TEST YOUR KNOWLEDGE 1.6

a How does health service governance differ from corporate governance?
b What are Nolan's seven principles of public life?
c What might be the consequences of bad governance practice in a charity?
d For what reasons have governance guidelines and codes of practice been developed for the voluntary sector?

CHAPTER SUMMARY

- Governance refers to the way in which an organisation is led, mainly by its directors. It is not concerned with executive management or business operations.
- Principles of good governance are fairness, accountability, responsibility and transparency.
- The main issue in governance is the effectiveness of the board of directors in promoting the long-term success of the organisation. Other key issues in governance are financial reporting and auditing, the remuneration of senior executives, relationships between an organisation and its stakeholder groups, risk management and internal control, communication between an organisation and its stakeholders, ethics and CSR.
- Health service governance operates on two levels: first, the manner in which the government department (DH) is held to account by the electorate for the way it manages the provision of healthcare; and second, the way in which individual parts of the NHS are governed and to what purpose.
- This text focuses on the aspects of health service governance that are concerned with the practices and procedures for ensuring that the individual parts of the NHS are run in such a way that they achieve their objectives and are in line with public sector values such as VFM and providing universal and free healthcare benefits to all those in need.

- Health service governance can be defined as a process for monitoring and control to ensure that management runs the organisation in the interests of those stakeholders, which, quite rightly will also include the DH as well as patients and employees.
- This is an interesting contrast to the objectives in the private sector where a company may decide to maximise the wealth of its owners (the shareholders), subject to various guidelines and constraints and with regard to other groups or individuals with an interest in what the company does.
- The UK has a history of mainly voluntary corporate governance practice. Its first governance code was the Cadbury Code (1992). The Combined Code (1998–2010) was revised and renamed the UK Corporate Governance Code in 2010. The *UK Code* and related guidelines are the responsibility of the FRC. Other countries have developed their own corporate governance regimes, mainly based on voluntary codes of practice for listed companies. The USA relies more on a regulatory system of corporate governance.
- Concepts of good governance practice have been extended from companies to the public sector and also the voluntary sector.
- In the UK, *Good Governance Standard for Public Services* was published in 2004, building on Nolan's Seven Principles of Public Life (selflessness, integrity, objectivity, accountability, openness, honesty and leadership).
- Similar codes of governance may be issued for the voluntary sector. In the UK, 'Good Governance: a code for the voluntary and community sector – Second Edition' was published in 2010.
- Although there are some significant differences, concepts of good health service governance are similar to concepts of best practice in corporate governance.

2 The NHS landscape

■ **CONTENTS**

1 History and context
2 Principles and values of the NHS
3 Rights and pledges provided by the constitution
4 Statement of NHS accountability
5 Other NHS bodies
6 Relationships with stakeholders and local accountability
7 Health and Social Care (HSC) Act 2012

■ **INTRODUCTION**

This chapter explains the nature and scope of the NHS Constitution, the principles and values that it codifies and the rights and pledges that are made to patients and staff. The system of responsibility and accountability for taking decisions in the NHS is explored. An overview of the regulatory system is outlined as well the structures that are in place to support local accountability. Finally, the chapter sets out a summary of the changes brought into force by the Health and Social Care (HSC) Act 2012.

1 History and context

The 'NHS constitution for England' is a formal constitution which, in one document, lays down the objectives of the NHS, the rights and responsibilities of the various parties involved in healthcare in England (patients, staff, trust boards) and the guiding principles that govern the service.

The constitution was first published on 21 January 2009 and was one of a number of recommendations in Lord Darzi's report 'High Quality Care for All', which provided a ten-year plan to provide the highest quality of care and service for patients in England.

Previously these rights and responsibilities had evolved in common law or through UK or EU law, or were policy pledges by the NHS and government. They have now been written into the constitution and from January 2010 under the Health Act 2009 all providers and commissioners of NHS care are under a new legal obligation to have regard to the NHS Constitution in all their decisions and actions.

The constitution is a concise document written in an accessible form and is simple to understand. Alongside the constitution is a handbook that gives more information to patients and staff about the constitution and a Statement of NHS accountability, which gives a clear account of the NHS system of accountability and responsibility.

The constitution grants patients 'rights' that are intended to be legally enforceable and also makes other non-binding 'pledges'. These are in the areas of access; quality of care and environment; access to treatments, medicines and screening programmes; respect, consent and confidentiality; informed choice; patient involvement in healthcare and public involvement in the NHS; and complaints and redress.

The constitution also sets out the 'rights' of NHS staff and makes other non-binding pledges to staff, recognising that high quality care requires high quality workplaces.

The constitution will be renewed every ten years, with the involvement of the public, patients and staff. The *Handbook to the NHS Constitution* will be renewed at least every three years, setting out current guidance on the rights, pledges, duties and responsibilities established by the constitution, and an updated version of the Constitution was issued in March 2012. These requirements for renewal are legally binding and guarantee that the principles and values that underpin the NHS are subject to regular review and recommitment; and that any government that seeks to alter the principles or values of the NHS, or the rights, pledges, duties and responsibilities set out in this constitution, has to engage in a full and transparent debate with the public, patients and staff.

The constitution provides an overriding strategy that is then underpinned at a local level by each NHS organisation as it actively considers its own specific local strategy.

2 Principles and values of the NHS

2.1 Principles of the NHS

- The NHS provides a comprehensive service, available to all irrespective of gender, race, disability, age, sexual orientation, religion or belief. It has a duty to each and every individual that it serves and must respect their human rights. At the same time, it has a wider social duty to promote equality through the services it provides and to pay particular attention to groups or sections of society where improvements in health and life expectancy are not keeping pace with the rest of the population.
- Access to NHS services is based on clinical need, not an individual's ability to pay. NHS services are free of charge, except in limited circumstances sanctioned by Parliament.
- The NHS aspires to the highest standards of excellence and professionalism – in the provision of high-quality care that is safe, effective and focused on patient experience; in the planning and delivery of the clinical and other services it provides; in the people it employs and the education, training and development they receive; in the leadership and management of its organisations; and through its commitment to innovation and to the promotion and conduct of research to improve the current and future health and care of the population.
- NHS services must reflect the needs and preferences of patients, their families and their carers. Patients, with their families and carers, where appropriate, will be involved in and consulted on all decisions about their care and treatment.
- The NHS works across organisational boundaries and in partnership with other organisations in the interest of patients, local communities and the wider population. The NHS is an integrated system of organisations and services bound together by the principles and values now reflected in the constitution. The NHS is committed to working jointly with local authorities and a wide range of other private, public and third sector organisations at national and local level to provide and deliver improvements in health and wellbeing.
- The NHS is committed to providing best value for taxpayers' money and the most effective, fair and sustainable use of finite resources. Public funds for healthcare will be devoted solely to the benefit of the people that the NHS serves.
- The NHS is accountable to the public, communities and patients that it serves. The NHS is a national service funded through national taxation, and it is the government that sets the framework for the NHS and which is accountable to Parliament for its operation. However, most decisions in the NHS, especially those about the treatment of individuals and the detailed organisation of services, are rightly taken by the local NHS and by patients with their clinicians. The system of responsibility and accountability for taking decisions in the NHS should be transparent and clear to the public, patients and staff. The government will ensure that there is always a clear and up-to-date statement of NHS accountability for this purpose.

2.2 Values of the NHS

These values have been developed with patients, public and staff with the intention that they should inspire passion in the NHS and guide it in the twenty-first century. Individual NHS organisations are expected to develop and refresh their own values, tailored to their local needs, however, these NHS values provide common ground for co-operation to achieve shared aspirations.

- a Respect and dignity. We value each person as an individual, respect their aspirations and commitments in life, and seek to understand their priorities, needs, abilities and limits. We take what others have to say seriously. We are honest about our point of view and what we can and cannot do.
- b Commitment to quality of care. We earn the trust placed in us by insisting on quality and striving to get the basics right every time: safety, confidentiality, professional and managerial integrity, accountability, dependable service and good communication. We welcome feedback, learn from our mistakes and build on our successes.
- c Compassion. We respond with humanity and kindness to each person's pain, distress, anxiety or need. We search for the things we can do, however small, to give comfort and relieve suffering. We find time for those we serve and work alongside. We do not wait to be asked, because we care.
- d Improving lives. We strive to improve health and wellbeing and people's experiences of the NHS. We value excellence and professionalism wherever we find it – in the everyday things that make people's lives better as much as in clinical practice, service improvements and innovation.
- e Working together for patients. We put patients first in everything we do, by reaching out to staff, patients, carers, families, communities and professionals outside the NHS. We put the needs of patients and communities before organisational boundaries.
- f Everyone counts. We use our resources for the benefit of the whole community, and make sure nobody is excluded or left behind. We accept that some people need more help, that difficult decisions have to be taken – and that when we waste resources we waste others' opportunities. We recognise that we all have a part to play in making ourselves and our communities healthier.

3 Rights and pledges provided by the constitution

The constitution grants patients 'rights', which are intended to be legally enforceable and also makes other non-binding 'pledges'.

3.1 Access to healthcare

The constitution defines 'RIGHTS' regarding 'access to healthcare', which will be:

- free of charge
- non-discriminatory
- never refused on unreasonable grounds
- obtainable from any UK NHS provider or with pre-approval from any European Economic Area or Swiss public provider
- assessed by the local NHS to meet locally assessed needs
- within maximum waiting times, or for the NHS to take all reasonable steps to offer you a range of suitable alternative providers if this is not possible.

The NHS also makes pledges:

- that access to healthcare will be convenient and easy to access within defined waiting times, based on decision making that will be clear and transparent
- that transfers from one provider to another will be as smooth as possible and that patients will be involved in all relevant discussions.

3.2 Quality of care and environment

The constitution defines 'RIGHTS' regarding 'quality of care and environment' as follows:

- Treatment with a professional standard of care, by appropriately qualified and experienced staff, an organisation that meets required levels of safety and quality.
- Patients can expect NHS organisations to monitor, and make efforts to improve, the quality of healthcare they commission or provide.

The NHS also makes pledges that:

- services will be provided in a clean and safe environment that is fit for purpose, based on national best practice
- there will be a continuous improvement in the quality of services, identifying and sharing best practice.

3.3 Approved treatments, drugs and programmes

The constitution defines 'RIGHTS' regarding 'approved treatments, drugs and programmes' as patients have the right to:

- drugs and treatments that have been recommended by the National Institute for Health and Clinical Excellence (NICE) for use in the NHS, if their doctor says they are clinically appropriate for them
- expect local decisions on funding of other drugs and treatments to be made rationally following a proper consideration of the evidence. If the local NHS decides not to fund a drug or treatment that you and your doctor feel would be right for you, the local NHS must explain that decision
- receive the approved vaccinations under an NHS-provided national immunisation programme.

The NHS also makes pledges:

- to provide screening programmes as recommended by the UK National Screening Committee.

This statement made it clear that NICE decisions rule nationally and override local NHS management and in the absence of other guidance from local NHS management then responsibility lies with the doctor and patient together. NICE was originally established to guide national policy where there were significant differences of opinion between the different local NHS organisations over certain drugs and treatments – the so-called **postcode lottery**, but local managements have generally had powers over budgets and coverage in their local area.

3.4 Respect, consent and confidentiality

The constitution defines 'RIGHTS' regarding 'Respect, consent and confidentiality' as follows:

- to be treated with dignity and respect
- able to accept or refuse treatment that is offered, and not to be given any examination or treatment without valid consent
- to be given information about their proposed treatment in advance, including any significant risks and any alternative treatments that may be available, and the risks involved in doing nothing
- to privacy and confidentiality and to expect the NHS to keep their confidential information safe and secure
- access to their own health records, which will always be used to manage treatment in the patient's best interests.

The NHS also makes pledges:

- that it will share with patients any letters sent between clinicians about their care.

3.5 Informed Choice

The constitution defines 'RIGHTS' regarding 'informed choice' as including the right to:

- choose their own GP practice, and to be accepted by that practice unless there are reasonable grounds to refuse
- express a preference for using a particular doctor within their GP practice, and for the practice to try to comply
- make choices about their NHS care and to information to support these choices.

The NHS also makes pledges:

- to inform patients about the healthcare services available locally and nationally
- to offer easily accessible, reliable and relevant information to enable patients to participate fully in their own healthcare decisions and to support them in making choices. This includes information on the quality of clinical services where there is robust and accurate information available.

3.6 Involvement in one's own healthcare and in the NHS

The constitution defines 'RIGHTS' regarding 'Involvement in their own healthcare and in the NHS' as rights to:

- be involved in discussions and decisions about one's own healthcare, and to be given information to enable one to do this
- be involved, directly or through representatives, in the planning of healthcare services, the development and consideration of proposals for changes in the way those services are provided, and in decisions to be made affecting the operation of those services.

The NHS also makes pledges:

- to provide the information needed for the people to influence and scrutinise the planning and delivery of NHS services
- to work in partnership with patients, their family, carers and their representatives.

3.7 Rights of redress

Under the constitution, when complaining or seeking redress, patients are given 'RIGHTS' to:

- have any complaint made about NHS services dealt with efficiently and to have it properly investigated
- know the outcome of any investigation into a complaint
- take a complaint to the independent Health Service Ombudsman, if they are not satisfied with the way their complaint was dealt with by the NHS
- make a claim for judicial review if they think they have been directly affected by an unlawful act or decision of an NHS body
- compensation where they have been harmed by negligent treatment.

The NHS also makes pledges:

- to ensure patients are treated with courtesy and receive appropriate support throughout the handling of a complaint, and the fact that they have made a complaint will not adversely affect their future treatment
- that when mistakes happen, the NHS promises to acknowledge them, apologise, explain what went wrong and put things right quickly and effectively
- that the organisation will learn lessons from complaints and will use them to improve NHS services.

TEST YOUR KNOWLEDGE 2.1

a The NHS Constitution enshrines a variety of objectives, rights, responsibilities and principles – what were the original sources of these?
b What is the difference between rights and pledges as set out in the Constitution?
c What legal obligation was created by the Health Act 2009?

4 Statement of NHS accountability

The NHS Constitution commits the government to providing a statement of NHS accountability, which describes the system of responsibility and accountability for taking decisions in the NHS. This document accompanies the NHS Constitution and provides a summary of the current structure and functions of the NHS in England.

The NHS is a system of organisations responsible for organising and providing a comprehensive health service. The funding for running the NHS is granted to the DH by Parliament out of national taxation. There is therefore a continuous thread of accountability to the government running throughout the NHS.

The Secretary of State for Health is accountable to Parliament, and through Parliament to the voters, for the promotion of a comprehensive health service and for the use of public money. Any decision taken by ministers about health policy can be scrutinised by Members of Parliament.

The NHS in England currently spends around £106 billion a year (2011/2012) – equivalent to nearly £2,000 per person on average. The majority of the funding granted to the DH by Parliament is currently allocated directly to local organisations known as PCTs, which use it to commission services for their population from provider organisations such as hospital trusts, mental health trusts, ambulance trusts, GP practices, dental practices, community pharmacies, optical practices and NHS Direct. PCTs will be replaced by Clinical Commissioning Groups in due course.

All organisations that provide care for NHS patients are responsible for ensuring that their services meet appropriate levels of safety and quality.

Essentially the provision of healthcare by NHS is divided into two sections: primary and secondary care. **Primary care** is the first point of contact for most people and is delivered by a wide range of independent contractors, including GPs, dentists, pharmacists and optometrists. **Secondary care** is known as acute healthcare and can be either elective care or emergency care. **Elective care** means planned specialist medical care or surgery, usually following referral from a primary or community health professional such as a GP. Most of these services are provided by 'NHS bodies', which are part of the public sector.

There are, however, also many other types of organisation involved in providing NHS care, including providers from the independent sector or third sector. For example, pharmacies tend to be independent sector organisations, and most GPs and dentists have traditionally worked as contractors for the NHS, either individually or in partnerships. The third sector includes organisations such as local community groups, voluntary groups, registered charities, social enterprises and co-operatives. All organisations contracted to provide NHS services must meet the NHS's required levels of care.

The Statement of Accountability describes how the NHS in England currently works and who is responsible for its different parts. It is being updated as a result of the HSC Act 2012.

Until the HSC Act 2012 is fully implemented, there are two main ways in which organisations providing care for NHS patients are held to account for the quality of their services – PCTs and regulators.

4.1 Primary care trusts (PCTs)

Until April 2013 the PCT is the key organisation responsible at the local level for ensuring there is a comprehensive range of health services for the local population. PCTs tend to call themselves by the name of their local area. For example, NHS Oxford is the PCT responsible for ensuring the provision of NHS services in the Oxford area. PCTs commission healthcare services for their area. They often also directly provide some NHS services, such as community health services. Overall, they control the vast majority of the NHS budget.

PCTs are responsible for improving the health and wellbeing of their local population. To achieve this, they are under a legal duty to work with the local authority to assess what kind of health services people need. They then commission services to meet those needs. This is done in partnership with local clinicians, who are involved in service planning and commissioning decisions.

PCTs can commission services from a range of different organisations. Any service a PCT commissions will always be NHS-funded but it can be provided by voluntary or independent sector organisations as well as NHS organisations. PCTs generally hold the providers of these services to account via contracts. PCTs can ask the regulators to step in if the providers are not meeting the expected standards.

The health of the public, however, is not solely the responsibility of the NHS. The wider local public sector, as well as employers, and voluntary and community groups, all have a vital contribution to make. PCTs work directly with other local partners such as local authorities, including children's services and housing services, to promote and protect the health and wellbeing of the local population.

All PCTs are also part of a body called a local strategic partnership, which is led by the local authority. This body brings together at a local level the different parts of the public sector as well as the private, community and voluntary sectors, for example, police, fire and rescue services, charity groups, local businesses and more, to coordinate plans and make sure the right services are delivered.

It is important that PCTs engage with their local populations and their partner organisations to take account of local views. There are a number of ways in which they can do this, in addition to their work with Local Involvement Networks (LINks) and the local authority's overview and scrutiny committees (see Section 6 below).

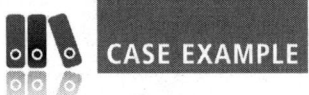

CASE EXAMPLE 2.1

The PCT in Leeds serves a population of 720,000 and has an annual budget of almost £1 billion. It commissions services from over 100 GP practices, as well as dental practices and community pharmacies. Many community health services, such as district nursing, are commissioned from the PCT's arm's-length provider. NHS Leeds commissions hospital and specialist care from a range of providers, including:

- Leeds Teaching Hospitals Trust;
- Leeds Partnership NHS Foundation Trust;
- Harrogate and District NHS Foundation Trust;
- Mid Yorkshire Hospitals NHS Trust; and
- the independent sector.

The government's White Paper in July 2010, **Equity and Excellence: liberating the NHS** set out the planned abolition of the PCTs from April 2013 with the intention of replacing them with clinical commissioning consortia. As a result PCTs have been required to form into regional clusters in preparation for this transition.

PCTs are held to account by SHAs. The board of the PCT is accountable to the board of the SHA covering that region (see Section 4.4).

4.2 Regulators

The NHS is underpinned by a system of regulation, which is independent from government and from the NHS itself. It is there to ensure that the care patients receive is safe and of acceptable quality. The regulators also make sure the bodies or healthcare professionals they regulate are sound and fit for purpose.

The national level – The Department of Health

The DH is a government department. Its overall aim is to improve the health and wellbeing of the people of England. To do this it:

- develops the strategy and direction for the healthcare system
- develops the legislative framework
- secures and allocates resources for healthcare services.

The Department is accountable to Parliament and the public. The Department does not lead on the day-to-day running and organisation of health services.

The DH is made up of civil servants who advise the Secretary of State for Health and other ministers on health policy. The Secretary of State is a politician and is the Cabinet minister responsible for health in England. He or she takes decisions on national health policy.

The chief executive of the NHS sits in the DH and is responsible for delivery and leadership in the healthcare system on behalf of the Secretary of State. The chief executive is the chief policy adviser to ministers on NHS matters.

The Department also has responsibilities beyond the NHS, including:

- setting the strategic framework for adult social care, and
- taking the lead on issues such as environmental hazards to health, infectious diseases, health promotion and education, the safety of medicines, and ethical issues in health and social care.

The regional NHS: strategic health authorities

Until the recent reforms, **SHAs** were the regional headquarters of the NHS and carry out functions delegated to them by the Secretary of State. They were accountable for the performance and management of the healthcare system. Each SHA was responsible for ensuring that patients had access to high-quality services in its area, overseeing the performance of PCTs and NHS trusts, and responsible for supporting NHS trusts to reach foundation trust status. They held PCTs to account and were directly accountable to the DH.

Until recently there were ten SHAs covering regions across England. For example, NHS Yorkshire and Humber was responsible for overseeing all the NHS services in that region. These ten SHAs have been moved into clusters ahead of their abolition under the government's reforms. The resulting four SHA Clusters are NHS North of England, NHS Midlands and the East, NHS South of England and NHS London.

Care Quality Commission

From April 2009, the safety and quality regulator for all health services has been the **CQC**, which is also responsible for the regulation of adult social care services. The CQC's principal functions in relation to healthcare is to:

- register healthcare providers (whether or not they provide services for the NHS)
- monitor compliance with registration requirements and, if necessary, use its enforcement powers to ensure all service providers meet those requirements
- review and publish comparative information on organisations providing and commissioning healthcare, and undertake reviews or studies of particular types of care
- monitor the operation of the Mental Health Act and Mental Capacity Act.

The CQC publishes independent assessments of how organisations are performing by drawing on a range of sources of information, including what patients and the public tell them. It also reports annually to Parliament on how the health and social care systems are working overall.

The CQC has the power to inspect all registered healthcare providers and to suspend services, impose fines, prosecute or deregister organisations if it has evidence that suggests a serious problem that may be putting patients at risk.

Monitor

Unlike NHS trusts, which are overseen by SHAs, NHS foundation trusts (see Section 5) are regulated by Monitor, an independent regulator. NHS foundation trusts are assessed by the CQC in the same way as other hospitals.

NHS trusts have to apply to become NHS foundation trusts. Monitor assesses and decides on their applications. It also ensures that NHS foundation trusts meet the conditions it sets for the way they operate so that they are well managed and financially robust. It has powers to intervene in the running of an NHS foundation trust to safeguard NHS patients and services.

Monitor is accountable to Parliament but independent of the Secretary of State.

Professional regulators

There are a number of regulatory bodies that are responsible for the regulation of healthcare professionals. An example is the General Medical Council, which regulates doctors, and the Nursing and Midwifery Council, which regulates nurses and midwives.

The professional regulators are independent bodies responsible to Parliament that register and regulate the training and practice of health professionals. They safeguard the safety and the quality of the care that patients receive from health professionals. This includes dealing with concerns about misconduct raised by patients, their families or other professionals. Professional regulators certify new practitioners and ensure that they maintain standards and remain fit to practice.

Health professionals can be reported to the relevant professional regulator and guidance is available on the website of the Council for Healthcare Regulatory Excellence, which provides an oversight role on professional regulation.

5 Other NHS bodies

5.1 Special health authorities

There are a number of national bodies involved in the provision or organisation of NHS services. They have responsibility for things that are best done or coordinated at the national level. Some examples are as follows:

- The NHS Blood and Transplant Authority is responsible for the supply of blood, organs, plasma and tissues across the NHS.
- The Medicines and Healthcare Products Regulatory Agency is responsible for ensuring that medicines work and are acceptably safe.
- NICE is responsible for producing national guidance on which drugs and treatments are clinically and cost effective, as well as guidance on promoting good health.

Special health authorities are health authorities that provide a health service to the whole of England, not just to a local community. They have been set up to provide a national service to the NHS or the public under section 9 of the NHS Act 1977. They are independent, but can be subject to ministerial direction in the same way as other NHS bodies.

5.2 NHS foundation trusts

NHS foundation trusts are part of the NHS. High-performing NHS trusts can apply for foundation trust status and the government intends for all NHS trusts to become NHS foundation trusts over time. They must be well managed and financially robust to be granted NHS foundation trust status.

NHS foundation trusts provide the same kind of services as any other hospital, mental health or ambulance trust but are accountable in a different way and have greater freedoms. They were created to move decision-making from central government to local organisations and communities so that services could become more responsive to the needs and wishes of local people. This means that, unlike other NHS bodies, NHS foundation trusts are not overseen by SHAs or the DH but are instead regulated by an independent body called Monitor.

Like all NHS bodies, NHS foundation trusts are accountable to the PCTs that commission services from them. They are also accountable to their local populations through a board of governors: members of the public, patients and staff can become members of their NHS foundation trust. The membership elects the board of governors, which is made up of patients, the public and staff through locally run elections. Local stakeholders are also represented on the board of governors. The governors' role is to represent the interests of patients and the local community in the way the trust is managed.

NHS foundation trusts are financially independent organisations with greater freedom over the way they shape the healthcare services they provide. They are free to manage their own budgets. However, national standards and the legal framework for the NHS are the responsibility of ministers and apply to NHS foundation trusts just as they do to other parts of the NHS.

A much fuller description of the health service governance relating to foundation trusts can be found in Chapter 6.

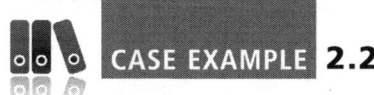
CASE EXAMPLE 2.2

Heart of England NHS Foundation Trust provides over 40 different healthcare services and is based across four sites: Birmingham Heartlands Hospital; Solihull Hospital; Good Hope Hospital; and Birmingham Chest Clinic.

The services provided by the trust include general medical, surgical and accident and emergency services, as well as specialist services, such as cardiology, dermatology, orthodontics, paediatrics, radiology, and speech and language therapy.

6 Relationships with stakeholders and local accountability

While the NHS is a national system that is primarily held to account nationally, there is also a range of ways in which it is accountable to patients and the public at a local level. Some of the main ways are described here.

6.1 Duty to involve and report to the public

NHS bodies are under a legal duty to involve people who use health services or their representatives in decisions about those services. This duty applies to SHAs, PCTs, NHS trusts and NHS foundation trusts. The duty applies to the planning of health services, proposals for changes in the provision of services and decisions that will affect the way services operate.

SHAs and PCTs are also under a legal duty to report publicly on how they have involved people in their activities and on the impact of the consultation on their decisions. Members of the public are also able to attend the board meetings of SHAs, PCTs and NHS Trusts.

There are also opportunities to give feedback on local services through regular patient surveys.

6.2 Local Involvement Networks (LINks)

LINks give the public a voice in how their health and social care services are planned and delivered. LINks are made up of individuals and community groups who work together to improve local health and social care services. Local authorities are responsible for making arrangements to establish LINks but LINks operate independently.

The role of LINks is to find out what people want, allow them to suggest ideas for improving services, monitor local services and look into specific issues of concern to the community. PCTs, NHS trusts and NHS foundation trusts are legally obliged to allow LINks representatives to enter and view their services.

NHS organisations are required to respond to recommendations made by LINks and be clear about what actions they will take as a result.

As part of the government reforms announced in July 2010, the government announced plans to set up an independent champion for health and social care consumers called HealthWatch England. LINks will become local HealthWatch Committees in due course.

6.3 Overview and scrutiny committees

The public's opinion can also influence local health services through the overview and scrutiny committees of local authorities. Overview and scrutiny committees (OSCs) are made up of elected local councillors, supported by council officials. They allow democratically elected community leaders to voice the views of their constituents and require local NHS bodies to listen and respond.

OSCs have the power to scrutinise the operation and planning of local health services. They can require the NHS to provide information and explanations about how the needs of the local population are being addressed.

As part of the government NHS reforms, Health and Wellbeing Boards will be established to support the work of these committees by providing the views of the local constituents.

6.4 Parliamentary and health service ombudsman

The ombudsman conducts independent investigations into complaints that government departments, a range of other public bodies in the UK, or the NHS in England have not acted properly or fairly, or have provided a poor service.

The ombudsman can look at complaints about the actions of providers of NHS care, as well as PCTs and SHAs. The ombudsman can also look at complaints about the DH, the CQC and Monitor.

The ombudsman is accountable to Parliament and independent of government and the NHS.

TEST YOUR KNOWLEDGE 2.2

a What does the Statement of NHS Accountability describe?
b Who are the key regulators within the NHS?
c How does governors provide local accountability for foundation trusts?
d What other arrangements are there to create local accountability for NHS organisations?

7 Health and Social Care (HSC) Act 2012

The Health and Social Care Bill was introduced into Parliament on 19 January 2011. It took forward the government White Paper **Equity and Excellence: liberating the NHS** (July 2010) and the subsequent government response **Liberating the NHS: legislative framework and next steps** (December 2010). It also included provision to strengthen public health services and reform the Department's arm's-length bodies. The Bill received Royal Assent at the end of March 2012. The Act is intended to create an independent NHS Board, promote patient choice and to reduce NHS administration costs.

The key areas of the Act are:

1 Establishing an independent NHS Board to allocate resources and provide commissioning guidance.
2 Increasing GPs' powers to commission services on behalf of their patients.
3 Strengthening the role of the CQC.
4 Developing Monitor, the body that currently regulates NHS foundation trusts, into an economic regulator to oversee aspects of access and competition in the NHS.
5 Cutting the number of health bodies to help meet the government's commitment to cut NHS administration costs by a third, including abolishing PCTs and SHAs.

The main aims of the Act are:

- to change how NHS care is commissioned through the greater involvement of GPs and a new Commissioning Board
- to improve accountability and patient voice
- to give NHS providers new freedoms to improve quality of care
- to establish an economic regulator to promote efficiency.

In addition, the Bill will underpin the creation of Public Health England, and take forward measures to reform health public bodies.

After the Health and Social Care Bill had passed through the Committee stage in the House of Commons the government launched a Listening Exercise to pause, listen and reflect on how to improve the NHS modernisation plans. Following this, a number of significant amendments were made to the Bill. These changes included:

1. Legal responsibility of the health secretary for the NHS to be reinstated.
2. Relaxation of the 2013 deadline for new GP commissioning arrangements.
3. Greater power for health and wellbeing boards with patients given a greater role on them.
4. Other professionals such as hospital doctors and nurses to be involved in commissioning consortia.

These were in addition to the significantly diluted focus on competition, with the regulator, Monitor, instead focusing on improving patient choice.

Figure 2.1 sets out the new structure.

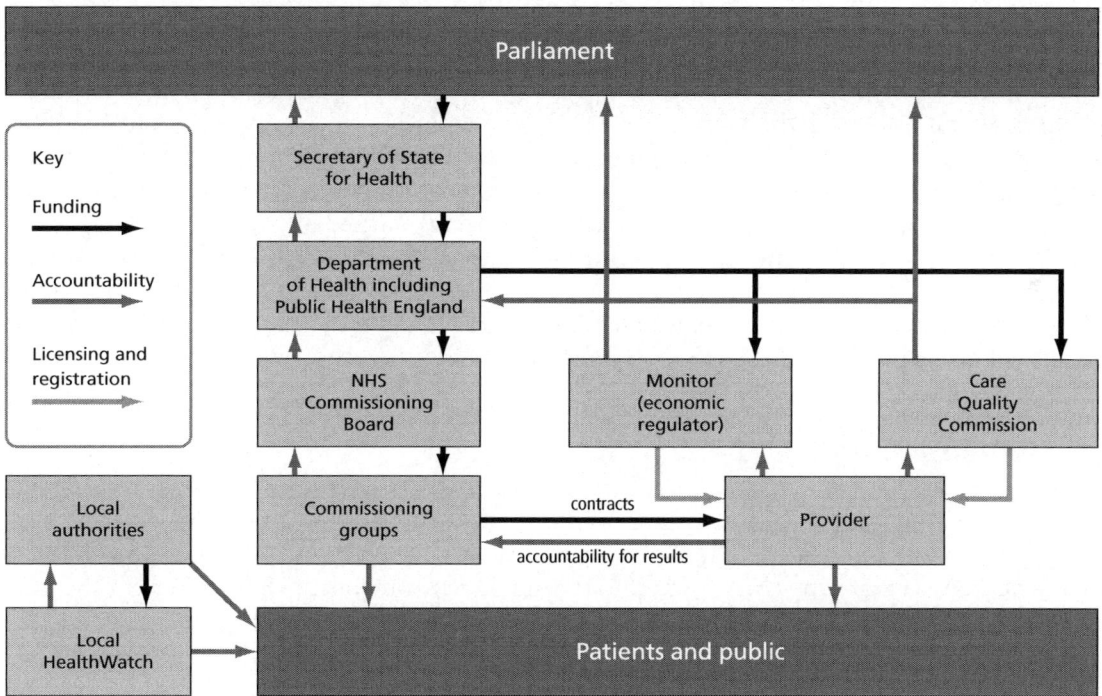

FIGURE 2.1 NHS structure under the Health and Social Care Act 2012
(Source: www.nhshistory.net)

7.1 Impact on NHS structure of accountability

The ten existing SHAs, which have moved into four clusters ahead of their abolition in 2012, will provide the basis for subnational arrangements of the NHS Commissioning Board.

The 150 or so PCTs to be abolished in April 2013 will be replaced by new **CCGs** of GPs and other professionals such as hospital doctors and nurses. The total number of consortiums is unclear and they may have different boundaries to those of local councils, or cover several local authority areas.

Clinical Commissioning Groups (CCGs)

These new consortiums will commission most but not all healthcare. They will be responsible to a new independent NHS Commissioning Board (NHSCB), which will itself commission some services, such as dentistry. The board will also hold the consortiums to account for the quality of the health outcomes they help to produce and their financial performance, given they will be responsible for a substantial slice of all public spending.

As statutory bodies, CCGs will assume significant responsibilities in terms of governance and accountability for taxpayers' money. The government intends consortia 'once established, [to] be statutory bodies, with powers and responsibilities set out through primary and secondary legislation. By that time, each consortium [will] need to have chosen its own accountable officer and chief financial officer'.

In NHS organisations the **accountable officer** role is normally fulfilled by the CEO. The accountable officer for a CCG will be accountable both to the NHSCB and within the commissioning group. The accountable officer will be selected by the commissioning group itself but formally appointed by the NHSCB at the time of authorisation. When established, commissioning groups will have a formal duty to cooperate with other NHS bodies. This will include providers of healthcare, PCTs and associated clusters (until they are formally abolished), and other commissioning groups.

The government has stated that each commissioning group will have a governing body with independent membership via at least two lay members (equivalent to NEDs), as well as further clinical representation through one registered nurse and one doctor who is a secondary care specialist. The two lay members will be key appointments with specific responsibilities, namely patient and public involvement and oversight of the governance arrangements. In addition, one of the lay members will undertake the role of chair or the deputy chair. The governing body will also be required to hold its meetings in public and publish the minutes of those meetings.

NHS Trust Development Agency

This agency will take over the role of the SHAs and is due to be legally established in June 2012, operating in shadow form from September 2012 and operational by April 2013. It will provide governance and oversight of NHS trusts, supporting them to NHS foundation trust status. It will bring together the functions that are currently carried out within the DH, by the SHA clusters and by the Appointments Commission (see Chapter 9). It will performance manage NHS trusts, manage the FT pipeline, assure clinical quality, governance and risk in NHS trusts and manage the appointments of chair and NEDs. The NTDA will remain responsible for the oversight of the performance of NHS trusts until the final NHS trust application for FT status has been authorised by Monitor.

NHS Commissioning Board

The NHSCB will be nationally accountable for the outcomes achieved by the NHS, and provide leadership for the new commissioning system outlined above. Responsibility for local commissioning will rest with CCGs, but they will be supported and overseen by the NHSCB, which will hold the groups to account for the quality of outcomes they achieve. The new architecture will take on many of the roles and responsibilities currently discharged by the DH, SHAs and PCTs.

Health and Wellbeing

Each local authority will have to set up a health and wellbeing board to oversee the quality of local services, present local people's views and draw up a health and wellbeing strategy for the area. Health and wellbeing boards will be a forum for local commissioners across the NHS, public health and social care, elected representatives, and representatives of HealthWatch to discuss how to work together to better the health and wellbeing outcomes of the people in their area.

It is intended that by involving democratically elected representatives and patient representatives, and bringing them together with local commissioners across health, public health and social care, it will significantly strengthen the democratic legitimacy of commissioning decisions, as well as providing a forum for challenge, discussion and the involvement of local people. The boards will need to work together regionally and with other national structures such as the NHSCB and Public Health England. They will also need to build credibility and trust with local communities.

Healthwatch England

This new public health organisation will help patients complain and also guide them when they have to choose where to go to receive healthcare. There will also be a local branch of HealthWatch in each local council area offering advocacy, advice and information and in due course these will replace the existing LINks.

NHS trusts

All hospital trusts will have to become foundation trusts by 2014, and therefore will not be overseen by SHAs or the DH. They will continue to be regulated by Monitor, whose role will be expanded to that of an economic regulator who will oversee aspects of access, competition and price-setting in the NHS.

Monitor

Under the Act, Monitor becomes the sector regulator for health and, at a later date, for adult social care. Monitor's core duty will be to protect and promote patients' interests. In the medium term it would also have a continuing role in assessing NHS trusts for foundation trust status, and for ensuring that foundation trusts are financially viable and well-led, in terms of both quality and finances. In carrying out its sector regulator role, Monitor would license providers of NHS services in England thus requiring any organisation wishing to provide NHS-funded services, to be jointly licensed by Monitor and the CQC. The licence would set out the way providers would have to operate, while licensing would enable Monitor to carry out its other roles in three key areas:

1 **Regulating prices**. Monitor would be responsible for designing a pricing methodology and calculating the efficiency requirements for the sector. This would then be used to set prices, in agreement with the NHS Commissioning Board.
2 **Enabling integrated care and preventing anti-competitive behaviour**. Monitor's role as the sector regulator would be to work with others, particularly commissioners, to remove any barriers and consider how to enable integrated care provision where this is in the interests of patients.
3 **Supporting service continuity**. Monitor would take on a new role in supporting commissioners to ensure that, in the rare event of the failure of a healthcare provider, patients could continue to access the care that they need.

The fact that Monitor will continue to authorise and regulate foundation trusts creates a potential conflict of interests with the proposed sector-wide role, which Monitor intends to address in the design of the organisation. Section 63 of the Act sets out that it is Monitor's duty to ensure that no conflicts arise in the exercise of its main functions, including those related to foundation trusts.

TEST YOUR KNOWLEDGE 2.3

a What key government papers are reflected in the HSC Act 2012?
b What are the main aims of the Act?
c What are the new NHS organisations are created under the Act?
d How will Monitor's role be extended?

STOP AND THINK 2.1

What are the significant governance risks that are posed by the NHS reforms?

Foundation Trusts

The key changes from the Health and Social Care Act 2012 that impact foundation trusts include:

- Monitor acting as a license provider, thus eliminating FT terms of authorisation.
- extended powers and responsibility for governors.
- clarification on the role of directors.
- requirement to hold board meetings in public.

These changes are set out in more detail in Chapter 6.

CHAPTER SUMMARY

- The NHS Constitution sets out the overall objectives for the NHS, as well as codifying its principles and values. It also sets out the rights of patient and staff.
- The constitution grants legally enforceable rights in the areas of access; quality of care and environment; access to treatments, medicines and screening programmes; respect, consent and confidentiality; informed choice; patient involvement in healthcare and public involvement in the NHS; and complaints and redress.
- The constitution provides an overriding strategy that is interpreted and implemented at a local level by NHS organisations.
- The constitution is also accompanied by the NHS Statement of Accountability, which describes the system of responsibility and accountability for taking decisions in the NHS.
- The funding for running the NHS is granted to the DH by Parliament out of national taxation. There is therefore a continuous thread of accountability to the government running throughout the NHS.
- The current system of accountability involves PCTs, provider trusts and SHAs.
- The NHS is also held to account by its regulators, i.e. the CQC, the respective professional regulatory bodies and Monitor.
- The HSC Act 2012 abolishes PCTs and SHAs and establishes CCGs, a NHS Trust Development Agency and a National Commissioning Board.

Governance, the law and the company secretary

■ CONTENTS

1 Governance and the law
2 UK healthcare law
3 Company law and other legislation
4 Compulsory regulation and voluntary best practice
5 The role of the company secretary

■ INTRODUCTION

This chapter considers the extent to which best practice in both health service governance and corporate governance is imposed on organisations by the law or other regulations. There are two different approaches to establishing a system of best practice in governance. One approach is to establish voluntary principles and guidelines, and invite (or expect) organisations to comply with them. A second approach is to establish laws and other regulations for governance that organisations must obey. In practice, many countries combine legal and regulatory requirements with voluntary principles and codes of conduct. The chapter concludes with an explanation of the role of the company secretary in applying best practice in governance, including complying with governance principles and provisions.

The chapter should enable you to identify both aspects of health service and corporate governance practice that may be regulated by law or regulations. It will demonstrate that laws and regulations on governance vary, so that some sectors and indeed some countries adopt a 'rules-based' approach to governance, while others rely more on a 'principles-based' approach.

1 Governance and the law

Governance is concerned with the way in which organisations are led. The directors of an organisation should be responsible for safeguarding its assets and for protecting the rights and interests of the stakeholders. In corporate governance this results in a significant level of accountability to the shareholders. It is inevitable that some aspects of governance practice should be regulated by law, and that organisations should be required to comply with 'best practice'. Regulations on governance may be found in:

- public law
- laws on transparency of information
- laws on consultation
- laws on counter fraud
- company law, insolvency law and laws regulating financial markets and services, insider dealing and money laundering.

There is no corporate governance law in any country: rather, some aspects of corporate governance are regulated by sections of different laws. Other aspects of governance are not regulated by law at all, or are regulated only partially. Even in the USA, where there is greater emphasis on regulation of corporate governance, many elements of 'best practice' in corporate governance are voluntary.

Similarly, there is no health service governance law for the NHS. Some aspects of health service governance are regulated by different aspects of public law as well as national legislation. There is also a raft of guidance and voluntary codes that have been established for use within the NHS.

2 UK healthcare law

The NHS was established in 1948 by the National Health Service Act 1948. Since that time there have been significant amendments and additions to the legislation, which has resulted in a very fragmented and piecemeal approach to NHS healthcare law. Rather than list each amendment and addition since 1948 this text sets out the main items of legislation that result in the current form and structure of the NHS.

The NHS Reorganisation Act 1973 provided for lines of authority from NHS providers up to the Secretary of State through the creation of 90 area health authorities (AHAs), which managed both hospitals and community health services. The AHAs were also given joint planning responsibilities with the local authorities. Beneath the AHAs were District Management Teams, which managed hospitals and family practitioner committees (FPCs) that took responsibility for administering contracts for GPs, dentists, pharmacists and opticians. The AHAs were under the supervision of 14 regional health authorities (RHAs), which operated from 1974 to 1996.

The National Health Service Act 1977 set out the obligations of the Secretary of State to promote a comprehensive health service. His national responsibilities were delegated to special heath authorities such as the National Blood Authority and NICE. His local responsibilities were delegated to AHAs. Management of these functions was carried out by regional health authorities on behalf of the Secretary of State.

The Health Services Act 1980 abolished the AHAs and District Management Teams and replaced them with district health authorities (DHAs) in 1982.

The National Health Service and Community Care Act 1990 set out how the NHS should assess and provide for patients based on their needs, requirements and circumstances. This Act established the split between 'purchasers' (health authorities and some family doctors, under the GP fundholding scheme), who were given budgets to commission healthcare, and 'providers' (acute hospitals, organisations providing care for the mentally ill, people with learning disabilities and the elderly, and ambulance services). The Act introduced the concept of the internal market, i.e. the relationship between the purchasers and the providers was a contractual one. These contractual relationships operated at a common law level but were not judicially enforceable. As a result of the internal market, the state became an 'enabler' rather than a supplier of health and social care provision. The functions of NHS trusts (the 'providers') were partly determined by the 1990 Act and partly through each individual trust's establishment order. The Act also set out key statutory financial obligations such as the obligation to break even, to carry out functions effectively, efficiently and economically, and to hold a public meeting at which the annual report and audited accounts were presented.

The NHS Trusts (Membership and Procedures) Regulations 1990 set out the composition of the board for NHS trusts, the criteria for appointment and tenure of the chairman and NEDs. It sets out the rules regarding the meetings and proceedings of NHS trusts and the appointment procedures for executive directors.

The Health Authorities Act 1995 abolished regional health authorities, district health authorities and family health services authorities and established a single tier of health authorities.

The Health Act 1999 abolished GP fund-holding in England, Wales and Scotland. The Act amended the National Health Service Act 1977 to make provision for the establishment of new statutory bodies in England and Wales to be known as PCTs, and provided for NHS trusts in Scotland to take on additional functions.

The Health and Social Care (HSC) Act 2001 was designed to deliver many of the aspects of the NHS Plan 2000 that required changes to primary legislation. The Act outlined a new delivery system for the NHS, which provided for the commissioning of health and social care by Care Trusts under partnership arrangements. It also strengthened the arrangements for public and patient involvement in the NHS by providing for local authority OSCs, whose role was to scrutinise the NHS and to represent local views on the development of local health services. It also created a duty on NHS organisations to have arrangements for involving patients and the public in decision making about the operation of the NHS.

The Act also legislated for

- the Healthcare Commission to be set up
- regulations to be made about complaints procedures in both health and social services
- the Health Service Ombudsman to consider complaints about the handling of NHS complaints by any person or NHS body.

The act also provided for a new form of trust, Care Trusts, to provide closer integration of health and social services.

The National Health Service Reform and Health Care Professions Act 2002 provided for amendment of the structural framework of the NHS. The Act renamed health authorities as SHAs and conferred most of their functions onto PCTs. NHS resources were to be allocated directly to the PCTs by the Secretary of State. Service planning would be undertaken by the PCTs, with the SHAs providing the performance management function for the health services provided within their boundaries. The Act also provided for the creation of an independent 'Patients' Forum' for every NHS trust and PCT in England, to perform an inspection, monitoring and representation role on behalf of patients and the public. The national Commission for Patient and Public Involvement in Health was created to oversee this.

The Health and Social Care (HSC) Act 2003 provided for the establishment of NHS foundation trusts that have the right to enter into legally enforceable contracts. The Act also established a new regulatory body for healthcare – the Commission for Healthcare Audit and Inspection (the CHAI).

The National Health Service Act 2006 redefined the structure of the NHS in England by consolidating much of the existing legislation concerning the health service. The consolidation repealed and re-enacted in its entirety the National Health Service Act 1977, which was itself a consolidation. It also incorporated provisions from:

- National Health Service and Community Care Act 1990.
- Health Authorities Act 1995
- Primary Care Act 1997
- Health Act 1999
- Health and Social Care Act (HSC) 2001
- National Health Service Reform and Health Care Professions Act 2002
- Health and Social Care (Community Health and Standards) Act 2003
- Health Act 2006.

The Local Government and Public Involvement in Health Act 2007 reformed the existing arrangements ('Patients Forums') for patient and public involvement in the provision of health and social care services with the creation of LINks.

The Health and Social Care (HSC) Act 2008 established a single, integrated regulator for health and adult social care – the CQC to replace the Healthcare Commission (health and adult social care regulator in England), the Commission for Social Care Inspection (social care regulator) and the Mental Health Act Commission (monitoring of Mental Health Act 1983).

The Health Act 2009 set out the framework for how the NHS Constitution would operate, including a new legal duty on providers of NHS services in England and other relevant bodies to have regard to the Constitution; and a duty on the Secretary of State to consult on, review and re-publish the Constitution at least every ten years, and to report on its impact. The Act also placed a duty on NHS providers to produce Quality Accounts and gave the Secretary of State power to set out in regulations the content (including locally agreed elements), format and timing of Quality Accounts (see Chapter 10).

The **Health and Social Care (HSC) Act 2012** – the significant reforms introduced by this Act have already been set out in detail in Chapter 2.

2.1 Freedom of Information Act (FOIA) 2000

The FOIA 2000 is an Act of Parliament that creates a public 'right of access' to information held by public authorities. The full provisions of the Act came into force on 1 January 2005.

The Act led to the renaming of the Data Protection Commissioner (set up to administer the Data Protection Act), who is now known as the Information Commissioner. The Office of the Information Commissioner oversees the operation of the Act.

The Act requires public authorities to have an approved publication scheme, which is a means of providing access to information that an authority proactively publishes.

The Information Commissioner's Office has developed and approved a model publication scheme that all public authorities must adopt.

The scheme:

- sets out the types of information that must be routinely published
- explains the way the information is provided
- states what charges can be made for providing information
- commits the authority to providing and maintaining a guide to the information provided, how it is provided and any charges.

All public authorities should have:

- adopted the model publication scheme
- produced a guide to information using either definition documents or template guides to information provided by the Information Commissioner's Office.

The definition documents for the main public sectors give sector-specific guidance on the type of information that authorities are expected to publish and list in their guide to information. The template guides to information are for smaller authorities and are downloadable guides that can be printed off, completed and used without further modification. They have been produced for local councils, schools and NHS practitioners.

The FOIA means that public authorities must disclose official information when people ask for it (unless there is a good legal reason not to), and they must reply within 20 working days.

This model publication scheme for NHS organisations gives examples of the kinds of information that they are expected to provide to meet their commitments under the model publication scheme. They are required to make the information available unless:

- they do not hold the information
- the information is exempt under one of the FOI exemptions or Environmental Information Regulations (EIRs) exceptions, or its release is prohibited under another statute
- the information is archived, out of date or otherwise inaccessible
- it would be impractical or resource-intensive to prepare the material for routine release.

Case example 3.1 sets out the kind of information that is required for NHS organisations in England.

Freedom of Information requests may be refused if:

- it would cost too much to comply
- the request is vexatious or repeated
- the information is exempt from disclosure under one of the exemptions in the Act.

If any of these criteria apply then the requester must be sent a written refusal notice.

The exemptions

The Act also recognises that there may be valid reasons for withholding information by setting out a number of exemptions from the right to know, some of which are subject to a public interest test. There are 23 exemptions in the FOIA, divided as follows:

Those that apply to a whole category (or class) of information, for example:

- information about investigations and proceedings conducted by public authorities
- court records
- trade secrets.

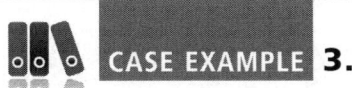

CASE EXAMPLE 3.1

Model Publication Scheme for NHS organisations

Who we are and what we do
Organisational information, structures, locations and contacts.

- How we fit into the NHS structure
- Organisational structure
- Lists of and information relating to organisations with which the authority works in partnership
- Senior staff and management board members
- Location and contact details for all public-facing departments

What we spend and how we spend it
Financial information relating to projected and actual income and expenditure, procurement, contracts and financial audit.

- Annual statement of accounts
- Budgets and variance reports
- Financial audit reports
- Standing financial instructions
- Capital programme
- Staff and board members' allowances and expenses
- Staff pay and grading structures
- Funding (including endowment funds)
- Procurement and tendering procedures
- Details of contracts currently being tendered
- List and value of contracts awarded and their value

What are our priorities and how are we doing
Strategies and plans, performance indicators, audits, inspections and reviews.

- Annual Report
- Annual business plan
- Targets, aims and objectives
- Strategic Direction document (five year)
- Performance against targets (KPI)/performance
- Clinical
- CQC reviews
- Audit reports
- Service user surveys

How we make decisions
Decision-making processes and records of decisions for at least the current and previous three years.

- Board papers – agenda, supporting papers and minutes
- Patient and public involvement (PPI) strategy
- Public consultations (for example, concerning closures/variations of services)
- Internal communications guidance and criteria used for decision making, i.e. process systems and key personnel

Our policies and procedures
Current written protocols, policies and procedures for delivering services and responsibilities.

- Policies and procedures relating to the conduct of business and the provision of services
- Policies and procedures relating to human resources (including Race, Disability, Age and Gender, Equal Opportunities)
- Policies and procedures relating to recruitment and employment

- Standing financial procedures
- Standing orders
- Complaints and other customer service policies and procedures
- Data protection/information governance/Caldicott Guardian
- Estate management
- Charging regimes and policies

List and registers

- Any information currently required by law to be held in publicly available registers
- List of main contractors/suppliers
- Assets registers and Information Asset Register
- Any register of interests kept in the authority
- Register of Gifts and Hospitality provided to board members and senior personnel
- Disclosure Log

The services offered
Information about the services offered, including leaflets, guidance and newsletters.

- Clinical services provided and/or commissioned
- Non-clinical services
- Services for which the authority is entitled to recover a fee together with those fees
- Patient information leaflets and other booklets and newsletters
- PALS
- Advice and guidance
- Corporate communications and media releases

Those that are subject to a 'prejudice' test, where disclosure would, or would be likely to, prejudice, for example:

- the interests of the United Kingdom abroad
- the prevention or detection of crime
- the activity or interest described in the exemption.

Information covered by one or more of the exemptions does not have to be disclosed. However, the decision has to be made as to whether the information should nevertheless be released in the public interest. This is called the public interest test and this involves considering the circumstances of each case with the exemption that covers the information. The information must be released unless the public interest in maintaining the exemption outweighs the public interest in releasing it.

Under the FOIA, an authority must apply the public interest test separately to each exemption. When the test does apply, these are called qualified exemptions. Those to which the test does not apply are called absolute exemptions.

There are also exemptions for personal information:

- If personal information relates to the applicant, the request must be dealt with as a 'subject access request' made under the Data Protection Act 1998.
- If the information requested relates to a third party, a decision on whether to release it must be based on whether releasing it would contravene the Data Protection Act.

When refusing a request for information, it is not possible to withhold an entire document because some of the information contained within it is exempt. A redacted version of the document must be provided along with a refusal notice stating why some of the information cannot be released. When refusing an information request the exemption or exemptions applied must be set out, why they have been applied and, where appropriate, the public interest factors for and against disclosure fully explained.

2.2 The 'duty to consult' legislation

NHS bodies have two separate legal duties to consult on the way that the NHS is operating and about any proposed changes. The duties focus on:

- consulting patients and the public; and
- consulting the local authority Overview and Scrutiny Committee (OSC).

If a legal duty to consult arises, in practice it means that:

- the public (and OSC) must be informed of the issues when the plans are at a formative stage
- the option(s) must be put to the public
- the views of the public and those affected by the changes must be sought on the proposals and their impact
- there must be a genuine consultation where the views of the public are taken into account when making the decision
- the NHS body must be open to objections being put up to the proposals and/or to other plans being put forward even if not included in the consultation options
- no final decisions – even decisions in principle – must be taken until the public has been consulted and the results of the consultation have been considered by the NHS body.

A public body that fails to consult leaves itself open to a challenge by way of Judicial Review and may not lawfully be able to take decisions and thus implement the changes until consultation has occurred.

The courts may also award legal costs against the NHS body. The duty to consult arises whether the changes in health service provision are required in response to financial pressures, clinical requirements or other reasons, or a combination of two or more factors. Changes made to comply with DH policy decisions are also subject to the duty to consult.

Patients and the public

Section 242(1B) of the National Health Service Act 2006 ('2006 Act'), as amended by the Local Government and Public Involvement in Health Act 2007 ('2007 Act'), provides as follows:

> 'Each relevant English body must make arrangements, as respects health services for which it is responsible, which secure that users of those services, whether directly or through representatives, are involved (whether by being consulted or provided with information, or in other ways) in –
>
> a the planning of the provision of those services
> b the development and consideration of proposals for changes in the way those services are provided, and
> c decisions to be made by that body affecting the operation of those services.'

The application of subsections (b) and (c) are only relevant if the proposals under consideration would have an impact on the manner in which the services are delivered to users of those services or the range of health services available to those users.

The legal duty to consult both patients and the wider public falls both on the commissioner of health services and on to those providing services.

The DH guidance on the section 242 consultation duty called **'Real Involvement: working with people to improve health services'** consists of two parts, the first containing statutory guidance, which must be followed, and the second that contains recommendations only.

'Real Involvement' is defined as describing good involvement practice that:

- happens early and continues throughout the process
- is inclusive
- is informed
- is fit for purpose
- is transparent
- is influential – it makes a difference
- is reciprocal – includes feedback
- is proportionate to the issue.

The DH guidance confirms that it is for the NHS body to decide which is the best method for the proposal in question and its community.

The Local Authority Overview and Scrutiny Committees

The HSC Act 2001 extended the scope of these committees to review and give opinions on the health services in their area and this was then included within Section 244 of the National Health Service Act 2006.

The DH guidance outlines the following areas where major change may lead to a duty to consult the OSC:

- outdated buildings and facilities
- new standards (such as National Service Frameworks)
- evidence of what works
- workforce pressures
- advances in technology and technique
- new thinking about how services are designed
- the needs of local people.

The role of the Local Involvement Networks

Until 1 April 2008 Patient and Public Involvement Forums (PPI Forums) existed in NHS trusts (including foundation trusts) to bring to trusts and PCTs the views and experiences of patients, their carers and families. However, Section 230 of the Local Government and Public Involvement in Health Act 2007 abolished PPI Forums and replaced them with 'LINks'. The role of LINks is to give communities a stronger voice in how their health and social care is delivered. They cover all publicly funded health and social care services in an area, irrespective of who provides them. They will be replaced by HealthWatch groups when the Health and Social Care Act 2012 is fully implemented.

The Local Involvement Network Regulations 2008, strengthened the role of LINks by establishing a right of response from any service provider (NHS trust, foundation trust, PCT or local authority), who had received a request for information or a report or recommendation from a LINk. The response must be made within 20 days of receipt, and must explain the actions the service provider intends to take in light of the request or report. If no action is to be taken they must explain why this is the case. If the LINk was not satisfied that the issue had been resolved they had the power to escalate the matter to the local council Overview and Scrutiny Committee.

In addition, the Local Involvement Networks (Duty of Services-Providers to Allow Entry) Regulations 2008 impose a duty on services providers to allow entry by authorised persons of LINks to certain premises owned or controlled by service providers so that the activities carried on there can be observed.

2.3 Directions to NHS bodies on Counter Fraud Measures 2004

These measures set out that each NHS organisation must take all necessary steps to counter fraud in the NHS in accordance with the Directions and according to:

- the NHS Counter Fraud and Corruption Manual;
- the policy statement **'Applying appropriate sanctions consistently'** published by the Counter Fraud and Security Management Service (CFSMS), now known as NHS Protect;

and having regard to guidance or advice issued by NHS Protect.

Each NHS organisation must require its chief executive and Director of Finance to monitor and ensure compliance with these Directions and must cooperate with NHS Protect to enable the CFSMS efficiently and effectively to carry out its counter-fraud functions.

Each NHS organisation must also designate a person to undertake specific responsibility for the promotion of counter fraud measures; in the case of an NHS trust this is to be one of the trust's NEDs and in the case of an NHS body other than an NHS trust, it must be one of that organisation's non-officer members.

> **TEST YOUR KNOWLEDGE 3.1**
>
> a What key pieces of legislation regulate health service governance in the NHS?
> b What is the relevance of the law on freedom of information to health service governance?
> c What is the relevance of counter fraud to good health service governance practice?
> d Give an example of a situation where it may not be clear where the duty to consult exists for an NHS organisation.

3 Company law and other legislation

While the NHS is not governed by UK company legislation it provides a useful backdrop for understanding health service governance. There are other aspects of UK legislation that do apply, such as money laundering and bribery legislation.

In the UK, the main item of company legislation is the Companies Act 2006. This includes regulations relating to:

1 The preparation and auditing of annual financial statements, for approval by the shareholders.
2 The powers and duties of directors.
3 Other disclosures to shareholders, such as the requirement for companies to publish an annual business review.
4 The disclosure of information about directors' remuneration.
5 General meetings of companies, and shareholder rights to call a general meeting.
6 Shareholder voting rights at general meetings, including the right to re-elect directors.

Similar regulations are included in the company legislation of other countries; however, this study text will concentrate mainly on UK company law. The impact of this legislation has been felt in health service governance and is covered in the relevant chapters within this text.

There have also been a number of EU Directives relating to company law. A proposal for a new or amended EU Directive is initiated by the **European Commission** in Brussels. Legislation is then agreed by the European Council and the European Parliament in a process known as the 'co-decision procedure'. When a Directive has been agreed, its contents must be implemented by all EU member states within a stated timeframe, either in a law or other regulation, if suitable legislation does not already exist. EU Directives on company law have included a requirement for companies to publish an annual business review and, for companies whose shares are traded on a regulated exchange, there have been:

1 A Shareholder Rights Directive.
2 Requirements to publish an annual corporate governance statement.
3 Requirements to have an audit committee.
4 Requirements to introduce measures that provide for the independence and ethical conduct of their external auditors.

The EU has therefore been responsible for the extension of legislation for aspects of corporate governance, and in doing so it has been influenced by the rules-based approach adopted in the USA (see below 'The USA and the Sarbanes-Oxley Act (SOX) 2002').

Insolvency law and governance

Companies become insolvent for reasons unconnected with corporate governance. Occasionally, however, the directors of a company may allow it to continue in business when they are aware that it is insolvent and will be unable to pay its creditors or employees. In the UK, the Companies Act 2006 includes provisions that make fraudulent trading a criminal offence and the Insolvency Act 1986 makes wrongful trading a civil offence.

Financial markets and services

Countries with regulated stock markets and markets for other financial products and services need legislation to regulate the conduct of participants in the markets. Financial markets should be regulated to give investors confidence to invest. Customers are important stakeholders in banks, and some elements of financial services legislation are intended to provide consumer protection. In the UK, following the crisis in the banking industry in 2007–2009 the Financial Services Authority (FSA; the UK financial markets regulator) recognised serious weaknesses in corporate governance in banks, particularly inadequate risk management systems, and its responsibility for enforcing improvements.

Insider dealing

Some aspects of 'bad' corporate governance practice are illegal and therefore subject to criminal law.

Directors and other individuals may possess price-sensitive 'inside' knowledge about a company to buy or sell shares in the company with the intention of making a profit (or avoiding a loss). **Insider dealing** is related to corporate governance because it is often carried out by a director or professional adviser of a company. It is also a criminal offence. (In the UK, insider dealing is a criminal offence under Part V of the Criminal Justice Act 1993.)

Money laundering

Money laundering is the process of disguising the source of money that has been obtained from serious crime or terrorism, so that it appears to come from a legitimate source. Companies are often used for the purpose of money laundering, which is a criminal offence in most countries, and the owners or directors of the companies concerned are often involved in the money laundering activity themselves.

Bribery Act 2010

Section 1 of the **Bribery Act** makes it an offence for a person to offer, promise or give a financial or other advantage to another person in one of two cases:

- Case 1 applies where the intention is to bring about the improper performance by another person of a relevant function or activity or to reward such improper performance.
- Case 2 applies where the intention is that the acceptance of the advantage offered, promised or given in itself constitutes the improper performance of a relevant function or activity.

The Act creates a new offence under section 7, which can be committed by commercial organisations that fail to prevent persons associated with them from bribing another person on their behalf. An organisation that can prove it has adequate procedures in place to prevent persons associated with it from bribing will have a defence to the section 7 offence. A 'relevant commercial organisation' is defined at section 7(5) as a body or partnership incorporated or formed in the UK irrespective of where it carries on a business, or an incorporated body or partnership that carries on a business or part of a business in the UK irrespective of the place of incorporation or formation. The key concept here is that of an organisation that 'carries on a business' and so is directly applicable to NHS organisations.

The UK Listing Regime and corporate governance

In every country where there is a regulated stock market, companies whose shares are traded on the market are required to comply with certain rules of conduct. In the UK, these are contained in the United Kingdom Listing Authority Rules. These include the **UK Listing Rules** and also **Disclosure Rules and Transparency Rules** (DTR). These rules are the responsibility of the FSA, the UK financial services regulator. All companies that have a listing for their shares on the main UK stock market (the main market of the London Stock Exchange) must comply with the rules.

A few of the UK Listing Rules are concerned with corporate governance. Briefly, however, most listed companies in the UK – including non-UK companies with a **premium** (UK) **listing** – must comply with all aspects of the *UK Corporate Governance Code* or explain their non-compliance in their annual report and accounts. Another rule requires listed companies to provide a 'going concern statement' in their annual report and accounts.

A section of the **DTR** set out regulations relating to audit committees and corporate governance statements by listed companies.

CHAPTER 3 Governance, the law and the company secretary

TEST YOUR KNOWLEDGE 3.2

a What aspects of corporate governance are regulated by company law (the Companies Act 2006) in the UK?
b What is the relevance of the law on insider dealing to corporate governance?
c What is the relevance of money laundering to good corporate governance practice?
d Give an example of a situation where insider dealing might occur.
e Can you identify any overlap with health service governance?

The USA and the Sarbanes-Oxley Act (SOX) 2002

A different approach to the regulation of corporate governance was taken in the USA, following a number of financial scandals and corporate collapses in 2001–2002 involving major corporations such as Enron, WorldCom and Tyco. Previously, corporate governance issues had not been considered a matter of any significance. As a result of Enron and the other corporate scandals, there was an immediate recognition of a need to protect investors, mainly by improving the accuracy and reliability of financial reporting and other disclosures by companies.

The USA took a regulatory approach to dealing with the problems that were recognised at the time, and a number of corporate governance measures were included in the **Sarbanes-Oxley Act 2002** (sometimes referred to as SOX). The law applied to all public companies in the USA and also to all non-US companies that had shares or debt securities registered with the SEC. CEOs and CFOs were made personally liable for the accuracy of the financial statements of their company, and new rules on financial reporting were introduced including a requirement to publish an internal audit report with the annual financial statements. Several other corporate governance measures were included in the Act, such as a requirement for legal protection for whistleblowers (explained in Chapter 12).

With the enactment of SOX, the USA was considered to have adopted a rules-based approach to corporate governance, different from the 'principles-based' approach in most other countries (described in Chapter 3). However, SOX is not a comprehensive law on corporate governance, and many aspects of corporate governance are not covered by the Act. For example, SOX does not contain any rules about the composition of the board of directors, remuneration of senior executives or dialogue between companies and their shareholders.

TEST YOUR KNOWLEDGE 3.3

Identify two of the main requirements of the SOX 2002 in relation to corporate governance practice in corporations (companies) registered with the Securities and Exchange Commission in the USA.

4 Compulsory regulation and voluntary best practice

This chapter has identified aspects of governance where laws or regulations might apply both in health service governance and corporate governance. In many countries there are voluntary codes of corporate governance, based mainly on principles of good governance rather than detailed and specific rules. Each of these approaches to governance – compulsory regulation and voluntary best practice – has limitations and advantages.

4.1 Advantages of compulsory regulation of governance issues

There are areas of business where laws are essential to protect the interests of shareholders, employees and other stakeholders in organisations. For example, employment laws are needed to give protection to employees against unfair treatment by employers. There should be a legal requirement for organisations to prepare annual financial statements and have them audited, and the duties of directors should be subject to the law, in order to protect stakeholders. There may be different views about the extent of regulation that is required; however, the need for some regulation seems unquestionable.

Best practice in health service governance and corporate governance has some connection with ethical business practice. Some aspects of behaviour may be considered unethical but legal. Laws are needed to prevent or punish activities that are considered so unethical that they should be illegal. Bribery is an example of behaviour that has been tolerated in the past but which is now accepted as illegal by most countries.

Regulation may be needed to address public concerns and maintain public confidence in the capitalist system. This has probably been most evident in the USA. The SOX was a response to public outrage against the many corporate scandals that emerged after the collapse of Enron. Public fury against the banks following the financial crisis in 2007–2008 prompted demands for legislative action that would affect the governance of banks.

4.2 Advantages of voluntary governance systems

It is difficult to devise a set of rules that should apply to all organisations in all circumstances. Rules that are appropriate for one organisation might not be appropriate for another whose circumstances are very different. Although a voluntary system of governance (such as the corporate governance system in the UK) places an expectation on organisations to comply with the guidelines, it also allows them to breach the guidelines if it seems appropriate and sensible to do so.

The biggest concerns about corporate governance practice apply to large stock market companies with large numbers of shareholders. Governance is less of a problem in small organisations.

As a general rule, governance issues become greater as the organisation gets bigger. A voluntary code of best practice in governance can be targeted at the largest organisations and smaller organisations are able to choose whether they want to model their own governance systems on parts of the code for the larger organisations. Governance practices can therefore be adapted to the circumstances of the organisation.

There may be a risk that if different countries have their own corporate governance regulations, companies will migrate to those countries where the rules are less onerous. Governments may therefore compete to offer a corporate governance regime that is more attractive in their country than in other countries, in order to attract foreign companies. Excessive regulations may deter companies from becoming a listed company, particularly if the rules for listed companies are stricter than the rules for private companies.

In practice, good governance is a combination of regulation and voluntary best practice. In some countries there is more emphasis on regulation and in others there is greater reliance on voluntary codes of practice for large organisations. However, unless governance is regulated by law, it is probable that standards of governance will vary substantially between organisations.

Voluntary best practice is explained more fully in Chapter 5.

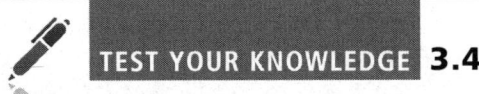
TEST YOUR KNOWLEDGE 3.4

Explain the disadvantages of a rules-based approach to corporate governance, compared with a principles-based approach.

5 The role of the company secretary

5.1 General responsibilities

Whatever the type of organisation, company secretaries are in a unique position to fulfil an important role in governance. They are not members of the board of directors, and so do not have direct responsibility for governance and accountability to stakeholders. Without being a director, they know about what is going on at board level in the organisation and can give advice and assistance, not only to the chairman but also to the board as a whole, board committees and individual directors.

Good governance relies on communication and the exchange of information, and the company secretary is able to help ensure that this happens. By attending board meetings and committee meetings, they should ensure that relevant information is passed from board to committee or from one committee to the board or another committee. By acting as a point of communication and contact for NEDs, the company secretary should also be able to contribute to the flows of information between NEDs and senior executive managers in the company:

> 'The company secretary should be responsible for advising the board through the chairman on all governance matters.'
>
> (UK Corporate Governance Code)

The company secretary should have a full understanding of governance requirements, and should be able to identify governance issues that arise and advise the board accordingly:

> 'All directors should have access to the advice and services of the company secretary, who is responsible to the board for ensuring that board procedures are complied with.'

The *Integrated Governance Handbook* attempted to establish this new role within the NHS and the authors had discussions with a number of FTSE 100 companies to look at the role of the company secretary, exploring, more importantly, whether these companies could exist without such an adviser. The evidence clearly pointed to the need for such integrated corporate support. Foundation trusts are already appointing such individuals and guidance is included in the *FT Code of Governance*. The significance of the role is to ensure that, for the first time in the history of NHS boards, the board *per se* can confidently assure itself that at the end of the 12-month cycle it has full evidence and is fully appraised before signing off the AGS.

The specific responsibilities of a company secretary for governance matters should be decided by the organisation. The 'ICSA Guidance Note on Corporate Governance Role of the Company Secretary' (2008) provides a list of responsibilities relating to corporate governance. These are divided into three main areas.

- specific responsibilities derived from the *UK Code*
- responsibilities relating to statutory and regulatory compliance
- corporate responsibility.

In health service governance, the ICSA have also worked alongside the NHS and have produced a sample job description outlining the responsibilities of an NHS PCT secretary and a foundation trust secretary.

ICSA Guidance Notes can be found on the ICSA website.

5.2 Specific responsibilities derived from the *UK Code*

For health service governance it is helpful to outline the responsibilities that can be assumed from the provisions of the *UK Code*. The broad headings below are the same as those in the Guidelines issued by the ICSA.

Board composition and procedures
- The company secretary should establish a list of matters reserved for decision-making by the board as a whole. Having established a list, the company secretary should ensure that the board deals with all the matters on it, and should not delegate responsibility for decision-making for any matter on the list to executive management or a board committee.

- The *UK Code* requires companies to establish certain board committees. The company secretary should ensure that the constitution and membership of committees of the board comply with the requirements of the Code, and that their membership is refreshed regularly.
- The company secretary schedules meetings of the board and its committees, and helps the chairman to set agendas for meetings. Much of this work is administrative and not directly related to governance, except that a properly functioning board is essential to good governance. The secretary should also ensure that information and papers for meetings are sent out to board members in advance.
- It should also be the responsibility of the company secretary to ensure that appropriate directors' and officers' liability insurance is available for the directors. The reason for this is explained in Chapter 5.
- A requirement of good governance is that there should be succession planning for major positions on the board, particularly for the positions of chairman and CEO. NEDs are usually appointed in the UK for periods of three years, after which time their contract is not renewed or they are invited to stand for re-election. The company secretary should provide assistance with succession planning by the board and should oversee the rotation of NEDs.

Board information, development and relationships

- The company secretary should contribute to the flow of information between the board and its committees, and between the board and executive management. Good governance also depends on fostering relationships.
- The secretary should therefore be responsible for facilitating information flows between board members and should help to develop good relationships between executive directors and NEDs.
- The company secretary should develop relationships with individual board directors, and act as a source of information and advice. The secretary should be the main point of contact for NEDs.
- The company secretary should arrange for directors to take independent professional advice at the company's expense, if they require it.
- The secretary should arrange for major shareholders to be offered the opportunity to meet with newly appointed NEDs, if they wish to do so.
- The company secretary should also have responsibility for the development of board directors, by:
  - building induction programmes for NEDs after being appointed to the board and
  - assisting with performance evaluations of the board, its committees and board members.

  (Performance evaluation is required by the *UK Code*, for which the chairman has most of the responsibility. The company secretary should provide support and assistance to the chairman.)

Remuneration

The *UK Code* contains provisions on the remuneration. These include a requirement for companies to have a **remuneration committee** to decide the remuneration of executive directors and other senior executives:

- The company secretary should be responsible for ensuring that the remuneration committee is familiar with the guidelines on remuneration in the Code and that the company's remuneration policies for directors and senior executives comply with the code.
- The secretary should also ensure that any new long-term incentive scheme is submitted to shareholders for approval.
- The chairman of the remuneration committee is required to make a report in the annual report and accounts. In addition there is a legal requirement in the UK for companies to include a directors' remuneration report in the annual report and accounts. The company secretary should help with the drafting of these reports.

Audit and internal control

- The *UK Code* contains provisions on the responsibility of the board for the review of internal control in the company. There is also a requirement for companies to have an audit committee. The company secretary should have a detailed knowledge of these requirements and should advise the board and audit committee on their application.
- The secretary should also ensure that the company's whistleblowing procedures are implemented, and should monitor their effectiveness.

Relationships with shareholders

The company secretary should ensure that the board keeps in touch with shareholders' opinions on a continuing basis and should manage relations with major institutional shareholders on corporate governance issues.

Disclosure and reporting

The *UK Code* requires that certain disclosures should be made on corporate governance matters, in the annual report and accounts or in circulars to shareholders or on the company's website. The company secretary should be responsible for ensuring that these disclosures are made.

5.3 Responsibilities of the company secretary for statutory and regulatory compliance

Compliance with laws and regulations is a requirement of good governance.

- The company secretary should be responsible for ensuring compliance with all the statutory and regulatory requirements relating to governance. For health service governance, these include the key pieces of NHS legislation and voluntary codes outlined in Chapters 3 and 5. For UK corporate governance, these include the requirements of the Companies Act 2006, and the Listing Rules, Prospectus Rules and **Disclosure and Transparency Rules** of the FSA.
- The company secretary should also be responsible for ensuring proper disclosures of information, e.g. quarterly disclosures to Monitor for foundations trusts and for companies, the dissemination of regulatory news announcements to the stock market, such as trading statements and information about share dealings by directors.
- The company secretary should also keep under review all legal and regulatory developments affecting the organisation's operations, and making sure that the directors are properly briefed about them.

In addition, in corporate governance, the Listing Rules require companies to comply with the **Model Code**, which sets out rules about when directors should not usually be permitted to buy or sell shares in the company. For example, directors should not deal in the company's shares during 'close periods' before an announcement of their financial results. The company secretary is responsible for making sure that directors understand the requirements of the Model Code and comply with them.

5.4 The company secretary and corporate social responsibility

The ICSA Guidelines refer to guidelines on CSR published by the ABI and NAPF on how to incorporate environmental, social and governance issues into investment decision-making. The ICSA Guidelines state that:

> '[T]he company secretary should share responsibility with relevant specialist functions for ensuring that the board is aware of current guidelines in this area and that it identifies and takes account of the significance of corporate responsibility issues in its stewardship and oversight of the company.'

The company secretary should therefore try to ensure that the interests of all important stakeholders are remembered when important business decisions are made, particularly those affecting employees.

The following Case example (3.2) is an illustration of the involvement of the company secretary in corporate governance matters, in this case where concerns were raised about illicit or improper share dealings by a director, and poor communications between the company and its shareholders. Issues of corporate governance are rarely clear-cut, as this case suggests. As a useful exercise, you should consider the role of the company secretary in these events and what the company should have done, if anything, differently from what it actually did do.

CASE EXAMPLE 3.2

In March 2000, the Anglo-French IT services company Sema acquired LHS, an Atlanta-based software company that sold mobile phone billing software. It was bought for £3 billion in March 2000, at a 75%premium to its current share price. Mr L, the founder of LHS and a major shareholder, became a non-executive director of Sema. The acquisition by Sema was seen as a strategic move by the company into the US market.

Investors started to become uneasy when Sema's interim results were announced in September 2000. These had very little to say about either the acquisition or Sema's expansion plans in the USA. Analysts were also annoyed by what they regarded as window dressing in the company's interim financial results. The company included in its profits a £14.3 million refund from its Swedish pension fund. Stripping out this one-off non-operational item would have left operating profits much lower. The share price fell by about 17% in the week the interim results were announced.

Unbeknown to Sema's board, in the week leading up to its interim results, Mr L had started selling shares in large quantities. He sold 1.8 million Sema shares for £24 million in the run-up to the Sema interim results, making three separate sales through a German bank. Each of these sale transactions was in breach of the Model Code requirement for UK listed companies that directors should not deal in shares of their company in a 'closed period', i.e. in the two months before the announcement of the company's results. Mr L sold a further 800,000 shares for £9 million on the day the results were announced. The average sale price for these transactions was about £12.70.

Sema's company secretary was reported as saying that he learned of the improper sales on 11 October, when he was contacted by an investment bank. It appears that when Sema purchased LHS, an arrangement in the transaction (intended to avoid German tax penalties) was that Mr L would hold on to his LHS shares after the acquisition, but with an option to exchange them for Sema shares from January 2002. From the investment bank, the Sema company secretary learned in October that Mr L had exercised his option over part of his stake, ahead of schedule and without notifying anyone at Sema.

The company secretary tried to obtain details of the share deals by Mr L, to make an announcement to the stock market. However, he needed the transaction dates, number of shares sold and price received for Sema to make a statement. He found Mr L obstructive and unhelpful and it took two weeks to get the information. Sema then informed the UK FSA.

Mr L apparently stated that he made the share transactions in all honesty, misunderstanding the stock exchange rules. Investors, however, were sceptical, since LHS had been quoted on the **Nasdaq** stock market in the US, and so its directors would have been familiar with the restrictions in the US on director share dealings.

A further problem for Sema was the poor trading performance of LHS after the acquisition. Far from growing, as the market had been led to expect when the acquisition was made in March, sales slumped from £42 million in the first quarter to £36 million in the second quarter and £24 million in the third. Profits were consequently well below expectations, and the company issued a profits warning on 25 November. The market suspected that Sema had known about the problem long before it issued the warning. The share price fell 44% on the day of the profits warning, and a further 10% (to 329 pence) on the following Monday. This was a long way below the level at which Mr L had sold his shares in September.

On 28 November, the *Financial Times* carried a report that the company was going to ask him to resign 'after concluding that he was damaging the company's standing with investors'. On 29 November, Sema announced that Mr L had resigned. The story of the share dealings by Mr L was given in the financial press, and it was reported that Mr L had apparently not followed Sema's formal compliance procedures and that an investigation was started by the FSA. Investors were said to be angry about the delay in informing the FSA, with questions asked about the company's compliance procedures. How could the company have remained ignorant for so long about the share dealings by Mr L?

With the profits warning as an additional problem, and the lack of adequate information from the company, the credibility of the company's senior management was at risk.

The *Daily Telegraph* commented on 3 December 2000: 'A botched acquisition, a profits warning and a share dealing scandal have shredded management credibility. After years of growth, the shares ended last week at a sixth of their February peak, threatening Sema's place in the **FTSE** 100 index.'

A stockbroker was reported to have said: 'The issue for everyone, and the reason the shares have been so weak since the profits warning, is that the market believes it has been misled for most of this year.'

The financial press identified a major problem as poor communications with investors by Sema's chief executive and finance director, caused to some extent by language difficulties. The report ended with a comment that the board needed strengthening, with someone who will 'fight the corner' of British investors, given the dominance of French directors at the moment.

On 4 December, the Sema share price fell to 271p and the company subsequently dropped out of the FTSE 100. This followed a decision by the company to postpone until January a scheduled meeting with analysts on 6 December. The company stated the postponement was 'appropriate' and that it had set up a board committee to investigate why the company did not warn earlier of the problems at LHS, and to examine the share dealings of Mr L. The board committee would consist of the company's chief executive officer, the board chairman, one other NED and the company secretary, and would be advised by solicitors Clifford Chance.

This immediately raised another corporate governance concern. One institutional investor, holding 2% of Sema shares, was reported to have said that an independent committee would have been more appropriate: 'We would prefer the involvement of independent accountants other than their auditors. This would give added credibility to the outcome of the process, and seems particularly necessary given the constitution of the committee. Clearly the cooperation of Sema's executives is important. But it would have been quite possible for the board to have set up a committee with the power to co-opt the views of the executives from time to time.'

The company's difficulties were not yet over. On 23 January 2001, it made another profits warning. The share price fell 47.5p. Its pre-tax profit forecast for the year was reduced to £90 million to £95 million, having been cut the previous November from £130 million to £100 million. Sema also announced that it had started the search for a new chief executive to replace 'in due course' the current CEO. The low level of Sema's share price was thought to make it vulnerable to a bid. France Telecom, the largest investor in Sema with a shareholding of 18%, stated that it did not regard its holding in Sema as 'core'.

5.5 The company secretary as the conscience of the company

In the context of **business ethics** and governance, the company secretary can be described as the 'conscience of the organisation'. There will often be situations where it is in the best short-term interests of an organisation to ignore best governance practice or even act in an unethical way. For example, the board of directors may want to 'window dress' the financial statements and make the performance of the organisation appear better than it really is. Or an organisation may wish to bribe a government official in order to win a major contract. The company secretary should speak out against bad governance and unethical practice, and remind the board and senior executives of the appropriate course of conduct and the principles of good governance that they should apply.

In order to act in this way, as a 'conscience' for the directors and senior executives, the company secretary must be independent-minded, and should not be under the influence of any other individual, such as the chairman or CEO.

5.6 Independence of the company secretary: appointment and removal

The role of the company secretary in governance is such that it is essential to ensure his or her independence from undue influence and pressure from a senior board member. An ICSA Guidance Note on Reporting Lines for the Company Secretary has commented:

'Boards of directors have a right to expect the company secretary to give impartial advice and to act in the best interests of the company. However, it is incumbent on boards of directors to ensure that company secretaries are in a position to do so, for example by ensuring that they are not subject to undue influence of one or more of the board of directors. If the board fails to protect the integrity of the company secretary's position, one of the most effective in-built internal controls available to the company is likely to be seriously undermined. The establishment of appropriate reporting lines for the company secretary will normally be a crucial factor in establishing that protection.'

The guidelines recommend that:

- In matters relating to their duties as an officer of the organisation, the company secretary should, through the chairman, be accountable to the board as a whole.
- If the company secretary has additional executive responsibilities to their core role, they should report to the CEO or appropriate executive director on such matters.
- the company secretary's remuneration should be set (or at least noted) by the board as a whole, or by the remuneration committee of the board on the recommendation of the chairman or CEO.

The *UK Code* also makes a specific provision about the appointment and removal of the company secretary. It states that: 'Both the appointment and removal of the company secretary should be a matter for the board as a whole.' In this way, the company secretary is not dependent on one individual, or a small group of board members, for their job.

Similar recommended practice is included in *King III*, which states that the board should appoint and remove the company secretary and empower the individual to enable them to fulfil their duties properly. It also recommends that the company secretary should have an 'arm's length relationship' with the board, emphasising the requirement for independence.

The *Integrated Governance Handbook* sets out the following points to establish the independence of the company secretary:

- The company secretary is appointed by the remuneration committee as opposed to either the chair or the CEO, in order to ensure neutrality of role.
- The company secretary is answerable to the board but will be line managed by the CEO in order to ensure personal development and accountability.
- The company secretary will also work closely with the chair, the CEO and the NEDs.
- The company secretary will be actively involved in or be a member of the executive team to ensure a full understanding of the organisation's business.
- The company secretary will not undertake executive activity in respect of having a specific role, but will be the neutral observer and adviser to the board or executive team.
- An NHS based company secretary should have sufficient knowledge of the NHS to gain the respect of the doctors in the organisation but need not necessarily be a clinician.
- The company secretary should be appropriately qualified to carry out his or her role and should ideally be accredited by a professional body such as the ICSA.

The *FT Code of Governance* also states that the appointment and removal of the trust secretary would be a matter for the chief executive and chairman jointly.

STOP AND THINK 3.1

The role of company secretary within many NHS organisations is a bolt-on role to an executive director's existing portfolio or is a role reporting to an executive director (who sometimes is not a board member themselves). By comparison the company secretary in a listed company is a senior role, on a par with being a board director and reporting directly to the chief executive and accountable to the chairman for governance arrangements.

What are the risks to NHS organisations in structuring the role in this way?

5.7 The company secretary and the in-house lawyer

Many of the governance duties of a company secretary have a legal aspect or involve compliance with regulations or a voluntary code of governance practice. It could be argued that many of these tasks could be performed better by an in-house lawyer working for the organisation, since corporate lawyers are specialists in company law and regulations.

However, as stated previously, independence is a critical aspect of the governance role of the company secretary. To perform the task effectively, the company secretary needs to be as independent as it is possible for a full-time employee to be.

In their legal work, an in-house lawyer must at times consider the specific interests of the organisation and individual directors, and may be required to advise them on the most appropriate way of dealing with legal issues that arise. In performing this role, the lawyer will often have to 'take sides' to represent a particular interest. This would be inconsistent with the requirement to be independent when advising on governance issues.

It would therefore be inappropriate for the organisation's in-house lawyers to take on the governance that are usually given to the company secretary. An individual who has trained and qualified as a professional lawyer could be a suitable candidate to act as company secretary or take on governance responsibilities within the organisation, but only if two key conditions are applied:

- the qualified lawyer does no legal work for the organisation, and also
- the independence of the individual can be protected in the same way as for a company secretary, with the board as a whole responsible for appointing and dismissing them and deciding their remuneration.

The *Integrated Governance Handbook* also clarifies this point by stating that it is not necessary for the company secretary to be either an accountant or a lawyer. Appointing a lawyer may increase the company secretary's responsibility and may make them responsible for some of the legal judgements, which is fundamentally not a company secretary role.

5.8 Core duties of an NHS primary care trust secretary

The following list includes both duties, which are legal obligations, as well as those that result from best practice. The trust secretary may also need to refer to other pertinent legislation and regulation:

Board meetings
- Facilitating the smooth operation of the PCT's formal decision making and reporting machinery.
- Organising board of directors meetings along with those of its committees (e.g. audit, remuneration, nomination, professional executive committees etc).
- Ensuring that there is proper and appropriate coordination of board meetings and committees and an effective flow of information.
- Formulating meeting agendas with the chairman and/or the chief executive and advising management on content and organisation of memoranda or presentations for the meeting.
- Collecting, organising and distributing such information, documents or other papers required for the meeting.
- Ensuring that all meetings are minuted and that the minute books are maintained with certified copies of the minutes; and that action is taken on matters arising.
- Communicating board decisions to those required to implement them and ensure that actions and tasks assigned are managed appropriately and to the required timetable, reporting back as required.
- Ensuring that the board of directors' meetings and all board committees are properly constituted and provided with clear terms of reference.
- Managing the PCT HQ secretariat ensuring the effective running of the board's support system including the production of board and committee papers.

Standing orders
Ensuring that the PCT complies with its standing orders and drafting and incorporating amendments in accordance with correct procedures.

- To lead the process of non-financial compliance with the trust's standing orders, including management of the public and staff membership and governance reporting requirements with the DH, professional bodies and other regulatory agencies.
- Review, propose and implement approved changes to the trust's standing orders.

Regulatory requirements
- To administer the Board Assurance Framework (BAF) for the PCT.
- To work with the chief executive and colleagues to identify and address the competency and capacity gaps in the directorate to meet the requirement of World Class Commissioning.
- Establishing and monitoring procedures to ensure that the PCT complies with the requirements of the National Health Service Act 2006.
- Ensuring all regulatory submissions are accurate and timely.
- Acting as initial point of contact between the PCT and NHS regulators.

Statutory registers
Maintaining the following statutory registers:

- Members of the board of directors.
- Directors' interests.
- Hospitality/gifts register.

Statutory returns
Ensuring that formal documentation is filed with appropriate bodies, as required, and to report certain changes regarding the PCT:

- Annual report and accounts.
- Amendments to the standing orders.
- Notices of removal or resignation of the auditors.

Annual report and accounts
Coordinating the preparation, publication, distribution and presentation of the annual report (including annual accounts), in consultation with the PCT's internal and external advisers.

Stakeholder relations
Communicating with stakeholders (e.g. through circulars, newsletters, consultations); maintaining good general relations with relevant parties and ensuring that the requisite public and patient involvement is met, when appropriate.

- Ensuring the public have access to timely information about the governance of the PCT (e.g. board papers) so as to strengthen public engagement.
- Make available, where appropriate, for public inspection copies of the latest annual accounts and auditor's report, annual report and latest information on forward planning.
- Be the executive liaison point with the OSC and the LINk, including maintaining appropriate relations with and representing the PCT at meetings of these fora.
- Develop links with appropriate agencies including local authority and other NHS organisations.

Health service governance
Continually reviewing developments in health service governance:

- Facilitating the proper induction of directors into their role.
- Advising and assisting the directors with respect to their duties and responsibilities.
- Advising and facilitating board performance evaluations and any ongoing development matters resulting from that exercise.

- Counselling directors when preparing presentations and memoranda.
- Ensuring the PCT has a robust framework for compliance with health service governance standards, and recommended best practice.
- Maintaining and reviewing procedures for the sound governance of the PCT and advising on developments in governance issues.
- Ensuring the PCT has adequate insurance arrangements (if the trust chooses to supplement the NHS Litigation Authority scheme cover).
- Ensuring standing orders, including standing financial instructions, a scheme of delegation, and schedule of matters reserved for the board of directors and associated procedures are reviewed updated and properly discharged.

NED development
- Acting as a channel of communication and information for NEDs.
- Management and development of the NEDs and their appropriate integration and interaction with the PCT, including appropriate organisational development.
- Arranging additional training and other support for all directors, as required.

Primary care trust seal
Ensuring the safe custody and proper use of common seal, where appropriate.

Primary care trust identity
Ensuring that all business letters, notices and other official publications of the PCT show the name of the trust and any other information as required by statute.

General compliance
Monitoring and implementing procedures that allow for compliance with relevant regulatory and legal requirements.

- Providing advice on the impact of PCT status on the terms and conditions of contracts with NHS bodies.
- Ensuring the PCT implements the structures associated with compliance and BAFs.
- Coordinating information and submitting relevant information to other regulatory bodies, as required.
- Arranging for the PCT to access a comprehensive legal service, where appropriate acting as the legal access gatekeeper by developing a written policy and procedures for the use of legal services and ensuring implementation and monitoring compliance against the policy.
- Reporting to the board of directors on any matters of non-compliance.

TEST YOUR KNOWLEDGE 3.5

a List 15 governance responsibilities that could be given to a company secretary.
b What is the meaning of 'conscience of the company'?
c Why is it important that a company secretary should be independent, and how can this independence be protected?
d Why is it inappropriate to give governance responsibilities to an individual who acts as the company's in-house lawyer?

CHAPTER SUMMARY

- Governance practices whether corporate or health service are guided partly by laws and regulations, and partly by voluntary adoption of codes of practice.
- In the NHS aspects of health service governance are set out in a number of key acts of parliaments, regulations and measures. These include accountability structures, rights of information and involvement for key stakeholders and protection of public monies.

- In many countries, including the UK, certain aspects of corporate governance are covered by the law. These include parts of companies' legislation and laws on corporate insolvency, insider dealing and money laundering.
- The UK has a voluntary system of both health service governance and corporate governance, but this voluntary system is enforced within each sector by a number of laws and regulations, e.g. the duty to consult in health service governance and the obligations placed on UK listed companies.
- The regulatory system of corporate governance in the USA provides a contrast with such a voluntary system, and it originated with the SOX in 2002.
- Company secretaries are in a unique position to fulfil an important role in governance. They are not members of the board of directors, and so do not have direct responsibility for governance and accountability to stakeholders.

The *UK Code* states that: 'Both the appointment and removal of the company secretary should be a matter for the board as a whole.' In this way, the company secretary is not dependent on one individual, or a small group of board members, for their job. This is mirrored in the *Integrated Governance Handbook* and the *FT Code of Governance*.

PART **TWO**

General principles of health service governance

■ **LIST OF CHAPTERS**

4   Issues in health service governance
5   The regulatory framework
6   Governance of foundation trusts

■ **OVERVIEW**

The second part of this study text looks further at the issues involved in health service governance and in particular at the regulatory frameworks that apply.

Chapter 4 explores in more detail the concept of health service governance and explains the possible consequences of poor governance in both the NHS and the wider commercial world. The different theoretical frameworks for an approach to best practice in governance are explained, and their application to health service governance considered. The close connection between governance and business ethics is explored. The chapter also highlights some of the key issues in governance, including the structure and balance of the board of directors, boardroom practice, the remuneration of senior executives and stakeholder relationships.

Chapter 5 builds on the legal frameworks established in Chapter 3 and explains the voluntary frameworks or codes that exist in health service governance. It will describe the nature and purpose of voluntary codes of health service governance, and compares a 'principles-based' approach to governance with a 'rules-based' approach. The chapter will also discuss the voluntary frameworks for corporate governance as these have influenced the development of health service governance frameworks significantly and describe the general principles of governance set out in some of the more well-known codes, and makes some comparisons between the various codes and frameworks. It will focus on the health service governance principles contained in guidance issued by the DH, Monitor and the Audit Commission. The chapter then explores the relationship between codes of ethics and governance.

Chapter 6 highlights the specific health service governance issues for foundation trusts and explores the roles played by governors and trust members. It considers the legislative background to the introduction of foundation trusts within the NHS and goes on to explore the specific governance structure that applies to foundation trusts including the particular role played by the board of governors. The role of Monitor as the regulator for foundation trusts is set out before the chapter finishes with the impact of the HSC Act 2012 and an exploration of the governance issues raised by the creation of foundation trusts.

■ LEARNING OUTCOMES

Part Two should enable you to:

- understand that health service governance is key to ensuring that there is effective leadership, responsible stewardship of public assets and services and public accountability
- define governance as a system that allows organisations to be effective in the delivery of their strategic objectives
- consider the impact for organisations where the separation between stakeholder interests and management is wider, particularly in relation to the NHS
- identify the underlying differences between health service governance in the NHS and corporate governance
- explain the different approaches to governance, which vary according to the extent to which the interests of stakeholders other than the company shareholders are recognised
- define who a stakeholder is and how they influence the organisation
- understand the interplay of regulation and **voluntary codes of governance**
- explain the difference between 'comply or explain' and 'apply or explain' regimes
- identify the key voluntary codes that apply to health service governance
- identify the key voluntary codes from corporate governance that underpin health service governance
- understand the role played by ethics and codes of conduct in underpinning good governance
- understand the close relationship between the health service governance that is required of foundation trusts and corporate governance
- identify how foundation trust membership and council of governors redefines the involvement of stakeholders in the governance of the NHS.

PART 2 CASE STUDY

Frampton Moor NHS Foundation Trust has been authorised as a FT since January 2009. The board is composed as follows:

Frank Smith, Chairman
Miranda Tabnorth, CEO
Dan Morden, NED, Chair of Audit Committee
Louise Melchett, NED, Deputy Chair
Cara Norton, NED
Andrew Birch, NED
Jack Wheeler, Director of Finance
Wilson Ford, Director of Nursing and Operations
Dr Lee Jesson, Medical Director
Helen Wrightford, Director of Corporate Affairs and Company Secretary

The last board evaluation carried out by an external assessor was part of the FT application process in 2008. As a result the board has recently commissioned a board evaluation process led by 'Stating the obvious' consultancy firm.

An observation of behaviours and process at board meetings identifies that the Chair is very passive and does not summarise discussion at board meetings or ensure that all members contribute. It has become apparent that the NEDs meet before every board meeting without the Chair being present to discuss the board papers and agree the approach they will take. They often request further information at board meetings and postpone decision making claiming that there is insufficient detail in the board papers to be properly assured.

The CEO is a very strong character who answers most questions posed by the NEDs and rarely let's her EDs respond to the challenges being presented. If they do respond they only deal with matters that relate to their portfolio.

Conversations with the CEO demonstrate that she sets the board agenda and vets all board papers before they are submitted. A recent CQC unannounced visit had resulted in a report that outlined a number of minor concerns but this had been prevented from being presented at the next board meeting by the CEO as she was not willing for it to be considered before a detailed action plan had been worked up by the Director of Nursing and Operations.

The feedback meeting from 'Stating the obvious' is chaired by the CEO and a very strong steer is given that as the trust's Financial Risk Rating and Governance Risk Rating are at 4 and green the concerns being expressed within the report are irrelevant.

The report also highlights the current NED vacancy that exists but the CEO makes it clear that the ex-audit partner from the Trust's auditors is being considered as a slot in for the role as the current Chair of Audit Committee has no financial experience or background.

Issues in health service governance

■ CONTENTS

1 Defining health service governance
2 Consequences of poor health service governance
3 Consequences of poor corporate governance
4 Common themes in poor governance
5 Theoretical frameworks
6 Stakeholders
7 Approaches to governance

■ INTRODUCTION

Chapter 4 explores in more detail the concept of health service governance and explains the possible consequences of poor governance in both the NHS and the wider commercial world. The different theoretical frameworks for an approach to best practice in governance are explained, and their application to health service governance considered. The close connection between governance and business ethics is also explored. The chapter highlights some of the key issues in governance, including the structure and balance of the board of directors, boardroom practice, the remuneration of senior executives and stakeholder relationships.

1 Defining health service governance

The NHS often faces times of uncertainty with short- and long-term policy competing for attention. This is particularly true with the significant changes being introduced by the HSC Act 2012. Good governance will be vital for NHS organisations as they face another series of major changes and will be key to ensuring that there is effective leadership, responsible stewardship of public assets and services and public accountability. Health service governance is not a product in itself but is foundational to the delivery of the high quality for all that is envisaged in the Darzi report of 2008.

Governance can be defined as a system that allows organisations to be effective in the delivery of their strategic objectives. Health service governance is a system that enables effective delivery of the healthcare rights and pledges set out in the NHS Constitution, which is tailored for the local communities in which it is delivered.

2 Consequences of poor health service governance

The importance of good governance is often only highlighted in circumstances where an organisation has failed or is in crisis. It tends to be seen in organisations where the separation between stakeholder interests and management is wider. This is a significant risk for NHS organisations, e.g. government spending on healthcare for 2011/2012 is approximately £106 billion and yet the recipients of the healthcare provided are often very distant from the holders of the healthcare budget. Health service governance in NHS organisations therefore must be resilient enough to hold NHS organisations to account for the responsibility of managing this expenditure. The separation between NHS stakeholders and Parliament is vast and it is only through the health service governance regimes of the individual parts of the NHS that NHS stakeholders can exercise the relatively limited powers they have to hold the boards of directors to account.

In public companies that have raised capital on the stock markets, their institutional investors hold vast portfolios of shares and other investments, and investors need to know that their money is reasonably safe. Should there be any doubts about the integrity or intentions of the individuals in charge of an organisation, the value of the organisation's shares will be affected and the organisation will have difficulty raising new capital should it wish to do so. If there is weak corporate governance in a country generally, the country will struggle to attract foreign investment.

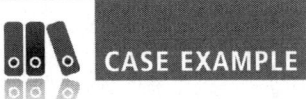

CASE EXAMPLE 4.1

Children's heart surgery at the Bristol Royal Infirmary (1984–1995)

In the early 1990s, it became clear to parents of very sick children who had been treated at Bristol Royal Infirmary that the rate of death or brain damage in or after heart surgery was abnormally high. Following an earlier, separate enquiry by the GMC, in 1998 health secretary, Frank Dobson, announced a public inquiry into events at Bristol under the chair of Sir Ian Kennedy. The Inquiry, which reported in 2001, found a number of significant governance failings including:

- unsafe arrangements for caring for the children
- no requirement for consultants to keep their skills and knowledge up to date
- no agreed standards of care
- no openness about clinical performance
- no systematic mechanism for monitoring the clinical performance of healthcare professionals or hospitals.

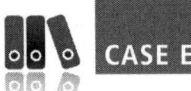

CASE EXAMPLE 4.2

Dr Harold Shipman

Dr Harold Shipman, a GP in Hyde, near Manchester, was convicted at Preston Crown Court on 31 January 2000 of the murder of 15 of his patients and of one count of forging a will. He was sentenced to life imprisonment. Following the trial, a public inquiry was set up that reported over the next five years.

The inquiry identified a number of significant gaps in governance processes that enabled Dr Shipman to continue to murder his patients over a long period of time without detection. Among other issues, the need to share information about complaints and concerns raised, and the requirement to investigate them systematically, and the importance of establishing strong governance processes and culture.

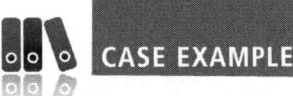

CASE EXAMPLE 4.3

Mid-Staffordshire NHS Foundation Trust Public Inquiry (2010)

The Healthcare Commission's 2009 investigation into Mid-Staffordshire NHS Foundation Trust (where multiple management failures led to high mortality rates) found that the trust, which was seeking to make financial savings in order to apply for foundation trust status, appeared to 'have lost sight of its real priorities'. The initial report by Robert Francis QC on Mid-Staffordshire (2010) revealed that deficiencies in staffing and governance extended over a period of more than five years and yet remained un-remedied by those responsible.

While poor governance within the NHS may not lead to its complete disappearance, it will lead to the continual pressure to move towards greater centralisation of control by the government. Political opinions will differ as to whether this is in the best interests of the recipients of a publicly funded healthcare system. Similarly lessons in good practice have generally resulted from misconduct and poor decision making and it is the reputation of the NHS that suffers as a consequence:

> 'Good governance should not be an end in itself and should not be the preserve of "governance specialists". Effective governance is not about processes. It is about successful leadership and making manifest the values of the organisation. It is sometimes regarded as an obscure subject, not necessarily visible in its own right, but it becomes a high profile reputation issue when it is found lacking.'
>
> The foundations of good governance: a compendium of best practice, FTN and Beachcroft LLP

The consequences for the NHS when health service governance goes wrong are often catastrophic for the patients and families involved and very public. The above case examples are just a few examples.

3 Consequences of poor corporate governance

The consequences of poor corporate governance are easily highlighted in the comments made by Arthur Levitt, a former chairman of the SEC, following the numerous corporate scandals in the US in 2001 and 2002:

> 'If a country does not have a reputation for strong corporate governance practice, capital will flow elsewhere. If investors are not confident with the level of disclosure, capital will flow elsewhere. If a country opts for lax accounting and reporting standards, capital will flow elsewhere. All enterprises in that country, regardless of how steadfast a particular organisation's practices, may suffer the consequences. Markets exist by the grace of investors. And it is today's more empowered investors who will determine which companies and which markets stand the test of time . . .'

Bad corporate governance is a problem for any country with large companies and capital markets. As noted in the context of the NHS, it often takes a scandal to focus the attention of the regulators as can be found in the following examples:

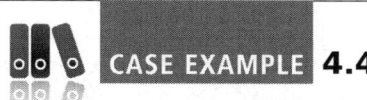

CASE EXAMPLE 4.4

Maxwell Corporation consisted mainly of Maxwell Communication Corporation and Mirror Group Newspapers. As its chairman and chief executive officer, Robert Maxwell had a position of dominant power on the board of directors. He was also a domineering personality, who bullied the people working with him; he was able to run his companies in whatever way he liked. He apparently made no clear distinction between his privately owned companies and the public Maxwell Corporation. In the early 1990s, his companies got into serious financial difficulties. Maxwell drowned falling off his yacht in 1991; after his death it emerged that his companies had accumulated debts of £4 billion, and an unauthorised 'hole' of more than £400 million existed in the pension fund of Mirror Group Newspapers. Maxwell's ability to accumulate unsustainable debts and to raid the pension fund was attributed to a combination of his domineering personality and position of power, a weak board of directors and questionable accounting practices. The Maxwell 'empire' collapsed.

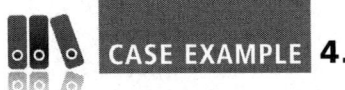

CASE EXAMPLE 4.5

Parmalat, which specialises in dairy and food manufacture and is one of the largest companies in Italy, was declared insolvent in December 2003. There was a fraud, which the organisation's internal controls and the external auditors failed to identify. Forged documents indicated that there was a substantial amount of cash held by one of the organisation's subsidiaries, but this money did not exist. The scandal, as in the case of Enron, suggested a need for more effective external audits and for a whistleblowing system within companies. At Parmalat, several employees had suspected wrongdoing, but no one reported their suspicions.

The USA was much slower than the UK to recognise problems of bad corporate governance, but in 2001 and 2002 there were a number of major corporate collapses that could be attributable partly to governance issues and fraud. The most well-known case is probably Enron Corporation (see Case example 1.1).

TEST YOUR KNOWLEDGE 4.1

a Why is good governance particularly crucial within the NHS?
b How would you define health service governance?

STOP AND THINK 4.1

What are the key issues for health service governance that can be identified in the corporate governance case examples?

4 Common themes in poor governance

The issues involved in governance are described in more detail throughout this text. Briefly, however, aspects of poor governance include:

- a board of directors that fails to perform its duties properly, perhaps because it is dominated by one or more individuals, or because it fails to carry out the tasks that it is supposed to
- a poor relationship between the board and the main stakeholders
- failure to deliver the appropriate returns or services required by either statute or by regulators
- ineffective systems of risk management, and exposure to errors and fraud due to inadequate internal control systems
- inappropriate remuneration and reward systems for directors and senior executives
- unethical business practices.

And specifically for companies, misleading financial reporting to shareholders and other investors, and perhaps inadequate auditing of the financial statements.

A key issue in governance is the relationship between the board of directors, its main stakeholders (e.g. DH or shareholders) and other important stakeholders.

TEST YOUR KNOWLEDGE 4.2

Give six examples of bad governance practice including both NHS organisations and other corporate bodies.

5 Theoretical frameworks

In order to understand the underlying differences between health service governance in the NHS and corporate governance in the private sector it is useful to consider the theoretical justification for a system of rules or guidelines on governance. There are a number of different frameworks to consider:

- stakeholder theory
- stewardship theory
- agency theory
- transaction cost theory
- policy governance theory
- generative governance theory.

5.1 Stakeholder theory

Stakeholder theory takes the view that the purpose of governance should be to satisfy, as far as possible, the objectives of all key stakeholders – employees, investors, major suppliers and creditors, customers, the government, local communities and the general public. The board of directors should therefore consider the interests of all the major stakeholders. However, some stakeholders are more important than others, so management should give priority to their interests above the interests of other stakeholder groups.

In the introduction to its principles of corporate governance, the **OECD** comments that an aim of government policy ('public policy') should be 'to provide firms with the incentives and discipline to minimise divergence between private and social returns and to protect the interest of stakeholders'.

The **OECD Principles of Corporate Governance** recognise the role and rights of stakeholders; they state that the corporate governance framework should:

- recognise the rights of stakeholders that are recognised in law or through mutual agreements
- encourage active cooperation between organisations and stakeholders in creating wealth, jobs and the **sustainability** of financially sound enterprises.

Stakeholder theory states that the organisation's managers should make decisions that take into consideration the interests of all the stakeholders. This means trying to achieve a range of different objectives, not just the aim of maximising the value of the organisation for its shareholders. This is because different stakeholders each have their own (different) expectations of the organisation, which the organisation's management should attempt to satisfy.

Stakeholder theory also considers the role of organisations in society, and the responsibility that they should have towards society as a whole. It could be argued that some organisations are so large, and their influence on society so strong, that they should be accountable to the public for what they do. The general public are taxpayers and as such they provide the economic and social infrastructure within which organisations are allowed to operate. In return organisations should be expected to act as corporate citizens and act in ways that benefit society as a whole. This aspect of stakeholder theory is consistent with the arguments in favour of CSR.

5.2 Agency theory

Agency theory is based on the separation of ownership and control in an organisation – the ownership of an organisation by its shareholders and control over the organisation's actions by its directors and senior executives. The agency relationship is a form of contract between an organisation's owners and its managers, where the owners (as principal) appoint an agent (the managers) to manage the organisation on their behalf. As part of this arrangement, the owners must delegate decision-making authority to the management. This gives rise to an inherent conflict of interest between the organisation's owners and managers.

- The shareholders want to increase their income and wealth over the long term. The value of their shares depends on the long-term financial prospects for the organisation. Shareholders

are therefore concerned not only about short-term profits and dividends; they are even more concerned about long-term profitability.
- The managers run the organisation on behalf of the shareholders. If they do not own shares in the organisation, managers have no direct interest in future returns for shareholders or in the value of the shares. They have an employment contract and earn a salary. Unless they own shares, or unless their remuneration is linked to profits or share values, their main interests are likely to be the size of their remuneration package and their status within the organisation.

Ideally, the 'agency contract' between the owners and the managers of an organisation should ensure that the managers always act in the best interests of the owners. However, it is impossible to arrange the 'perfect' contract because any decisions managers make affect their personal welfare as well as the interests of the owners.

Agency conflicts are differences in the interests of owners and managers. They arise in several ways:

- **Moral hazard**. A manager has an interest in receiving benefits from his position in the organisation. These include all the benefits that come from status, such as a car, use of a plane, a house or flat, attendance at sponsored sporting events, and so on. A manager's incentive to obtain these benefits is higher when he has no shares, or only a few shares, in the organisation. For example, senior managers may pursue a strategy of growth through acquisitions, in order to gain more power and 'earn' higher remuneration, even though takeovers might not be in the best interests of the organisation and its shareholders.
- **Level of effort**. Managers may work less hard than they would if they were the owners of the organisation. The effect of this lack of effort could be smaller profits and a lower share price.
- **Earnings retention**. The remuneration of directors and senior managers is often related to the size of the organisation (measured by annual sales revenue and value of assets) rather than its profits. This gives managers an incentive to increase the size of the organisation, rather than to increase the returns to the organisation's shareholders. Management are more likely to want to reinvest profits in order to expand the organisation, rather than pay out the profits as dividends. When this happens, companies might invest in capital investment projects where the expected profitability is quite small, or propose high-priced takeover bids for other companies in order to build a bigger corporate empire.
- **Time horizon**. Shareholders are concerned about the long-term financial prospects of their organisation, because the value of their shares depends on expectations for the long-term future. In contrast, managers might only be interested in the short term. This is partly because they might receive annual bonuses based on short-term performance, and partly because they might not expect to be with the organisation for more than a few years.

Agency costs are the costs of having an agent make decisions on behalf of a principal. Applying this to corporate governance, agency costs are the costs of monitoring the actions and performance of management, to ensure that management is acting in their best interests, bonding costs that may be incurred in providing incentives to managers to act in the best interests of the shareholders (e.g. remuneration packages) and the residual loss is the cost to the shareholder, which occurs when the managers take decisions that are not in the best interests of the shareholders but are in the interests of the managers themselves (e.g. when managers pay too much for a large acquisition).

The key elements of agency theory

Agency theory is based on the view that the system of corporate governance should be designed to minimise the agency problem and reduce agency costs. One approach to reducing the agency problem is to make the board of directors more effective at monitoring the decisions of the executive management. Another approach is to design schemes of remuneration for directors and senior managers that bring their interests more into line with those of the shareholders.

Agents should also be accountable to their principals for their decisions and actions. **Accountability** means reporting back to the principals and giving an account of what has been achieved, and the principal having power to reward or punish an agent for good or bad performance. Greater accountability should reduce the agency problem, because it provides management with a greater incentive (obtaining rewards/avoiding punishments) to achieve performance levels that are in the best interests of the shareholders.

Agency theory may therefore be summarised as follows:

- In large companies there is a separation of ownership from control. Professional managers are appointed to act as agents for the owners of the organisation.
- Individuals are driven by self-interest.
- Conflicts of self-interest arise between shareholders and managers.
- Managers, because they are driven by self-interest, cannot be relied on to act in the best interests of the shareholders. This creates problems in the agency relationship between shareholders and management.
- These agency problems create costs for the shareholders.
- The aim should be to minimise these costs, by improving the monitoring of management and/or providing management with incentives to bring their interests closer to those of the shareholders.

5.3 Stewardship theory

Stewardship theory has its roots in psychology and sociology and is concerned with the behaviour of executives and directors who act as stewards to protect and maximise shareholders wealth, and in so doing, the stewards maximise their own potential. In this theory, stewards are organisation executives and directors working for the shareholders, who protect and make profits for the shareholders. Unlike **agency theory**, stewardship theory stresses not the perspective of individualism, but rather the role of top management acting as stewards, integrating their goals as part of the organisation. The stewardship theory suggests that stewards are satisfied and motivated when organisational success is attained.

This theory also sees the need to engage with a range of interests but prioritises a positive connection between public bodies and civil society. The key role of those who govern is to create a framework of shared values and then to engage with key stakeholders and a suitably skilled and autonomous workforce, all of whom benefit from helping the organisation to achieve its goals.

Whereas agency theory assumes that being a manager or employee suppresses an individual's own aspirations, stewardship theory requires organisational structures that empower the steward and offers maximum autonomy built on trust. It stresses the position of employees or executives to act more autonomously so that the shareholders' returns are maximised.

Stewardship theory can also be seen in the behaviour of executives and directors when decisions are made to maximise financial performance as well as shareholders' profits in order to protect their reputations as decision makers in organisations. In other words, executives and directors are also managing their careers in order to be seen as effective stewards of their organisation.

5.4 Transaction cost theory

Transaction cost theory provides a different basis for explaining the relationship between the owners of an organisation and its management. Although it is an economic theory, it also attempts to explain companies not just as economic units, but as an organisation consisting of people with differing views and objectives.

The operations of an organisation can be performed either through market transactions or by doing the work in-house. For example, an organisation could obtain its raw materials from an external supplier or it could make the materials itself. Similarly, an organisation could hire self-employed contractors to do work or it could hire full-time employees. In economic terms, a firm's decision about whether to arrange transactions in the open market or whether to do the work in-house (itself) should depend on which is cheaper. When a firm does work in-house, it needs a management structure and a hierarchy of authority with senior management at the top. According to transaction cost theory, the structure of a firm and the relationship between the owners of a firm and its management depends on the extent to which transactions are performed in-house.

Total costs are defined as the sum of production costs and transaction costs:

- Production costs are the costs that would be incurred by the organisation in an ideal economic market. In an ideal economic market, production costs are minimised.

- Transaction costs are additional costs incurred whenever the perfect economic market is not achieved. For example, an organisation might buy goods from a supplier who is not the cheapest available, because it is not aware of the existence of the cheapest supplier. An organisation might sell goods on credit to a customer, not knowing that money owed will become a bad debt.

Transaction costs are sometimes higher when a transaction is arranged in the market, and they are sometimes higher when the transaction is done in-house. Carrying out activities in-house rather than arranging contracts externally is referred to as vertical integration. Total costs are minimised when transaction costs are minimised. This should determine the optimal size of the firm and the size of the management hierarchy in the firm. The way in which an organisation is organised, and the extent to which it is vertically integrated, also affect the control the organisation has over its transactions. As a general rule, it is in the interests of an organisation's management to carry out transactions internally, rather than in the external market. Performing transactions internally:

- removes the risks and uncertainties about prices of products and product quality
- removes all the risks and costs of dealing with external suppliers.

Traditional economic theory is based on the assumptions that all behaviour is rational and that profit maximisation is the rational objective of all businesses. Transaction cost economics changes these assumptions by trying to allow for human behaviour, and the fact that individuals do not always act rationally. The theory is based on two assumptions about behaviour:

- bounded rationality
- opportunism.

Bounded rationality

Human beings act rationally, but only within certain limits of understanding. This means, for example, that the managers of an organisation will in theory act rationally in seeking to maximise the value of the organisation for its shareholders, but their bounded rationality might make them act differently. Business is very complex, and large businesses are much more complex than small businesses. However, in any business, there is a limit to the amount of information that individuals can remember, understand and deal with. No one is capable of assessing all the possible courses of action and no one can anticipate what will happen in the future. In a competitive market, no one can anticipate with certainty what competitors will do.

Playing chess has been used as an example of **bounded rationality**. The game is very complex and there are many different possible moves. The actions of the opponent in a game of chess cannot be predicted, so it is impossible to predict what the opponent will do in response to a particular move. The same problem applies to managing an organisation. It is impossible to predict with certainty what will happen, because there are too many factors and too many possibilities to consider.

When individuals reach the boundaries of their understanding, because a situation is too complex or too uncertain there is a greater tendency to carry out transactions in-house and to have vertical integration.

Opportunism

The theory also assumes that individuals will act in a self-interested way and 'with guile'. They will not always be honest and truthful about their intentions. Opportunism is defined as 'an effort to realise individual gains through a lack of candour or honesty in transactions'. An individual might try to take advantage of an opportunity to gain a benefit at the expense of someone else. Managers are opportunistic by nature. Given the opportunity, they will take advantage of any way of improving their own benefits and privileges.

A problem with opportunism is that external parties (e.g. contractors and suppliers) cannot always be trusted to act honestly. As a result, there may be a tendency for an organisation to carry out transactions itself, rather than to rely on external suppliers. However, there is also a risk that by taking control of transactions internally, managers will have opportunities to take decisions and actions that are in their personal interests. This self-interested behaviour needs to be controlled. In this respect, transaction cost theory has similarities with agency theory.

Although they are based on different assumptions, both agency theory and transaction cost theory support the need for controls over corporate governance.

5.5 The policy governance theory

The **policy governance theory** sharply distinguishes between the role of 'owners' (in the public service context, the local public) and 'operators' (those who deliver the service). According to John Carver, in this theory, boards act as 'owner representatives' who set objectives but fully delegate the running of the organisation to operators through the chief executive as the main point of contact. A framework of policies limits the freedom of the management, ensuring that the effectiveness of an activity is not prioritised over its being ethical or prudent.

Under this theory good governance will enable the board ('owner representatives') to:

- cradle the vision and explicitly address fundamental values
- force an external focus
- enable an outcome-driven organising system
- force forward thinking
- enable proactivity
- facilitate diversity and unity in board composition and opinion
- describe relationships to relevant constituencies
- delineate the board's role in common topics (ensuring the board's specific contribution to any topic is clear)
- determine what information is needed
- balance over-control and under-control.

5.6 The generative governance model

Recently a new approach has emerged from the experience of not-for-profit boards in the USA and described by Richard Chait, William Ryan and Barbara Taylor as Governance as Leadership or generative governance. They set out three modes in which the board should be effective: fiduciary, strategic and generative. The main contribution of this tri-modal model is to emphasise the role of 'generative thinking' in producing a sense of what knowledge, information and data mean. This requires an active process of dialogue and engagement between the board, staff and service users.

The fiduciary mode is where boards are concerned primarily with the stewardship of tangible assets that makes up the core of governance – the fiduciary work is intended to ensure that nonprofit organisations are faithful to their mission, accountable for performance, and compliant with the relevant laws and regulations. Without this, the organisation, including its stakeholders, could be harmed.

The strategic mode is where boards develop strategy with management to set the organisation's priorities and course, and to deploy resources accordingly. Without this, there is little power or influence and governance would be primarily be about staying on course than setting the course.

The generative mode, is where boards, along with executives, frame problems and make sense of ambiguous situations – which in turn shapes the organisation's strategies, plans and decisions.

The claim of this theory of governance is that most organisations lack the frameworks and practices for this work.

TEST YOUR KNOWLEDGE 4.3

a Name the different theoretical frameworks of governance that are outlined in this text.
b Which theories are more relevant to health service governance?
c In agency theory, what are agency costs and what are the three main elements?
d Why is this theory an appropriate framework for corporate governance?
e What controls are there within the NHS to manage opportunism?
f Who are the 'owner representatives' in the policy governance theory?

6 Stakeholders

A stakeholder in an organisation is someone who has an interest or 'stake' in it, and is affected by what the organisation does. A stakeholder, in turn, has an influence on what the organisation does. Each stakeholder or stakeholder group may expect the organisation to behave or act in a particular way with regard to the stakeholders' interests. A stakeholder can also expect to have some say in some of the decisions an organisation makes and some of the actions it takes. The **balance of power** between different stakeholder groups, and the way in which that power is exercised, are key issues in governance.

One of the major distinctions between health service governance and corporate governance is that a corporate body has a number of different stakeholder groups, which can be divided into financial stakeholders and other stakeholders. In these companies the main focus of their attention will be on meeting the expectations of their financial stakeholders. While an NHS organisation has a wide number of stakeholders only a small minority will have a purely financial interest. This minority are likely to be banks or lenders who have supplied funding for capital projects such as Private Finance Initiative schemes. Any other financial interest will be driven by a requirement for efficient and effective use of public assets rather than an expectation of wealth accumulation. By exploring the expectations of financial stakeholders this distinction becomes quite apparent.

6.1 Stakeholders specific to health service governance

Stakeholders specific to health service governance include PCTs (and subsequently the CCGs) who hold provider trusts to account and who themselves are held to account by SHAs. Regulators such as the CQC and Monitor, as well as the regulatory bodies that are responsible for the regulation of healthcare professionals, are also stakeholders within health service governance.

NHS foundation trusts will be stakeholders for PCTs/CCGs and other provider trusts that they work collaboratively with. In foundation trusts their governors and members will be stakeholders as well as specifically Monitor.

SHAs are currently the stakeholders for PCTs and the DH will be one of their stakeholders.

The DH as the government department with overall responsibility to the Secretary of State is a key stakeholder for NHS organisations.

Other stakeholders include or will include in the future:

- LINks
- OSCs
- Health and Wellbeing Boards
- Local authorities
- Clinical commissioning groups
- The NHS Commissioning Board
- Healthwatch England.

6.2 Stakeholders specific to corporate governance

As stated above, much of the attention of public companies is focused on their financial stakeholders. These consist mainly of shareholders and lenders. Lenders may be banks or investors in bonds.

- An organisation's members or equity shareholders are the owners. In a small organisation, the owners may also be directors. In a large public organisation, the directors may own some shares, but are not usually the largest shareholders. The interests of the shareholders are likely to be focused on the value of their shares and dividend payments. However, the powers of shareholders in large public companies are usually fairly restricted and shareholders have to rely on the board to act in their best interests.
- A different situation arises when there is a **majority shareholder** or a significant shareholder. A shareholder with a controlling interest is able to influence decisions of the organisation through an ability to control the composition of the board of directors.

- A distinction can also be made between long-term and short-term institutional investors. Short-term investors buy shares with the expectation of making a short-term profit from an increase in the price before selling the shares in the market. This includes, for example, hedge funds which buy shares in what they consider to be an undervalued and badly managed organisation with potential for a significant increase in value if the management problems can be resolved (or if the organisation becomes a takeover bid target). Long-term investors are more interested in the longer-term returns from an organisation than short-term profit.
- Lenders and bondholders provide debt capital to an organisation but are not owners. Even so, they have a financial interest in the organisation, and expect payment of interest and repayment of capital on schedule. Excessive borrowing by an organisation might put lenders as well as shareholders at risk financially; therefore, lenders have an interest in preventing the financial gearing or leverage of the organisation from getting too high. Loan covenants might set limits on borrowing by the organisation.

6.3 The influence of other stakeholders

Other stakeholders in an organisation could have significant influence, e.g. regulators, employees, suppliers, customers/patients. The list of stakeholders must also include the board of directors, although in public companies some directors might also be large shareholders.

The board of directors

The board has the responsibility for giving direction to the organisation. It delegates most executive powers to the executive management, but reserves some decision-making powers to itself, such as decisions about strategy, raising finance, paying dividends and making major investments.

In the NHS there are six key functions, for which an organisation will be held accountable by the DH on behalf of the Secretary of State. These are:

- To ensure effective financial stewardship through VFM, financial control and financial planning.
- To ensure that high standards of health service governance and personal behaviour are maintained in the conduct of the business of the whole.
- To appoint, appraise and remunerate senior managers.
- To ratify the strategic direction of the organisation within the overall policies and priorities of the government and NHS, define its annual and longer term objectives and agree plans to achieve.
- To oversee the delivery of planned results by monitoring performance against objectives and ensuring corrective action is taken when necessary.
- To ensure effective dialogue between the organisation and local community on its plans and performance, and that these are responsive to the communities' needs.

Executive management is also held accountable to the board for the organisation's operational performance.

A board of directors is made up of both executive directors and **NEDs**. Executive directors are individuals who combine their role as director with their position within the executive management of the organisation. NEDs perform the functions of director only, without any executive responsibilities. Executive directors combine their stake in the organisation as a director with their stake as a fully paid employee, and their interests are therefore likely to differ from those of the non-executives.

The board may take decisions collectively, but it is also a collection of individuals, each with personal interests and ambitions. Some individuals are more likely to dominate the decisions by a board and to exert strong influence over their colleagues. The most influential individuals are likely to be the chairman, who is usually a non-executive but may occasionally have executive powers and responsibilities, and the CEO. The chairman is responsible for the functioning of the board. The chief executive officer (CEO) is the senior executive director, and is accountable to the board for the executive management of the organisation. The term 'chief executive officer' derives from the USA, but is now widely used in the UK (where the term 'managing director' is also used).

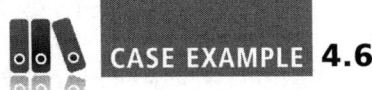

CASE EXAMPLE 4.6

At a board meeting of a well-established foundation trust, which was being held in private session, the chairman proposed that a significant donation be made to a local charity that was working alongside one of the healthcare areas delivered by the trust. The chairman was an aggressive person, who bullied and dominated the people working with him; and he often attempted to run the trust regardless of the role of the CEO. The chair was also a trustee of the charity in question. He apparently made no clear distinction between his own private activities and the public sector.

It was only the concerted effort of the **senior independent director (SID)** in conjunction with the finance director that enabled the board to turn down the request.

Management is responsible for running the business operations and is accountable to the board of directors (and more particularly to the CEO). Individual managers, like executive directors, may want power, status and a high remuneration. As employees, they may see their stake in the organisation in terms of the need for a career and an income.

Employees

Employees have a stake in their organisation because it provides them with a job and an income. They too have expectations about what their employer should offer them, e.g. security of employment, good pay and suitable working conditions. Some employee rights are protected by employment law, but the powers of employees are generally limited.

Suppliers

Major suppliers have an indirect interest in an organisation, because they expect to be paid what they are owed. If they deal with the organisation regularly or over a long period of time, they will expect the organisation to do business with them in accordance with their contractual agreements. If the organisation becomes insolvent, unpaid creditors will take a more significant role in its governance. For example, in the private sector, a creditor might take legal action to take control of the business or its assets.

Representative bodies

In the corporate, commercial world, a number of representative bodies act in the interests of members of the investment community and can influence public companies whose shares are traded on a stock market. Representative bodies include the **ABI** and the **NAPF** in the UK, and the **ICGN**, an association of activist institutional investors around the world (insurance companies and pension funds are major investors in securities). These bodies may coordinate the activities of their members, e.g. by encouraging them to vote in a particular way on resolutions at the **AGMs** of companies in which they are shareholders. These bodies represent the opinions of the investment community generally.

In the NHS, there are a number of regulatory bodies that also act as representative bodies, for example, the General Medical Council, which regulates doctors and the Nursing and Midwifery Council, which regulates nurses and midwives.

And the HSC Act is introducing Health and Wellbeing Boards that will act as a forum for local commissioners across the NHS, public health and social care, elected representatives, and representatives of HealthWatch (the new public health organisation) to discuss how to work together to better the health and wellbeing outcomes of the people in their area.

General public

The general public are also stakeholders in large organisations, often because they rely on the goods or services provided by an organisation to carry on their life. For example, households expect utility companies to provide an uninterrupted supply to their homes, or a reliable telephone connection. Commuters expect a rail company to be under an obligation to provide a convenient and reliable transport service to and from work, and at a reasonable price. Pressure groups, such as environment protection groups, sometimes try to influence the decisions of companies in the interests of society in general.

In the NHS, LINks, which will, in due course, be replaced by local branches of HealthWatch in each local council area, act as representative bodies giving the public a voice in how their health and social care services are planned and delivered. Alongside this, foundation trusts are accountable to their local populations through their membership – members of the public, patients and staff can become members of their NHS foundation trust. The membership elects the board of governors, which is made up of patients, the public and staff through locally run elections. Local stakeholders are also represented on the board of governors. The governors' role is to represent the interests of patients and the local community in the way the trust is managed.

TEST YOUR KNOWLEDGE 4.4

a Name the different stakeholders that are specific to health service governance.
b How are these different to the stakeholders that are specific to corporate governance?
c Why is the board also classed as a stakeholder?

STOP AND THINK 4.2

Do you agree with the view that a board of directors should give more consideration to the interests of other NHS stakeholders rather than individual third sector groups? Give your reasons.

7 Approaches to governance

There has been considerable debate about what the objectives of sound corporate governance should be and the different views can be divided into broad approaches:

- the shareholder value or owner approach
- the **stakeholder approach**, also called the stakeholder inclusive approach or pluralist approach
- the **enlightened shareholder approach**
- an integrated approach, as recommended by the King Report (a report on recommended corporate governance practice for South Africa).

There are other approaches for governance in not-for-profit organisations, which should also be considered:

- the policy governance approach
- the governance as leadership approach.

While corporate governance may be restricted by company law, which underpins the primary role of shareholders as key stakeholders, nevertheless, there are some points of interest that would frame a wider remit for corporate governance. All of these broad approaches can be considered in respect of health service governance and indeed no one approach should be seen as providing the only approach to governance. It is more likely that the interplay of a number of these approaches will frame the development of good health service governance that is not bound by the company legislation that enshrines the legal rights of shareholders.

7.1 The shareholder value approach

The **shareholder value** or owner approach is the well-established view for corporate governance, supported by company law in advanced economies, that the board of directors should govern their organisation in the best interests of its owners, the shareholders.

This means that the main objective of an organisation should be to maximise the wealth of its shareholders, in the form of share price growth and dividend payments, subject to conforming to the rules of society as embodied in laws and customs. The directors should be accountable to their shareholders, who should have the power to remove them from office if their performance is inadequate. The shareholder view is closely linked to agency theory or transaction cost theory.

The OECD, in the introduction to its *Principles of Corporate Governance*, states that from an organisation's perspective, corporate governance is about 'maximising value subject to meeting the corporation's financial and other legal and contractual obligations. This inclusive definition stresses the need for boards of directors to balance the interests of shareholders with those of other stakeholders in order to achieve long-term sustained value.'

The strength of this approach to corporate governance is its general acceptance. Many people hold the view that public companies are in business to earn profits for the benefit of their shareholders. Successful companies are perceived as those paying dividends to shareholders and whose share price goes up. Within the broad objective of maximising shareholder values, the board of directors will also act fairly in the interests of employees, customers, suppliers and others with an interest in the organisation's affairs.

Despite its wide acceptance within corporate governance, this approach is of limited application within health service governance. As has already been established in this text, the role played by the shareholder or financial stakeholder is very limited within the NHS.

7.2 The stakeholder approach (pluralist approach)

An alternative approach is based on stakeholder theory. This argues that the aim of sound corporate governance is not just to meet the objectives of shareholders, but also to have regard for the interests of other individuals and groups with a stake in the organisation, including the public at large. This resonates more widely with health advice governance where the objectives of NHS organisations are influenced by a wide-ranging variety of stakeholders.

From a 'stakeholder view', governance is concerned with achieving a balance between economic and social goals and between individual and communal goals. Sound governance should recognise the economic imperatives organisations face in competitive markets and should encourage the efficient use of resources through sound investment. It should also require accountability from the board of directors to the stakeholders for the stewardship of those resources. Within this framework, the aim should be to recognise the interests of other individuals, companies and society at large in the decisions and activities of the organisation.

A problem with the stakeholder approach for corporate governance is that company law gives certain rights to shareholders, and there are some legal duties placed on the board of directors towards their organisation. However, the interests of other stakeholders are not reinforced to any great extent by company law. The stakeholder approach expects that co-operative and productive relationships will be optimised only if the directors are permitted or required to balance shareholder interests with the interests of other stakeholders who are committed to the organisation. For the approach to be more applicable to corporate governance then changes in company law would be required to introduce such an approach in practice.

This approach is also limited in its application to health service governance as the concept of competitive markets is limited within the NHS and while there is an increasing emphasis on a market economy with healthcare this is still limited in reality. The concept of individual goals for stakeholders is also tempered by the overriding objective of the NHS to provide healthcare at the point of need for all.

A further distinction for health service governance is that the rights of other stakeholders such as employees, suppliers and the general public, although not well protected by company law, are protected by health law (e.g. FOIA, NHS Constitution) as well as other aspects of law such as employment law, health and safety legislation, and environmental law.

7.3 The enlightened shareholder approach

The enlightened shareholder approach to corporate governance is that the directors of an organisation should pursue the interests of their shareholders, but in an enlightened and inclusive way. It is a form of compromise between the agency view and the stakeholder view.

The directors should look to the long term, not just the short term, and they should also have regard to the interests of other stakeholders in the organisation, not just the shareholders. Managers should be aware of the need to create and maintain productive relationships with a range of stakeholders having an interest in their organisation.

A criticism of the enlightened shareholder view is that most shareholders do not fit the image of enlightened investors. Most shares in public companies are owned by institutional investors, who themselves may be relatively unaccountable to their beneficiaries. When companies become a target for a takeover bid, speculative investors such as hedge funds may acquire large but short-term shareholdings, with a view to making a quick profit from their investment. However, the role of institutional investors in corporate governance is likely to evolve in the future, with institutions expected to be more proactive in promoting the rights and interests of shareholders.

This approach is of greater application to health service governance as it does address the need to balance the competing needs of the different stakeholders. Its limitation, however, is in its lack of clarity on how to balance the diverse and/or differing stakeholder interests. This is still largely a shareholder driven approach to governance and is limited in its application to health service governance.

7.4 The King Code – an integrated approach

The **King Code** or King Report developed by the Institute of Directors in South Africa, was first introduced in 1994. A revised Code (*King II*) was published in 2004 and a further revision (*King III*) was published in 2009. *King III* (and *King II* before it) rejected an enlightened shareholder approach to governance in favour of a 'stakeholder inclusive' approach.

In the introduction to the *King III Code*, this approach is explained in some detail. The enlightened shareholder model and the stakeholder inclusive model both take the view that the board of directors should consider the interests and expectations of stakeholders other than shareholders; however, the two models differ significantly in their emphasis.

In the 'enlightened shareholder' approach the legitimate interests and expectations of stakeholders only have an instrumental value. Stakeholders are only considered in as far as it would be in the interests of shareholders to do so.

In the case of the 'stakeholder inclusive' approach, the board of directors considers the legitimate interests and expectations of stakeholders on the basis that this is in the best interests of the organisation, and not merely as an instrument to serve the interests of the shareholder.

The King Code, therefore, states that a board of directors should consider what is best for the organisation and in doing so it should have regard to the legitimate interests and expectations of all stakeholders. It should then integrate these, or decide how they should be traded off against each other, on a case-by-case basis, with the aim of making decisions that are in the best interests of the organisation. The shareholder does not have any predetermined precedence over other stakeholders. The 'best interests of the organisation' are defined not in terms of maximising shareholder wealth, but 'within the parameters of the organisation as a sustainable enterprise and the organisation as a corporate citizen'.

7.5 The policy governance approach

The **policy governance approach** requires a clear direction from boards in setting the objectives of the organisation. These objectives need to be established in direct correlation with the wishes of the owners (or beneficiaries) of the organisation. Having established clear objectives the board then fully delegates the running of the organisation to the management team via the chief executive as the main point of contact. This form of governance can be seen clearly in charitable trusts where the trustees act as the owner representatives and the chief executive is held to account at the board meetings of the trustees. In this approach it would be unusual for members of the management team to also act as a trustee. The trustees are then responsible for establishing a framework of policies within which the chief executive and their management team operate, ensuring that the effectiveness of an activity is not prioritised over its being ethical or prudent.

This approach has been adopted by some foundation trusts within the NHS, although they would differ from the trustee model outlined above in that their executive directors are also voting members of the foundation trust board. One of the advantages of this approach is the direct focus on the objectives of the organisation with a clear set of policies within which the chief executive and team may operate. The success or otherwise of this approach for health service governance lies in the extent to which the board can define the objectives for the organisation and balance the competing interests of the diverse variety of the stakeholders.

7.6 The governance as leadership approach

The governance as leadership or 'generative' approach relies on the inter-play of three key roles for boards. This requires an active process of dialogue and engagement between the board, staff and service users.

The approach requires boards to understand their stewardship role in respect of the public assets of their organisation, to be accountable for performance and to ensure compliance with the relevant laws and regulations. At the same time boards need to work with the executive management to set the organisation's priorities for the future, and to deploy resources accordingly. None of which seems much different to the approaches already outlined and relies on the key relationship between the board and the executive management team. The final aspect to this approach is what distinguishes it from the others and relies on sharing knowledge, experiences, information and the analysis of organisational data. This final role for the board is to lead, along with executives, on framing problems and making sense of ambiguous situations – which in turn shapes the organisation's strategies, plans and decisions. This third role is of significant importance for health service governance as it provides an opportunity to manage the competing interests of a diverse stakeholder base.

TEST YOUR KNOWLEDGE 4.5

a Which approaches to governance are most applicable to health service governance?
b What will limit the integrated approach of the King Code in its application to corporate governance?

CHAPTER SUMMARY

- Health service governance is key to ensuring that there is effective leadership, responsible stewardship of public assets and services and public accountability.
- Governance can be defined as a system that allows organisations to be effective in the delivery of their strategic objectives.
- The importance of good governance is often only highlighted in circumstances where an organisation has failed or is in crisis. It is often seen in organisations where the separation between stakeholder interests and management is wider. The separation between NHS stakeholders and Parliament is vast and it is only through the health service governance regimes of the individual parts of the NHS that NHS stakeholders can exercise the relatively limited powers they have to hold the boards of directors to account.
- In order to understand the underlying differences between health service governance in the NHS and corporate governance in the private sector it is useful to consider the theoretical justification for a system of rules or guidelines on governance.
- There are different approaches to corporate governance, which vary according to the extent to which the interests of stakeholders other than the organisation shareholders are recognised. The differing approaches may be summarised as a shareholder approach, an enlightened shareholder or inclusive approach, and a stakeholder or pluralist approach. The approach taken by the directors of an organisation affects decision-making at a strategic level.
- A stakeholder in an organisation is someone who has an interest or 'stake' in it, and is affected by what the organisation does. A stakeholder, in turn, has an influence on what the organisation does. Each stakeholder or stakeholder group may expect the organisation to behave or act in a particular way with regard to the stakeholders' interests. A stakeholder can also expect to have some say in some of the decisions an organisation makes and some of the actions it takes.

The regulatory framework

■ CONTENTS

1. Voluntary frameworks for governance
2. Codes for health service governance
3. *UK Corporate Governance Code*
4. Other codes
5. Ethics and governance
6. The reality of health service governance

■ INTRODUCTION

Chapter 5 builds on the legal frameworks established in Chapter 3 and explains the voluntary frameworks or codes that exist in health service governance. It describes the nature and purpose of voluntary codes of health service governance, and compares a 'principles-based' approach to governance with a 'rules-based' approach. The chapter will also discuss the voluntary frameworks for corporate governance as these have influenced the development of health service governance frameworks significantly and describe the general principles of governance set out in some of the more well-known codes, and makes some comparisons between the various codes and frameworks. It will focus on the health service governance principles contained in guidance issued by the DH, Monitor and the Audit Commission. The chapter then explores the relationship between codes of ethics and governance.

At the end of this chapter you should have an appreciation of the general principles of good governance, but you should also be aware that differences in emphasis exist between the different codes.

1 Voluntary frameworks for governance

A voluntary code of governance is issued by an authoritative national or international body and contains principles or best practice in governance that major companies (listed companies) or organisations are encouraged to adopt and apply. The principles may consist of main principles with associated supporting principles, and for each principle, there may also be provisions or recommendations about how the principle should be applied in practice. Voluntary codes of corporate governance have been adopted in many countries, e.g. in all the countries of the Commonwealth and all the countries of the EU.

There is no statutory requirement for organisations to apply the principles or provisions of a voluntary code. However, a well-established code should attract the support of the significant organisations in that sector, and this develops an expectation that others should adopt the code unless their circumstances are such that non-compliance with some of the code's provisions is a more sensible option.

Although voluntary, organisations may be required (e.g. companies whose shares are traded on a major stock market by their listing rules or NHS foundation trusts by their terms of authorisation) to adopt the code of governance or to explain in their annual report and accounts their non-compliance with any aspect of the code and their reasons for non-compliance. This requirement, common in many countries, is known as 'comply or explain'.

The purpose of a voluntary code is to raise standards of governance. It is **principles-based**, because there is a recognition that the same set of rules is not necessarily appropriate in every way for all organisations, and that there will be situations where:

- non-compliance with provisions in the code is desirable, given the circumstances that the organisation faces
- implementing a principle of best practice is not always best achieved by following the detailed provisions or recommendations in the code, and some flexibility should be allowed.

It is also recognised that a code cannot provide detailed guidelines for every situation and circumstance. The preface to the *UK Corporate Governance Code* in 2010 points out:

> 'It seems that there is almost a belief that complying with the Code in itself constitutes good governance. The Code, however, is of necessity limited to being a guide only in general terms to principles, structure and processes. It cannot guarantee effective board behaviour because the range of situations in which it is applicable is much too great for it to attempt to mandate behaviour more specifically than it does.'

1.1 'Comply or explain' and 'apply or explain'

In the NHS, Monitor requires foundation trusts to comply with the NHS Foundation Trust Code of Governance or to explain any non-compliance. The same is true of the UK Listing Rules, which require listed companies to comply with the *UK Corporate Governance Code*. There is a view that the word 'comply' will encourage organisations to follow the provisions of a code in all its details, without considering the principles that underpin the code. This may encourage a **box-ticking approach**, and a view that the detailed provisions must be followed without considering whether the provisions might be appropriate or finding a suitable way of applying the governance principles in the actual circumstances.

For this reason, some countries have adopted what they call an **'apply or explain' rule** (or approach) such as, The King Code III the governance code for South Africa – see Section 4.2.

The *UK Corporate Governance Code* recognises the dangers of a 'box-ticking' mentality with 'comply or explain' and stresses that it is not intended to be a set of rules:

> 'The Code is not a rigid set of rules . . . It is recognised that [non-compliance with a provision] may be justified in particular circumstances if good governance can be achieved by other means.'

Likewise, Monitor in the introduction to its Code of Governance for foundation trusts makes it clear some foundation trusts may decide that the provisions are disproportionate or less relevant in their case and they should actively consider how to adopt the approach in the code in their particular circumstances.

TEST YOUR KNOWLEDGE 5.1

a What is the difference between principles and provisions in a code of governance?
b For foundation trusts, how does the 'comply or explain' rule apply?
c What is the difference between 'comply or explain' and 'apply or explain'?
d What is a box-ticking approach to compliance with governance requirements and how might such an approach be harmful for NHS organisations?

2 Codes for health service governance

Governance in the public sector, and specifically in the NHS, is the subject of several reports:

- **Nolan Principles (1995)**: covered in detail the standards of behaviour and principles in public life with particular focus on appointment on merit, with an independent element on all selection panels recommended as the way forward for public bodies.
- **The Intelligent Board (2006)**: looked at board level information needs.
- **The Integrated Governance Handbook (2006)**: looked in detail at the processes and information requirements of sound governance.
- **The Intelligent Board – Modernising Mental Health Services (2007)**: focused on the board in mental health trusts.
- **Taking it on Trust (2009)**: examines how the boards of NHS trusts and foundation trusts in England assure themselves that internal controls are in place and operating effectively.
- **The NHS Foundation Trust Code of Governance (2010)**: sets out the governance arrangements for foundation trusts.
- **The Healthy NHS Board: principles for good governance (2010)**: sets out the principles of high quality governance, and is supported by a regularly updated digital compendium, which puts the principles in an operational context.

The Nolan principles have already been covered in Chapter 1; however, the other reports are set out in more detail below. In addition other reports such as the **Audit Code for Foundation Trusts**, the **Guide for Governors: audit code for NHS Foundation Trusts** and **Your Statutory Duties: a reference guide for NHS Foundation Trust governors** will be set out in more detail in Chapter 6 as they relate specifically to foundation trusts.

2.1 The Intelligent Board

This report set out a set of principles and model framework for structuring information to support strategy development and oversight of business delivery and effectiveness. It also suggests practical ways in which boards might use the framework proposed.

The report outlines:

- **The information challenge**: discussion of the growing pressure on boards to raise their game and the need to improve the information they receive and how they use it.
- **Intelligent information for the board**: some key principles that should govern information for the board, together with a proposed framework and minimum data set for reviewing trust performance, supporting decision-making and considering strategy.
- **Putting the framework into practice**: improving the structure of agendas for the board; developing a 'dashboard' of routine performance indicators; informing the annual cycle of board meetings.

The Intelligent Board series, which includes guidance for mental health trusts, ambulance trusts and clinical commissioners outlines practical, focused advice for NHS board members on the kind of information they should be using to understand and oversee their organisations' performance.

All the reports in the series are based on these Intelligent Board principles:

- All information should cover locally defined priorities as well as national 'must do' requirements.
- All information should focus on outcomes, not systems and processes.
- All information should be available in a timely and understandable format.
- All information should be clearly and simply presented.
- All information should be forward-looking, presenting trends and anticipating future issues.
- All information should allow internal comparison between services and make use of external benchmarks.
- All information should provide interpretation and analysis as well as information.
- All information should provide a level of detail that is appropriate to the board's governance role.

2.2 Integrated Governance Handbook

The idea of integrated governance was developed by Professor Michael Deighan and Dr Roger Moore with support from Sir William Wells, Professor Sir Ian Kennedy and Bill Moyes and was first introduced to the NHS in a paper entitled 'Developing Integrated Governance', published by the NHS Confederation in May 2004. The handbook was published in 2006 by the DH to ensure that the basic building blocks of integrated governance were in place, with rollout and implementation planned over the following two years. The handbook was aimed at PCTs, NHS trusts, SHAs, care trusts and foundation trusts. The chief concern that the integrated governance sought to address was the risk of boards governing in silos (e.g. clinical governance, information governance) by moving to an integrated agenda that would enable boards to meet their responsibilities.

Integrated governance is defined as: 'Systems, processes and behaviours by which trusts lead, direct and control their functions to achieve organisational objectives, safety and quality of service and in which they relate to patients and carers, the wider community and partner organisations.'

The NHS chief executive at the time, Sir Nigel Crisp, said:

> 'Integrated Governance provides the umbrella for all NHS governance approaches. It combines the principles of corporate/financial accountability and it moves towards a single risk sensitivity process which covers all the trust's objectives, supported by a coordinated source of collecting information and subject to coordinated inspection.'
>
> (Chief Executive Bulletin, 13–18 November 2004, Issue 245, Item 7, Gateway number 4161)

The handbook built on previous guidance including *Governing the NHS* and the *Good Governance Standard for Public Services* (CIPFA, JRF and OPM 2005) as well as further afield in Europe (OECD Guidelines on the Corporate Governance of State-Owned, Enterprises, December 2004) and the US (The Sarbanes-Oxley (SOX) Act passed in 2002).

The handbook was also aligned to The NHS Foundation Trust Code of Governance 2005 produced by the regulator for foundation trusts, Monitor, and the *NHS Audit Committee Handbook* (2005) produced by the DH.

Integrated governance emphasised the critical importance of the board defining, within the overall goals established for the NHS, its own purpose and strategic direction, with clarity of purpose, objective setting and planning of the board's annual cycle of business. The handbook also focused on quality as the driver of change, examined the critical role of clinical governance at the heart of the Integrated Governance agenda, and covered the legal implications for boards and what they should to do to plan the journey towards good governance.

Integrated governance required an examination of a number of key areas:

- the need for boards to take account of a wide range of NHS requirements in determining overall priorities and drawing up annual operational plans
- a review of assurance arrangements, with particular reference to the Standards for Better Health (now superseded by the CQC)
- the 'intelligent' information required by boards integrating a wide range of perspectives, including finance, human resources, information systems, and research; and most importantly clinical governance
- the key role of the Assurance Framework, which should complement the strategic priorities identified during the annual business planning cycle
- the simplification of committee structures and supports in order to ensure they had clear terms of reference and understood the actions and behaviours expected of them.

It was envisaged that the board would then take corporate responsibility for all aspects of strategy setting, performance management and quality assurance, as a result of being assured that the appropriate systems were in place to manage the identified risks.

In particular, the handbook suggested a consideration of the 'company secretary' role within health organisations and a development of the role of the audit committee to scrutinise and streamline committee structures and agendas, ensuring all risks (activity, quality and resources) were anticipated, aligned and integrated.

The key task for integration was an examination of the role of the audit committee to ensure that it scrutinised all the subcommittees reporting to the board. At the time some boards had more than 40 committees, some of course were subcommittees; but they reported either through the audit committee or directly to the board. This was unworkable and did not allow the non-executives to fulfil their strategic role. The handbook proposed a phased transition to the following structure:

The handbook recommended that boards should be served by the following main standing committees:

- Audit
- Remuneration and Review
- Appointments.

Other committees that boards might find useful included:

- Risk Compliance and Assurance
- Clinical Governance
- Health and Safety.

This required a different reporting structure at board meetings to ensure that agendas were robust enough to deal adequately with the business from many of the committees that no longer existed and relied upon the strengthened audit committee clarifying much of the work prior to it being placed on the board's agenda.

The handbook set out a direction of travel for health service governance, which was developed further by a publication in 2007 by the HfMA called 'Integrated Governance: delivering reform on 2.5 days a month'. This later publication maintained the focus on the key controls assurance requirement of a **BAF** and on a Statement on Internal Control (now the AGS), but added additional useful guidance around board functioning and etiquette. This was subsequently updated and revised by a further publication 'Integrated Governance: a guide to risk and joining up the NHS reforms' in 2011, which sets out a governance development programme. The programme is set out in four parts that clarify the purpose and behaviours of the board, the board structures and systems, the review and improvement process and then sets out a number of exercises for board development.

2.3 NHS Foundation Trust Code of Governance

Monitor, as the regulator of foundation trusts, describes the legal framework for NHS Foundation Trusts as being closer to that of a commercial company, and as such adopts a much more 'commercial' approach to their regulation. NHS Foundation Trusts must comply with Monitor's terms of authorisation and reporting requirements and the Audit Code used by Monitor. Each NHS Foundation Trust needs to develop individual standing orders, giving authority to each organisation's standing financial instructions, schemes of delegation and matters reserved for the board.

The NHS Foundation Trust Code of Governance was first published in 2006. Following reviews in 2008 and 2009 of its application, and taking account of more recent developments in governance practices specific to NHS foundation trusts, the code was updated and applied from 1 April 2010. The code builds on the approach, principles and provisions of the *UK Corporate Governance Code* (and the Combined Codes before it) to bring best practice from the private sector to the NHS.

NHS foundation trusts are created as legal entities as **public benefit corporations** by the National Health Service Act 2006 ('the 2006 Act'). The legislation constitutes NHS foundation trusts with a new governance regime that is fundamentally different from NHS trusts. NHS foundation trust boards of directors have more autonomy to make financial and strategic decisions. They also have a framework of local accountability through members and a council of governors, which has replaced central control from the Secretary of State for Health.

In this regime, NHS foundation trust directors are ultimately and collectively responsible as a board for all aspects of the performance of the foundation trust. Therefore, they need to be able to deliver more focused strategic leadership and more effective scrutiny of the trust's operations.

The purpose of the Code of Governance is to assist NHS foundation trust boards in improving their governance practices by bringing together the best practices of corporate governance. The code sets out a common overarching framework for the governance of NHS foundation trusts and complements the statutory and regulatory obligations on them.

The emphasis on governance can be demonstrated from the example of Derbyshire Healthcare NHS Foundation Trust, which was authorised in 2011 after having been unsuccessful in two earlier assessments.

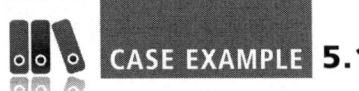

CASE EXAMPLE 5.1

Derbyshire Healthcare NHS Foundation Trust Strengthening the board

The trust first came to Monitor in 2007 and subsequently requested a deferral, which was agreed and imposed a number of conditions that would need to be resolved before assessment could recommence. These included concerns about the board's capacity to deliver the business plan, and a less than satisfactory working capital report.

When assessed again in 2008, Monitor were still not satisfied that the trust's board was able to deliver the business plan, or that the trust was financially viable in the medium term.

Monitor recommended that, among other actions, the trust re-examine the skill mix of the non-executive directors and how any gaps on the board could be addressed. The trust returned to Monitor for assessment in September 2010.

The actions the trust had taken in the intervening period, following Monitor's recommendations, were evident. A new chair had been appointed, along with four new non-executive directors. A new finance director had been recruited from an existing foundation trust, and a director of business strategy post had been created. The appointee brought in-depth knowledge of commissioning and an effective working relationship with the local PCT. Significant time had been committed to board development activities, focusing heavily on the principles of good governance and the characteristics of high performing boards. Monitor observed board meetings and held individual meetings at the trust, and the board was clearly very capable. The executive and non-executive teams worked effectively together, which was apparent throughout the assessment process, and from the outset the integrated business plan had been developed and owned jointly. The trust also demonstrated that it was very focused on quality.

Mike Shewan, Chief Executive of Derbyshire Healthcare NHS Foundation Trust said: 'From day one, Monitor's assessment team was very clear about their expectations and gave us every opportunity to provide the evidence they were looking for. We had learned a lot about the process from our previous assessments and had developed a keen awareness of what Monitor would be looking for. We knew that we needed to be operating as a foundation trust board before we became a foundation trust, and so spent a lot of time developing our board and a strong governance structure. We knew that a high performing unitary board was key to our success, not only in order to achieve foundation trust status, but to continue to deliver in the future.'

The trust's commitment to improving the board and strengthening organisational capacity, based on feedback from Monitor's assessment process, meant that it was authorised as a foundation trust on 1 February 2011.

Extract from Monitor's Annual Report and Accounts 2010/2011

This code is best practice advice. It is not mandatory guidance and accordingly, non-compliance with the provisions of the code does not in itself create a breach of the terms of authorisation. NHS foundation trusts are, however, strongly encouraged to take full account of the best practice provisions described in this code.

The code does impose some specific disclosure requirements upon NHS foundation trusts, which are similar to the requirements set out by the UK Listing Authority for listed companies. These relate to the reporting in the annual report of the application of the main and supporting principles of the code and confirming by way of a specific statement compliance with the provisions of the code or – where it does not – to provide an explanation.

The code adopts a similar structure to the UK Corporate Governance with a series of Main Principles, supported by a series of supporting principles, under the following broad headings:

- **Directors**: the responsibilities of the board directors, including the chair and chief executive.
- **Governors**: the role and responsibilities of the board of governors, including the role of the chairman.
- **Appointment, resignation and terms of office**: the appointments to and the composition of the board of directors, the election and re-election of directors, the role of the nominations committee and the appointment of the chairman.
- **Information, development and evaluation**: the provision of information to the board, the induction and training of directors and deals with the annual evaluation of directors individually and the board as a whole.
- **Director remuneration**: the role of the remuneration committee, disclosure, directors service contracts and developing a remuneration policy.
- **Accountability and audit**: the accountability of the board of directors and its responsibility for disclosure, and internal control.
- **Relationships with stakeholders**: the responsibility of the board to communicate and consult with key stakeholders such as members, patients and the local community. It also sets out the board's responsibility for cooperating with other stakeholders such as related NHS organisations and local authorities.

Key aspects emphasised in the code are:

- the unitary nature of the board of directors and the collective responsibility for all aspects of the performance of the foundation trust, including financial performance, clinical and service quality, management and governance
- at least 50% of board members to be independent non-executives
- a recommendation to appoint a SID
- an emphasis on actively developing the effectiveness of the board of directors through performance evaluation of the board, its committees and individual directors
- clarification on the committee structure of the board of directors and the roles of the remuneration, audit and nomination committees. This includes a recommendation for a clear nominations process
- clarification of the need for good quality information tailored to the board's duties and availability of access to external advice
- a recommendation to appoint a secretary of the board of directors and the board of governors
- the role of a nominated **lead governor**
- recommendations to be clear on the purpose and outcomes of the relationships of the NHS foundation trust with other stakeholders including members, patients, the local community, commissioners and other NHS and non-NHS bodies with an interest in the local health economy.

2.4 The *Healthy NHS Board: principles for good governance*

This document sets out the principles that will allow NHS board members to understand the:

- collective role of the board
- governance role within the wider health system
- activities and approaches that are most likely to improve board effectiveness
- contribution expected of them as individual board members.

The guidance is for boards of all NHS organisations, although some interpretation is required for organisations operating at a national or regional level. The guidance sets the three key roles of an effective board as:

- formulating strategy for the organisation
- ensuring accountability by holding the organisation to account for the delivery of the strategy and through seeking assurance that systems of control are robust and reliable
- shaping a positive culture for the board and the organisation.

These are underpinned by three building blocks that allow boards to exercise their role, namely that boards:

- Are informed by the external context within which they must operate.
- Are informed by, and shape, the intelligence that provides trend and comparative information on how the organisation is performing together with an understanding of local people's needs, market and stakeholder analyses.
- Give priority to engagement with key stakeholders and opinion formers within and beyond the organisation; the emphasis here is on building a healthy dialogue with, and being accountable to, patients, the public and staff, including clinicians.

The three roles of the board and the three building blocks all interconnect and influence one another. The guidance also sets out clear boundaries for the various roles within the board and outlines an established role for a company secretary.

2.5 *Taking it on Trust*

The Audit Commission Report **Taking it on Trust** was published in April 2009 and examined the rigour with which NHS trust boards operated the processes available to them and obtained the assurance they need.

The report highlighted discrepancies between trust declarations of compliance with Standards for Better Health and subsequent Healthcare Commission inspections; differences between SICs and core standards declarations; and some major failures in patient care, such as that at Maidstone and Tunbridge Wells NHS Trust and Mid Staffordshire NHS Foundation Trust. There were significant gaps between the processes on paper and the rigour with which they were applied. The report said that the introduction of foundation trusts had generally reinvigorated governance processes and resulted in the recruitment of non-executives with a greater knowledge of effective risk management and board challenge drawn from private sector experience. The report was critical of assurance processes that had become 'a paper chase' rather than a critical examination of the effectiveness of the trust's internal controls and risk management arrangements.

The report recommended that NHS trusts should:

- ensure that their strategic aims and objectives are clearly defined and few in number so they can be widely understood and clearly cascaded throughout the organisation, and that their strategic risks are identified and aligned to their strategic objectives
- review their risk management arrangements – including the way in which risks are reported to the board and consider how best to promote and demonstrate the value of risk management work to staff
- ensure they have systems in place to comply with all statutory, regulatory, clinical and contractual requirements
- consider cascading the **Statement of Internal Control** (now the AGS) through the organisation by sub-certification by managers, allied with a more effective compliance function, performance information and performance management
- review how they identify and then evidence assurances on the operation of controls and how these are then evaluated
- review and increase the assurances they receive from sources other than internal audit, including clinical audit, and in doing so ensure that their full portfolio of risk is covered
- maximise the assurance obtained from internal audit by reviewing the scope of internal audit plans and improving its commissioning
- better align clinical audit programmes to key strategic and operational risks to maximise the assurance provided by the clinical audit function
- strengthen their compliance mechanisms and distinguish them more clearly from internal audit, which should review the effectiveness of the compliance framework
- ensure they have robust arrangements for assuring the quality of their data and by developing systematic and formalised review programmes for their data, including checking accuracy back to records
- develop policies and guidance on data quality and assurance processes, including defining and allocating responsibility for data quality, to promote consistency and improve awareness of board members.

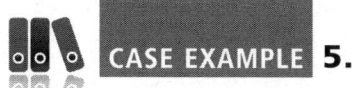 **CASE EXAMPLE 5.2**

An independent review into the board leadership of Maidstone and Tunbridge Wells NHS Trust

In the autumn of 2005 the trust suffered a significant outbreak (150 cases) of *Clostridium difficile* (*C. difficile*) infection, although it went unrecognised at the time. In April 2006 a second outbreak (258 cases) occurred and was recognised and reported to the SHA (NHS South East Coast) and the Health Protection Agency (HPA). The SHA arranged for an investigation by the Healthcare Commission.

The Commission's report was published in October 2007. As well as analysing the problem and the management of *C. difficile* specifically, the report also made general comments and criticisms about the leadership and governance of the trust.

One of the central issues was the role of the chairman and the non-executive directors and their ability to govern. The non-executive board members had struggled to gain a true understanding of what was going on in the organisation and to hold the chief executive and senior managers and clinicians of the trust to account in the period covered by the report. The report stated that the board could have been in a position to ensure the trust managed emergent control of infection issues better than they did if the non-executives had been better advised.

Other issues included the board not providing clear leadership to the organisation as a whole, in its culture and approach to its core business. Board members were reported as being remote and preoccupied with finance and targets.

It was also clear that the board was given information, rather than asking for it and most came with a recommendation only that it be noted. The reports to the board on nursing and cleanliness issues were long and academic and did not make clear the success or otherwise of the solutions relied on, such as the nursing quality assurance framework. There was no lack of information or data, but there was an apparent lack of analysis about what it showed. All information appeared to have been given the same weight.

The trust had an assurance framework throughout, but it was mostly not serviceable and not capable of identifying at board level the primary risks. There was no evidence in the minutes that the chairman and non-executives made sufficient attempts to clarify what they were being told, to consider the implications, or to identify the decisions that may be required of them.

The Commission estimated that about 90 patients 'definitely or probably' died as a result of the infection.

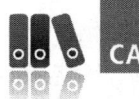 **CASE EXAMPLE 5.3**

Barking, Havering and Redbridge University Hospitals NHS Trust

The trust had experienced frequent changes to its board. Since February 2011 there had been a new chief executive in place. Since the chief executive was appointed, a medical director had been appointed following a number of years where non-permanent staff had provided this function. A number of new non-executive directors had also been appointed and an interim chair had been in place since 2010.

At the time of CQC registration, the trust had a high number of 'conditions' placed on it to require improvements in care. A series of unannounced inspections in 2010/2011 resulted in some of these being lifted, but also resulted in warning notices being issued to the trust (in March, June and July 2011) on staffing levels and maternity care.

CQC concluded their investigation into the quality and safety of care at the trust. One of the findings of that investigation were that trust governance systems were weak and health service governance was underdeveloped. Governance systems had recently changed, but lines of communication in the new structure were unclear and there was a risk of duplication or issues being missed. The trust was reliant on external reviews to identify issues, and while it held extensive performance information, this was not used to drive change. There was a lack of learning from incidents, with investigations identifying recurring themes.

> **TEST YOUR KNOWLEDGE 5.2**
>
> a What principles does The Intelligent Board guidance apply to the information that boards use to govern?
> b What risks was the *Integrated Governance Handbook* trying to address?
> c What specific disclosure requirements are imposed on foundation trusts under the *FT Code of Governance*?
> d What are the three key roles of an effective board according to The Health NHS Board guidance?
> e The report *Taking it on Trust* raised some key concerns about the NHS assurance process – what were these concerns?

3 UK Corporate Governance Code

There has been a code of corporate governance for listed companies in the UK since the Cadbury Code in 1992. From 1998 it was the Combined Code and in 2010 a revised code was re-named the *UK Corporate Governance Code*. The FRC has responsibility for the code.

It is useful to look at the main sections of the code, to see what the main areas of corporate governance are. The code has five sections:

- **Leadership**. This contains principles and provisions relating to the responsibilities of the board as a whole, its chairman and its NEDs.
- **Effectiveness**. This section is concerned with the effectiveness of the board of directors. It deals with issues such as the composition of the board of directors, the appointment and re-election of directors, induction and training for directors, and annual performance reviews for the board, its committees and individual directors.
- **Accountability**. This section deals with the accountability of the board of directors, and also its responsibility for risk and risk management, including internal control risk (see also Chapters 11 and 12).
- **Remuneration**. The fourth section of the code contains principles and provisions relating to the remuneration of directors and senior executives.
- **Relations with shareholders**. The final section of the code sets out the responsibilities of the board for establishing a dialogue with shareholders, and using the AGM to communicate with shareholders and encourage their participation.

The Combined Code, which was replaced by the *UK Corporate Governance Code* in 2010, used to have a section that was addressed specifically to institutional shareholders, and dealt with the responsibilities of institutional investors for good corporate governance. This has now been replaced by a separate UK Stewardship Code, which is also the responsibility of the FRC.

3.1 Additional guidance

When the Combined Code was published in the UK in 2003, there was some uncertainty about how some aspects of the code should be applied. This led to the development of three additional guidelines, which are all now the responsibility of the FRC.

A report was produced on the role of the chairman and independent NEDs, known as the Higgs Report (or the Higgs Guidance). This was updated in 2010 following a review on behalf of the FRC by the ICSA, and amended guidance was issued with the title 'Improving Board Effectiveness'.

Another report was published providing more detailed guidance on the role of the audit committee. It was originally called the Smith Report (after the name of the committee chairman) but is now called the FRC *Guidance on Audit Committees*.

A third report, known as the Turnbull Report, was published giving additional guidance on the responsibilities of the board for the systems of risk management and internal control in the company. This is still called the *Turnbull Guidance*.

All of this additional guidance underpins the various codes of health service governance that have been set out in this chapter. The clearest similarity exists between the Monitor Code of Governance and the *UK Corporate Governance Code* as can be seen by the common main principles.

4 Other codes

4.1 Organisation for Economic Co-operation and Development

In 1999, the OECD issued some non-binding principles on corporate governance, which were reviewed and amended in 2004. They are intended to serve as a reference point for countries to use when evaluating their legal, institutional and regulatory provisions for corporate governance. They also offer guidance and suggestions for stock exchanges, investors, companies and other bodies involved in developing good corporate governance practices.

Unlike national codes of corporate governance, such as the *UK Code*, the OECD Principles do not contain any detailed provisions about how the principles should be applied in practice. They are simply a set of main principles and supporting principles, with some additional explanations or 'annotations'. The principles deal with six aspects of governance, as follows:

- Ensuring the basics for an effective corporate governance framework.
- The rights of shareholders and key ownership functions.
- The equitable treatment of shareholders.
- The role of stakeholders in corporate governance.
- Disclosure and transparency.
- The responsibilities of the board.

The OECD Principles begin with a statement that the corporate governance framework should:

- promote transparent and efficient markets
- be consistent with the rule of law
- clearly articulate the division of responsibilities among different supervisory, regulatory and enforcement authorities.

In the UK these basics are probably accepted as 'normal' for public companies, but it is a useful reminder that this is not necessarily the case at all times or in all countries.

4.2 King Code

Most codes of corporate governance are based on a 'shareholder' approach or 'enlightened shareholder' approach to corporate governance. The *King III Code* (2009), which is the corporate governance code for South Africa, is distinctive because it adopts a 'stakeholder inclusive' approach to corporate governance. In taking this approach, *King III* includes some aspects of governance that are not found in other voluntary codes such as the *UK Code*. The 'stakeholder inclusive' approach of the King Code is described in Chapter 4.

The introduction to *King III* states that the 'philosophy of the (Code) revolves around leadership, sustainability and corporate citizenship':

- **Leadership**. Companies should be given effective leadership, which should be characterised by the ethical governance values of fairness, accountability, responsibility and transparency.
- **Sustainability**. This is the ability of a company to operate its business without compromising the needs of future generations, e.g. through excessive consumption of natural resources or irreversible environmental damage. *King III* refers to sustainability as a 'primary moral and economic imperative'.
- **Corporate citizenship**. A company is a person and like other people it should be aware of its role in society and the need to act as a good citizen. Companies should therefore consider social and environmental (sustainability) issues in the decisions that they make.

Another feature of the King Code is its requirement for 'integrated reporting'. This is reporting that integrates financial aspects of performance with sustainability aspects. (It also recommends forward-looking elements to reporting as well as reporting of historical performance.)

The *King II Code* (2004) recommended that companies should produce annual sustainability reports, in addition to their financial statements. *King III* goes further by calling for an integrated report that combines financial and sustainability issues.

An additional unique feature of *King III* is that it states specifically that, unlike its predecessor *King II*, it applies to all entities regardless of the form of their establishment or incorporation. This means that the code applies not only to companies, but also to public sector and not-for-profit organisations.

The code itself has nine sections. Some of these deal with the same issues as the *UK Code*; others are different or possibly unique:

- Ethical leadership and corporate citizenship. Compared with the *UK Code*, *King III* places more emphasis on ethical behaviour.
- Boards and directors.
- Audit committees.
- The governance of risk.
- The governance of information technology (**IT**). This was not included in the earlier *King II* Code. However, it was considered that directors should be made aware of their responsibilities for IT governance, including the formulation of IT strategy (having due regard for IT risk) and the need for a robust framework for internal control of IT systems.
- Compliance with laws, rules, codes and standards. *King III* states specifically that **compliance risk** (see Chapter 11) should be an integral part of the risk management process.
- Internal audit. *King III* states that there should be an effective risk-based internal audit, and an internal audit function.
- Governing stakeholder relationships. By taking an 'inclusive stakeholder' approach to governance, the board of directors should manage the 'gap' between the expectations of stakeholders and company performance. Relations with stakeholder groups should be managed, and decisions should be taken by the board in the best interests of the company, which means taking into account the legitimate interests and expectations of stakeholders.
- Integrated reporting. As stated earlier, companies should provide integrated annual reports, combining financial and sustainability aspects of performance.

TEST YOUR KNOWLEDGE 5.3

a What are the five sections of the *UK Corporate Governance Code*?
b What has replaced the section in the Combined Code relating to institutional shareholders?
c How is the OECD guidance different to the *UK Code*?
d Why is the King Code distinctive from other codes of corporate governance?

5 Ethics and governance

Ethics are the rules or codes of behaviour that individuals and organisations apply in their decision-making and actions. Personal ethics and business ethics underlie the regulations and codification in governance. The owners and leaders of organisations should establish the standards of ethical behaviour that they expect all their employees to follow, and this behaviour (and the attitudes associated with them) should be consistent with the way in which the organisation is governed.

There is a close connection between best practice in governance and ethical behaviour. Individuals have personal ethics and professional bodies require professional ethical behaviour from their members. Corporate ethics refer to the way in which an organisation conducts its business: companies may have a corporate code of ethics that employees are expected to comply with.

5.1 Personal ethics

Personal ethics are closely associated with morality and a view of what is right and what is wrong. Unethical behaviour by an individual is regarded as unacceptable. To some extent, the law can establish rules about what is 'wrong'. A breach of the criminal law is illegal. Other aspects of law, such as contract law and employment law, can also establish standards of behaviour that are required, and legal action can be taken against anyone in breach of the law.

However, standards of behaviour are determined by social attitudes of morality and good conduct, much more than by legal rules, even though the attitudes of individuals often differ about whether a particular action is 'wrong' and unethical. Ethical personal behaviour helps to build trust. In the context of governance, ethical personal behaviour is commonly associated with integrity and transparency.

Integrity is honesty and behaviour consistent with a clear set of moral rules. Ethical behaviour in this sense means telling the truth and carrying out promises. Transparency (as explained earlier) is openness, so that a person makes his views and intentions clear.

Unethical personal behaviour may be associated with selfishness, seeking personal satisfaction and the fulfilment of personal objectives. Organisational leaders are sometimes accused of this.

5.2 Business ethics

Business ethics are standards of behaviour in business. The way in which employees act can be influenced strongly by the way in which the employer expects them to act, and each organisation has its own ethical (or unethical) standards. This can affect the organisation's dealings with its employees, customers, suppliers and agents, as well as the government, local communities and society as a whole.

There is a connection between business ethics and the different approaches to governance. For example, if a company has a shareholder approach to corporate governance, it puts the interests of shareholders ahead of the interests of anyone else. If it adopts a stakeholder approach to governance, it will act in a way that considers the needs and concerns of other stakeholders.

5.3 Professional ethics

The professions, such as medicine, law and accountancy, are governed by professional bodies that require all members to comply with standards of professional ethics. Members of the accountancy profession, for example, are required to act with integrity, to be independent in their opinion and judgement, to be objective (avoid bias), and to comply with all relevant laws and regulations. In addition, they are required in most circumstances to maintain client confidentiality.

Six of the values that commonly apply to members of the medical profession are:

- **Autonomy**. The patient has the right to refuse or choose their treatment.
- **Beneficence**. A practitioner should act in the best interest of the patient.
- **Non-maleficence**. 'First, do no harm'.
- **Justice**. Concerns the distribution of scarce health resources, and the decision of who gets what treatment (fairness and equality).
- **Dignity**. The patient (and the person treating the patient) have the right to be treated with dignity.
- **Truthfulness and honesty**. The concept of informed consent has increased in importance.

Values such as these do not give answers to how to handle a particular situation, but provide a useful framework for understanding conflicts.

In the context of governance, it is essential that auditors should retain their independence, objectivity and integrity, because stakeholders rely on the opinion they provide about the company's annual financial statements. Unfortunately, a number of corporate scandals in the past, notably the collapse of Enron (see Case example 1.1), have raised questions about the integrity of the information in financial statements and the independence and judgement of the company's auditors.

The measures that should be taken to protect auditor independence are described more fully in Chapter 10.

5.4 A business code of ethics

In the private sector, a large number of companies have developed, adopted and disclosed a formal code of ethics that employees are required to apply. For example, in the USA, one of the requirements for a listing on the NYSE is that the company must adopt and disclose a code of business conduct and ethics for its directors and employees. Key features of a corporate code of ethics are that:

- it is a formal document, adopted by the board of directors
- it is disclosed to employees and to the public, including other stakeholders who have direct dealings with the company
- it is made clear to employees that they should comply with the code
- its application in practice should be monitored, and breaches of ethical conduct should be dealt with according to established rules and procedures.

The effectiveness of a code of ethics depends on the leadership of the company – its directors and senior managers. These individuals must be seen to comply with the ethical code, otherwise employees will see no purpose in complying with the code themselves. The culture of a company drives its ethical behaviour, and a code of ethics provides useful guidance.

There are no rules about what a code of business ethics should contain. The Institute of Business Ethics (IBE) identifies two styles of ethical code that could be developed: a stakeholder model code (focused on ethical behaviour towards stakeholder groups) and an issues model code, which focuses on specific issues relating to ethical or unethical behaviour.

5.5 The *NHS Code of Conduct*

This code sets out the core standards of conduct expected of NHS managers. It follows the consultation that ended on 12 July 2002 and aims to serve two purposes:

- to guide NHS managers and employing health bodies in the work they do and the decisions and choices they have to make
- to reassure the public that these important decisions are being made against a background of professional standards and accountability.

As Sir Nigel Crisp, as CEO of the NHS in 2002, said:

> 'The environment in which the Code will operate is a complex one. NHS managers have very important jobs to do and work in a very public and demanding environment. The management of the NHS calls for difficult decisions and complicated choices. The interests of individual patients have to be balanced with the interests of groups of patients and of the community as a whole. The interests of patients and staff do not always coincide. Managerial and clinical imperatives do not always suggest the same priorities. A balance has to be maintained between national and local priorities.'

The code requires NHS managers to observe the following principles:

- to make the care and safety of patients their first concern and act to protect them from risk
- to respect the public, patients, relatives, carers, NHS staff and partners in other agencies
- to be honest and act with integrity
- to accept responsibility for their own work and the proper performance of the people they manage
- to show their commitment to working as a team member by working with all their colleagues in the NHS and the wider community
- to take responsibility for their own learning and development.

The code should be seen in a wider context that NHS managers must also follow the 'Nolan Principles on Conduct in Public Life', the 'Corporate Governance Codes of Conduct and Accountability', the 'Standards of Business Conduct', the 'Code of Practice on Openness in the NHS' and standards of good employment practice. In addition, many NHS managers come from professional backgrounds and must follow the code of conduct of their own professions as well.

5.6 Implementation of ethical codes

A code of ethics should include an explanation of the process by which the code is issued and used, and how employees can obtain advice on dealing with ethical problems. Senior management must be satisfied that the code of ethics is applied by everyone in the organisation, including the directors. The quality of a system to implement and manage ethical behaviour depends on factors such as:

- employee training in ethical conduct and procedures
- a system for monitoring compliance
- whistleblowing procedures
- reporting breaches of the code and enforcement of suitable disciplinary action
- regular review of the code to ensure that it is still suitable and applicable.

TEST YOUR KNOWLEDGE 5.4

a What is accountability? What is transparency in governance, and why is it a feature of good governance practice?
b In what ways do personal ethics differ from business ethics?
c What are the typical contents of a code of business ethics?
d What are the main principles of the *NHS Code of Conduct*?

6 The reality of health service governance

The 'Mapping the gap' research project was initiated by ICSA in 2011 to examine the degree to which boards in the NHS understood issues of governance, and the extent to which actual boardroom behaviour reflected guidance on best practice. The aim of the research was to establish whether current board governance arrangements increased, or decreased, the likelihood of strategic objectives being met and, depending on the findings, to make observations concerning the challenges facing the existing NHS framework, as well as to inform proposed governance arrangements under the new NHS framework to be introduced under the HSC Act 2012. The research demonstrated that board members were aware of the importance of good governance and understood notions of best practice, but that there was a gap between the theory and the reality in all of the key areas:

Strategy
- there was little discussion relating to a board's vision for staff and stakeholders
- boards believed holding the executive team to account was a higher priority than strategy setting
- on average, 10% of agenda items were dedicated to strategic issues in contrast to best practice recommendations of 60%.

Decision-making
- observed boardroom behaviours evidenced a lack of appropriate challenge
- information presented to boards was of variable quality when assessed in terms of accuracy, timeliness and relevance, with a lack of cross-referencing, internal and external validation and data on future trends and market context
- boards were more frequently presented with items 'to note' than 'for decision'.

Clinical and quality matters
- only 5% of boards observed clearly aligned clinical and quality issues to strategic objectives
- clinical and quality issues took up between 4% and 13% of the top five agenda items, depending on the type of trust, in contrast with governance guidance recommending a minimum of 20%

- the acquisition of information on clinical and quality matters from a range of sources, including site visits and patient feedback, did not appear robust.

Probity and transparency
- 75% of board agendas included declarations of interest as an item
- open board meetings alone were not considered by interviewees to be satisfactory for meeting accountability and transparency obligations.

The research points to governance arrangements inside the NHS trust board as one of the main factors in improving NHS systems. The report's conclusion has implications for the way in which the NHS is currently governed, and for the design of governance systems under the NHS that will emerge from the anticipated reforms and subsequent restructuring.

CHAPTER SUMMARY

- A voluntary code of governance is issued by an authoritative national or international body and contains principles or best practice in governance that major companies (listed companies) or organisations are encouraged to adopt and apply.
- The purpose of a voluntary code is to raise standards of governance and is principles-based.
- In the NHS, Monitor requires foundation trusts to comply with the NHS Foundation Trust Code of Governance or explain any non-compliance.
- The *King III Code* is an 'apply or explain' regime that shows an appreciation for the fact that it is often not a case of whether to comply or not, but rather to consider how the principles and recommendations can be applied.
- There are several voluntary codes which relate to health service governance: the Nolan Code, The Intelligent Board, *The Integrated Governance Handbook*, The Intelligent Board – Modernising Mental Health Services, The NHS Foundation Trust Code of Governance, *The Healthy NHS Board: principles for good governance* and *Taking it on Trust*.
- There has been a code of corporate governance for listed companies in the UK since the Cadbury Code in 1992. From 1998 it was the Combined Code and in 2010 a revised code was re-named the *UK Corporate Governance Code*.
- The OECD has issued non-binding principles on corporate governance, intended to serve as a reference point for countries to use when evaluating their legal, institutional and regulatory provisions for corporate governance, they offer guidance and suggestions for stock exchanges, investors, companies and other bodies involved in developing good corporate governance practices.
- The King III Code is the corporate governance code for South Africa and is particularly distinctive because it adopts a 'stakeholder inclusive' approach to corporate governance.
- Ethics are the rules or codes of behaviour that individuals and organisations apply in their decision-making and actions. Personal ethics and business ethics underlie the regulations and codification in governance.
- The *NHS Code of Conduct* sets out the core standards of conduct expected of NHS managers and aims to guide NHS managers and employing health bodies in the work they do and the decisions and choices they have to make, as well as reassuring the public that these important decisions are being made against a background of professional standards and accountability.
- 'Mapping the gap' highlights the potential disconnect for NHS boards between governance best practice.

Governance of foundation trusts

■ CONTENTS

1. Foundation trusts overview
2. Regulation
3. Governance structure
4. Membership
5. Council of governors
6. Elections
7. Foundation Trust Network
8. The future for foundation trusts
9. The governance challenge

■ INTRODUCTION

This chapter considers the legislative background to the introduction of foundation trusts within the NHS. It goes onto explore the specific governance structure that applies to foundation trusts and the particular role played by the board of governors. The role of Monitor as the regulator for foundation trusts is set out before the chapter finishes with the impact of the Health and Social Care (HSC) Act 2012 and an exploration of the governance issues raised by the creation of foundation trusts.

1 Foundation trusts overview

The introduction of NHS Foundation Trusts (often referred to as 'foundation hospitals') in 2006 represented a significant change in the way in which hospital services were managed and provided in England. Foundation trusts were part of the government's plan for creating a patient-led NHS. The aim of the reforms was to provide high-quality care, with devolved decision making so that they were more responsive to the needs and wishes of patients and communities. They were also at the leading edge of many of the other reforms and improvements that aim to create a patient-led NHS.

NHS Foundation Trusts are not subject to direction from the Secretary of State for Health, and as part of their constitution they are required to establish stronger connections with their local communities by encouraging people living locally to become members of the trust. The membership of each NHS Foundation Trust is therefore made up of local people (including patients and carers) and staff.

Members are able to stand as, and vote to elect, representatives to serve on the council of governors. Governors are responsible for representing the interests of the members and partner organisations in the local health economy in the running of the NHS Foundation Trust. The intention is that local communities and staff working on the front line can influence the management and provision of NHS services in their area. This allows NHS Foundation Trusts to direct their services more closely to the needs of their communities, with freedom to develop new ways of working so that hospital services more accurately reflect the needs and expectations of local people.

Although run locally, NHS Foundation Trusts remain fully part of the NHS. They have been set up as **Public Benefit Corporations**, with a primary purpose to provide NHS services to NHS patients and users according to NHS principles and standards – free care, based on need and not ability to pay.

In the Government's White Paper 'Equity and Excellence: liberating the NHS' in July 2010 it was made clear that all NHS trusts would become or become part of a foundation trust by 2014 and NHS trusts would be abolished. Failure to meet this deadline, or achieve a credible plan for transition, would result in the Secretary of State for Health placing the NHS trust under a special administration regime. In more recent discussions, however, it would seem that this deadline may soften to allow trusts, with difficult long-term decisions to make around the remodeling of clinical services, to still achieve foundation trust status.

1.1 Foundation trust freedoms

As foundation trusts are not directed by government, they have greater freedom to decide, with their governors and members, their own strategy and the way services are run.

They have significantly greater freedoms over the way they conduct their finances. Unlike NHS trusts, NHS foundation trusts are able to:

- build up operational surpluses
- retain proceeds from asset sales
- raise capital in the public and/or private sectors
- manage their organisations and their resources – free from central government control.

Foundation trusts have the freedom to decide locally the capital investment needed in order to improve services and increase capacity. They are able to borrow to support this investment, as long as they can afford it, without needing to seek external approval. Access to Private Finance Initiative (PFI) and public capital for major schemes continues as before. The amount they can borrow is determined by a formula – the Prudential Code – directly linked to their ability to repay the debt from the revenue they raise. Each foundation trust calculates its borrowing limit based on this formula.

The limit that each NHS Foundation Trust can borrow is set out in its terms of authorisation and is subject to annual review by its Regulator, Monitor. Against this borrowing limit, NHS Foundation Trusts are allowed to raise finance to build new facilities and improve existing ones. They are able to borrow money from the government and from private sector lenders.

1.2 Terms of authorisation

Under the provisions of the National Health Service Act 2006, the functions of each foundation trust are set out in its terms of authorisation as granted by Monitor. The terms of authorisation cover such things as:

- a description of the health services that the foundation trust is authorised to provide
- a list of services that the foundation trust is required to provide to the NHS in England
- a requirement to operate to national standards and targets, based on the national standards for healthcare against which the CQC inspects
- the circumstances in which major changes to services (for example, in response to a changing local population) need to be discussed locally and agreed by Monitor
- a list of assets such as buildings, land or equipment that are designated as 'protected' because they are needed to provide required NHS services
- the amount of money the foundation trust is allowed to borrow
- the financial and statistical information the foundation trust is required to provide
- a limit on the amount of private work the foundation trust can carry out.

1.3 Accountability

Foundation trusts are accountable to:

- their local communities through their members and governors
- their commissioners through contracts
- Parliament (each foundation trust must lay its annual report and accounts before Parliament)

- the CQC (through the legal requirement to register and meet the associated standards for the quality of care provided)
- Monitor as their regulator.

The figure below sets out the accountability structure for foundation trusts prior to the implementation of the Health and Social Care Act 2012.

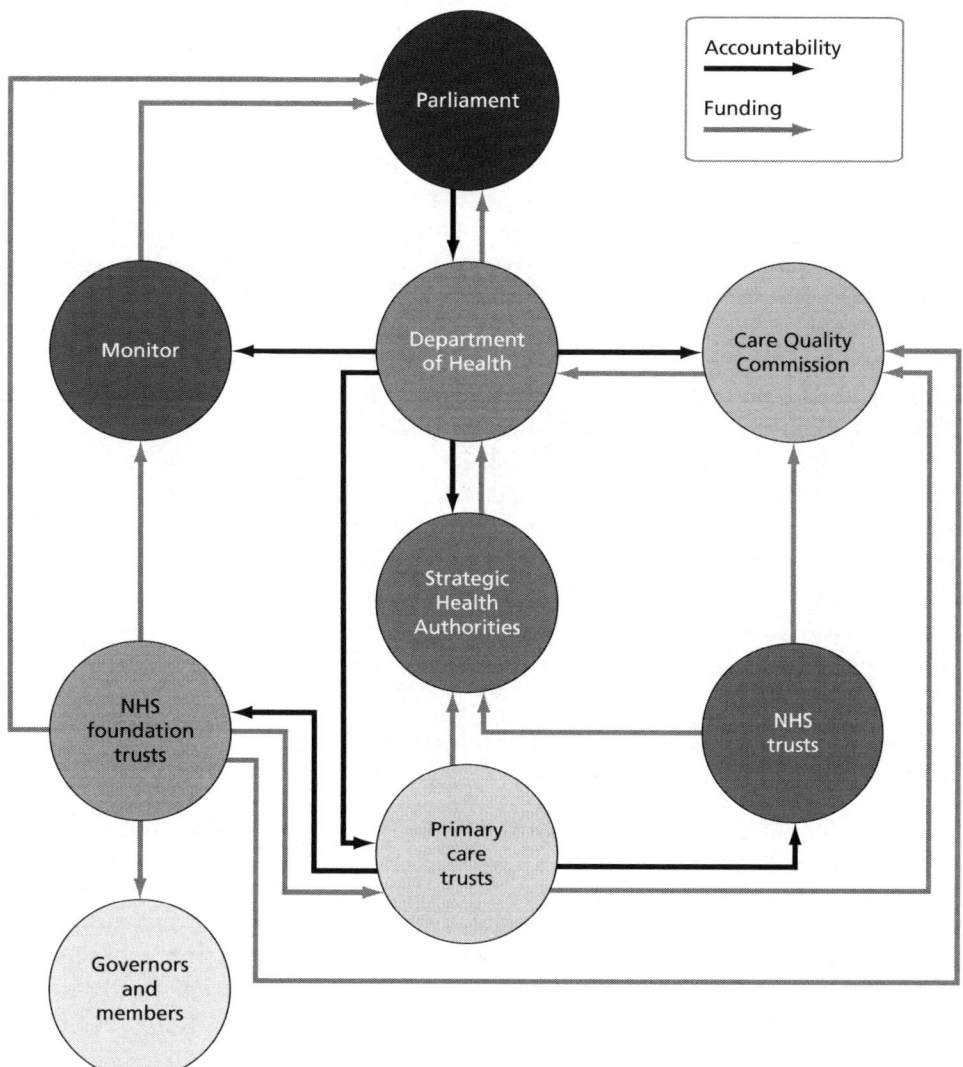

FIGURE 6.1 Accountability in foundation trusts

2 Regulation

Monitor is the independent regulator of NHS foundation trusts and was established in January 2004. Monitor is independent of central government and directly accountable to Parliament. Monitor has three specific areas of work:

- determining whether NHS trusts are ready to become NHS foundation trusts
- ensuring that NHS foundation trusts comply with the conditions they signed up to – that they are well-led and financially robust
- supporting NHS foundation trust development.

Monitor's functions and powers are currently set out in the National Health Service Act 2006.

One of Monitor's key roles at present is to assess applications by NHS trusts, authorise NHS trusts as NHS foundation trusts, issue terms of authorisation to every NHS foundation trust, oversee compliance against this and intervene if required only if there is significant non-compliance with the terms of authorisation, which in summary include:

- the general requirement to operate effectively, efficiently and economically
- requirements to meet healthcare targets and national standards
- the requirement to cooperate with other NHS organisations.

The board of directors is the first line of regulation in foundation trusts and Monitor requires foundation trusts to submit an annual plan and quarterly reports. If Monitor considers that problems are starting to develop then they will ensure that the trust has an action plan in place and will monitor progress against that plan. Monitor has powers to intervene in a foundation trust in the event of failings in its healthcare standards as judged by the CQC, or other aspects of its leadership, which result in a significant breach of its terms of authorisation.

Monitor's intervention powers are broad and range from closing a specific service, if there are serious concerns about it, or requiring a board to take – or not take – a specific action(s), requiring a board to obtain external advice on a particular issue, or, in extreme cases, removing any or all of the directors or governors and appointing replacements.

In the most serious cases, where intervention by Monitor cannot resolve the breach, an NHS Foundation Trust could be dissolved after consultation. If this were to happen, the Health and Social Care (Community Health and Standards) Act 2003 provides mechanisms to ensure that NHS patients and users continue to receive high quality treatment.

There are significant amendments to Monitor's role in the HSC Act 2012. The Act provides for Monitor to be the sector regulator for health and, at a later date, for adult social care. Monitor's core duty would be to protect and promote patients' interests. In the medium term it would continue to assess NHS trusts for foundation trust status, and to ensure that foundation trusts were financially viable and well led, in terms of both quality and finances.

In carrying out the health sector regulator role, Monitor would license providers of NHS services in England and exercise functions in three areas:

- regulating prices
- enabling integrated care and preventing anti-competitive behaviour
- supporting service continuity.

As a result of these changes the terms of authorisation will cease to exist and instead of assessing foundation trusts' compliance with their terms of authorisation, the new oversight function will assess the risk to foundation trusts fulfilling their Principal Purpose, namely the provision of goods and services for the purposes of the health service in England. Where Monitor identifies a significant risk to fulfilment of the Principal Purpose, they may impose additional conditions in the foundation trust's licence and, if those conditions were subsequently breached, they could take regulatory action. These proposals will be the subject of a full consultation process during 2012.

In addition it is proposed that Monitor will no longer set out a compliance framework for foundation trusts, check whether a constitution complies with statutory requirements nor approve changes or review significant or material transactions.

2.1 Becoming a foundation trust

NHS trusts wishing to become NHS foundation trusts must first obtain the support of the Secretary of State for Health before they can make an application to Monitor for consideration for authorisation as a foundation trust. In order to obtain the Secretary of State's support, applicant trusts must demonstrate that they have consulted staff, local NHS partners and the public on their proposals and that their proposals fit with the local vision for health services. Support is dependent on the development of a five-year business plan, HR strategy and governance proposals (e.g. membership arrangements, size and composition of the council of governors and board of directors).

The process of authorisation as an FT helps equip NHS trust boards more effectively to meet future challenges, by testing both clinical quality and financial viability. Not all boards pass these tests. Half of all aspirant NHS trusts whose FT application is deferred during the authorisation process do so due to a failure of governance. More expressly, it means that there have been issues with the capacity and capability of the board. As a result the DH has recently produced a Board Governance Assurance Framework that assists aspirant foundation trust boards through a combination of self and independent assessment processes to ensure that they are appropriately skilled, and prepared to achieve FT authorisation.

The Framework is designed to provide assurance in relation to various leading indicators of effective board governance. These indicators are:

1 **Board composition and commitment** (e.g. balance of skills, knowledge and experience).
2 **Board evaluation, development and learning** (e.g. the board has a development programme in place).
3 **Board insight and foresight** (e.g. Performance Reporting).
4 **Board engagement and involvement** (e.g. communicating priorities and expectations).
5 **Board impact case studies** (e.g. a case study that describes how the board has responded to a recent financial issue).

Once the Secretary of State has given support, applicants are asked to submit an application for authorisation to Monitor. The decision to authorise a trust as an NHS foundation trust is strictly a decision for Monitor after having satisfied itself of an applicant's preparedness and viability for foundation status.

Monitor will assess three areas in their decision to authorise:

1 Is the trust well governed with the leadership in place to drive future strategy and improve patient care?
2 Is the trust financially viable with a sound business plan?
3 Is the trust legally constituted, with a membership that is representative of its local community?

TEST YOUR KNOWLEDGE 6.1

a What are the main areas of Monitor's work?
b What intervention will Monitor exercise if a trust is at risk of breaching its terms of authorisation?
c What three areas will Monitor assess for NHS trusts applying for authorisation as a foundation trust?

3 Governance structures

The DH in its **Guide to NHS Foundation Trusts** (2002) set out that the governance of foundation trusts was to be based on experience in other sectors as the following extracts demonstrate:

> 'The new governance arrangements for NHS Foundation Trusts have been modelled on cooperative societies and mutual organisations. These combine community ownership with accountability.'
>
> (DH, 2002, 10)

> 'NHS Foundation Trusts will herald a new form of social ownership where health services are owned by and accountable to local people rather than central Government. In this way, much stronger connections will be established between providers of NHS services and their stakeholder communities . . . In a similar way to becoming a member of a co-operative society or mutual organisation, the members of an NHS Foundation Trust will become its owners, taking on responsibility for their local hospitals from national Government.'
>
> (DH, 2002, 15)

Earlier discussions in this text have highlighted the need to understand the lines of accountability in setting out appropriate forms of governance. The guidance for foundation trusts establishes that they are to be accountable to their members. This accountability is underpinned by the

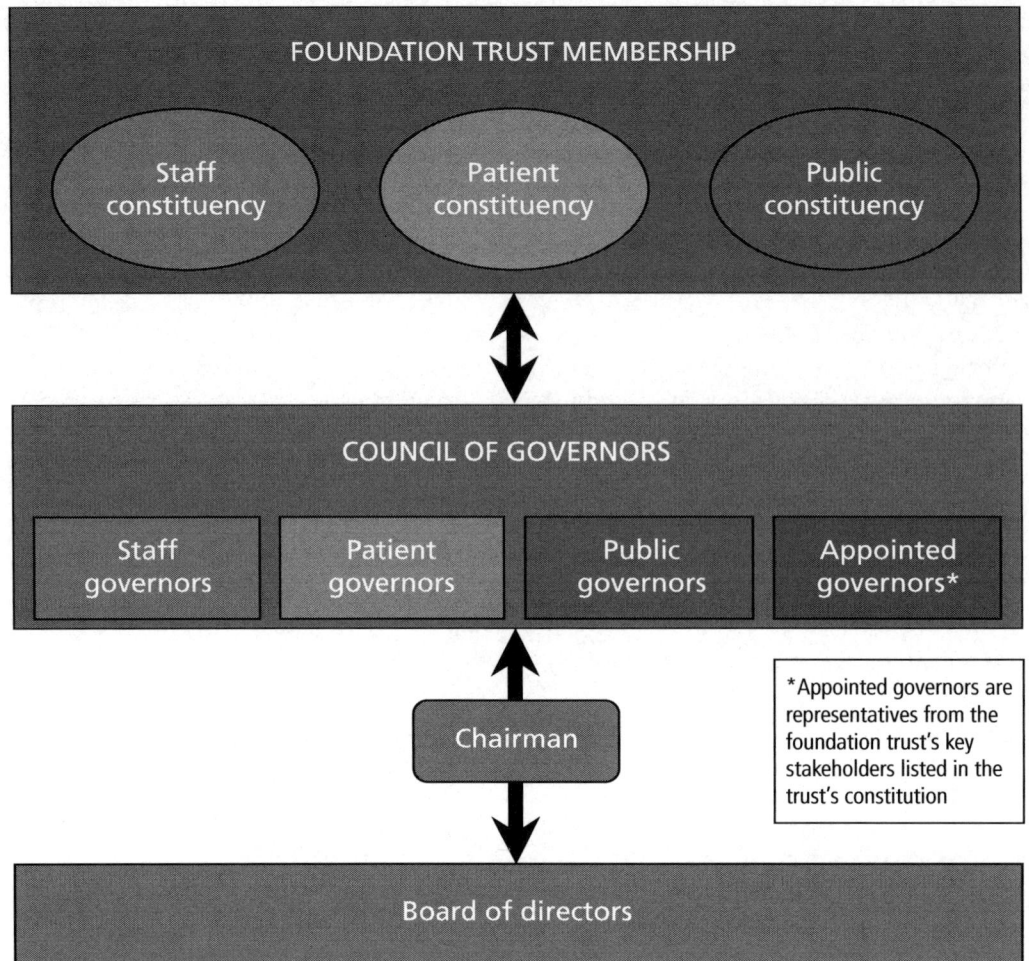

FIGURE 6.2 Governance structure in foundation trusts

two board structure required of foundation trusts as shown in Figure 6.2. This is set out in the individual foundation trust's constitution.

Every authorised foundation trust will have a constitution that has been approved by Monitor. The constitution will set out the governance arrangements for the foundation trust. Although each constitution will be unique to the foundation trust it relates to, there are legal requirements that apply to all NHS foundation trusts. The requirements are set out in Monitor's Model Core Constitution, on which all NHS foundation trust constitutions must be based.

The basic governance structure of all NHS foundation trusts includes:

- the membership
- the council of governors
- the board of directors.

Figure 6.2 sets out the governance structure for foundation trusts.

The board of governors is made up of elected governors and appointed governors. Elected governors are those members elected by the membership to represent the staff, patient and public constituencies that make up the membership of a foundation trust. The appointed governors are the representatives from certain key stakeholders, such as a PCT that commissions services from the NHS foundation trust, and a local authority – they are appointed to the board of governors to represent those stakeholder groups.

A model core constitution for foundation trusts has been prepared by Monitor to reflect the requirements of Schedule 7 of the 2006 Act. It sets out what Monitor considers 'otherwise appropriate', as set out in Appendix B8 of Monitor's publication, *Applying for NHS Foundation Trust Status: guide for applicants*. Monitor requires all applicant trusts for foundation trust authorisation to prepare their constitutions on the basis of this model core constitution.

Monitor have also prepared an updated Model Core Constitution, which reflects the legislative changes to be implemented by the HSC Act 2012, at a date to be determined. The revised constitution has been published for guidance purposes only and the current Model Core Constitution (dated September 2008) continues to apply for the time being.

Additions or amendments to the model core constitution may be made, however, Monitor requires that any departure from the model core constitutions:

- be in accordance with Schedule 7
- be clearly indicated as a tracked change
- be accompanied by an explanation for the intended departure from the model core.

The constitution sets out:

- who may be a member
- the make up of the council of governors
- how elections of governors will be carried out
- the statutory duties of the governors
- the grounds and procedures for the disqualification and removal of members and governors
- the requirement for open meetings of the council of governors
- the make up of the board of directors
- the requirement for statutory registers.

The constitution also includes a number of annexes as follows:

- the public constituency
- the staff constituency
- the patient constituency
- composition of the board of governors
- the Model Election Rules
- additional provisions – board of governors
- standing orders – board of governors
- standing orders – board of directors
- further provisions.

Until the full implementation of the HSC Act 2012 the foundation trust is required to obtain the approval of Monitor to any amendment to the trust's constitution or any of the accompanying annexes.

TEST YOUR KNOWLEDGE 6.2

a What is a public benefit corporation?
b What freedoms do foundation trusts have?
c Who is a foundation trust accountable to?
d Describe the governance structure for a foundation trust
e What are the key aspects of the Model Core Constitution?

4 Membership

Residents and patients in areas served by a foundation trust, with an interest in the wellbeing of their local hospital and health services, can register as members of the organisation. Patients who do not live locally, and their carers, may also become members, if provided for in the trust's constitution. Members of foundation trusts do not receive any special treatment as NHS patients and users. They have the same access to NHS services as anyone who chooses not to become a member.

The eligibility for membership of a foundation trust is open to local residents, patients and carers and staff employed by the trust, in the terms provided in each trust's constitution.

All foundation trust members can expect to receive regular information about their local trust and be consulted on plans for future development.

The model constitution sets out that a foundation trust membership will consist of two main groupings, namely staff and public members. In addition a third grouping of members may be included to represent patient members. These groupings are known as constituencies. Within each constituency there may be a number of classes, which differentiate between geographical areas for public members or between staff categories for staff members. For the public constituency the constitution must specify the area or areas and each of these areas must be an electoral area for the purposes of local government elections in England and Wales or an area consisting of two or more areas. The constitution may provide for automatic membership of the staff constituency by default.

If a foundation trust decides to have a patient constituency then it may also divide those members into descriptions or classes of individuals. There must, however, be at least three such classes and one must comprise the carers of patients. The constitution may provide for automatic membership of the patients' constituency (if there is one) by default.

If automatic membership for the staff and/or patient constituency is within the constitution, the foundation trust must consider how they will inform staff and/or patients that they are subject to automatic membership.

There is no limit on the number of people who can register as members, providing they meet the eligibility criteria. It is for foundation trusts to ensure they have a representative membership and sufficient members so that they can mount credible election processes. Governance arrangements for foundation trusts need to be reflective of local conditions and proposals that work best for them.

It is this membership body made up of local residents, patients and carers and staff employed by the trust, which are able to vote in the elections to appoint the council of governors of the foundation trust. Each member, if nominated, can stand for election as a governor.

5 Council of governors

The council of governors is responsible for representing the interests of the local community in the management and stewardship of the foundation trust, and for sharing information about key decisions with other foundation trust members. It is not responsible for the day-to-day management of the organisation such as setting budgets, staff pay and other operational matters – that is a matter for the board of directors. However, the council of governors allows local residents, staff and key stakeholders to influence decisions about spending and the development of services. The council of governors should hold the board of directors to account for the performance of the trust, including ensuring the board of directors acts so that the foundation trust does not breach the terms of its authorisation.

Typically the board of governors meets as a full council four or five times a year. The meetings are held in public and are open to all members and the general public. The council of governors is required to hold an AGM to receive the annual report and accounts and any report of the auditor. This meeting is often used to provide an overview of the year from the CEO.

Foundation trusts are allowed some local flexibility over the size and composition of their council of governors. However, every council must have:

- **Public governors**: a majority of governors elected by members in the public constituency.
- **Staff governors**: at least three governors representing staff.
- **Appointed governors**: at least one governor representing local NHS PCTs or their successor body plus at least one governor representing local authorities in the area, plus at least one governor appointed from the local university (if the trust's hospitals include a medical or dental school).
- **A chair**.

The chairman of the foundation trust is responsible for leadership of both the board of directors and for the council of governors. *The FT Code of Governance* sets out that it is the chair's responsibility to ensure that the board and the council work together effectively, but that the governors also have a responsibility to make these arrangements work and should take the lead in inviting the chief executive or other board members to their meetings, where they may raise questions about the affairs of the trust of the chair or other board members.

It is up to each foundation trust to determine the detail of the arrangements for the membership and election to the council of governors, although the election must follow the DH's Model Election Rules. These rules form part of the model core constitution. A foundation trust may also specify other organisations within its constitution as a partnership organisation who may also appoint a member of the council of governors.

5.1 Lead governor

Monitor have also recommended that the council of governors appoint a lead governor who would lead the council of governors where it is not considered appropriate for the chair or another one of the NEDs to do so. These occasions are likely to be infrequent but one example may be a meeting discussing the appointment of the chair.

The lead governor could also have a role in certain circumstances where it would not be appropriate for the chair to contact Monitor, or Monitor to contact the chair (for example, in relation to appointment of the chair). Communication would instead take place between the lead governor and Monitor in such circumstances. Routine communication from Monitor to governors is disseminated through the foundation trust secretary.

The main circumstances where Monitor will contact a lead governor are where Monitor has concerns as to the quality of the board leadership at a foundation trust, which may lead to Monitor's use of its formal powers to remove the chairman or non-executive directors. As the council of governors appoints the chairman and NEDs, Monitor would want to consult with the governors as to the capacity and capability of these individuals to lead the trust, to rectify successfully any issues, and also for the governors to understand Monitor's concerns.

Monitor suggests that: 'The lead governor should take steps to understand Monitor's role, the available guidance and the basis on which Monitor may take regulatory action. The lead governor will then be able to communicate more widely with other governors.'

The other situation where Monitor may wish to contact the lead governor is where it has concerns that the process for the appointment of the chairman or other members of the board, or elections for governors, may not have complied with the NHS foundation trust's constitution, or alternatively may be inappropriate.

The existence of a lead governor does not, in itself, prevent any governor from contacting Monitor directly if they feel it is necessary. The term lead governor is used to prevent confusion with the deputy.

The lead governor should be chosen by the council of governors. The lead governor should not deputise for the deputy chair of the board of directors.

5.2 Statutory duties

The statutory duties of foundation trust governors are set out in The National Health Service Act 2006 and expanded further in the Monitor guidance: *Your Statutory Duties: a reference guide for NHS foundation trust governors*. The statutory duties are to:

- appoint and, if appropriate, remove the chair
- appoint and, if appropriate, remove the other NEDs
- decide the remuneration and allowances, and the other terms and conditions of office, of the chair and the other NEDs
- approve the appointment of the chief executive
- appoint and, if appropriate, remove the NHS foundation trust's auditor
- receive the NHS foundation trust's annual accounts, any report of the auditor on them and the annual report.

In addition, in preparing the foundation trust's forward plan, the board of directors must have regard to the views of the council of governors.

Under The HSC Act 2012 governors have a greater role in monitoring effective governance at foundation trusts, as Monitor takes up the role of health sector regulator. It is proposed that Monitor will continue to have transitional powers over all foundation trusts until 2016 to maintain high standards of governance during the transition. This will give foundation trusts time to develop their governance arrangements, and will give governors time to learn how to use their powers effectively, which is in the best interest of patients.

Additional powers proposed for governors in the Bill include the power to require one or more directors to attend a meeting and the right to receive agendas and minutes of the meetings of directors. Approval of more than half of the members of the council of governors will also be needed for any amendment to the trust constitution or entry by the trust into a significant transaction, merger, acquisition, separation or dissolution.

Appointment or removal of a chair or non-executive director (NED)

In fulfilling the role to appoint (or remove) the chair and other NEDs the council of governors has a similar committee structure to that of the board of directors. *The FT Code of Governance* sets out that:

> 'The governors are responsible at a general meeting for the appointment, re-appointment and removal of the chairman and the other NEDs. They should agree with the nominations committee a clear process for the nomination of a new chair and NEDs. Once suitable candidates have been identified the nominations committee should make recommendations to the council of governors.'

The *FT Code of Governance* describes two scenarios for the role of the board of governors in the appointment of non-executives:

> 'In foundation trusts there may be one or two nominations committees. If there are two committees, one will be responsible for considering nominations for executive directors and the other for non-executive directors (including the chairman) . . . Where a foundation trust has two nominations committees, the nominations committee responsible for the appointment of non-executive directors should consist of a majority of governors. If only one nominations committee exists, when nominations for non-executives, including the appointment of a chairman or a deputy chairman, are being discussed, there should be a majority of governors on the committee and also a majority governor representation on the interview panel.'

A person may only be appointed as a NED or chairman if he is a member of the public constituency (or the patient constituency if there is one). Where the trust has a university medical or dental school, a person may be appointed as a NED if he exercises functions for that university.

Upon receiving a recommendation to appoint the council of governors should consider the qualifications, skills and experience required and for the appointment of a chairman they should also consider the time commitment required. The *FT Code of Governance* stipulates that 'no individual, simultaneously while being a chairman of an NHS foundation trust, should be the substantive chairman of another NHS foundation trust'.

In accordance with the foundation trust's constitution:

- appointment is by a majority of the governors attending the relevant meeting, and
- removal requires the approval of three-quarters of the members of the council of governors, not just those who attend the meeting.

Remuneration of a chair or non-executive director (NED)

The council of governors is also responsible for setting the remuneration of NEDs and the chairman. The council of governors should consult external professional advisers to market-test the remuneration levels of the chairman and other non-executives at least once every three years and when they intend to make a material change to the remuneration of a non-executive. Levels of remuneration for the chairman and other NEDs should reflect the time commitment and responsibilities of their roles. The council of governors may delegate the task of market-testing to a remuneration committee that would consist solely of governors. The chairing of this committee would often be the responsibility of the lead governor if one has been appointed; if not the council of governors may appoint a chair. The committee then makes its recommendation back to the council of governors for decision.

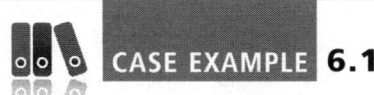

CASE EXAMPLE 6.1

The council of governors and board of directors had worked collaboratively in the process of appointing a new chairman. The nominations committee, consisting of the deputy chair and other non-executives had considered the make-up of the board and identified the key skills and experience required from the new appointment. They had made their recommendations to the Governor's Appointment Committee and these had been accepted.

The Governors Appointments Committee, led by the deputy chairman, appointed recruitment consultants to assist them with the search and consulted with executive and non-executive directors alike on the process for appointment.

The committee, again led by the deputy chairman and supported by the company secretary, director of HR and the recruitment advisers conducted the interviews and offered an opportunity for the candidates to be met by members of the board, the wider council of governors and members of staff.

When it came to a decision to appoint, the committee was divided in its view as to the best candidate for the post. One candidate was very experienced but had demonstrated less commitment to the trust, the other was less experienced but much more committed to the organisation. The committee agreed that both candidates were appointable and therefore invited the current CEO to offer her opinion as to which candidate would gain the support of the executive team. As a result the decision was taken to recommend the less experienced candidate to the council of governors for appointment as the new chairman.

The executive directors immediately rejected the decision of the committee and refused to support the proposal. The CEO demanded that the committee reconvene and reconsider its decision. The pressure on the committee was such that it subsequently decided not to appoint and to re-advertise the post. The committee complained to Monitor that the executive directors had undermined their statutory duty to appoint the chairman and the executive directors were formally reprimanded by Monitor. The committee was advised to appoint an independent adviser to work with them on the new recruitment process.

Approval of the appointment of the chief executive

It is for the NEDs to appoint and remove the chief executive; however, the appointment of a chief executive does require the approval of the council of governors.

Monitor's guide *Your Statutory Duties: a reference guide for NHS foundation trust governors* sets out a clear process for engaging with the council of governors to reduce the likelihood of the governors not giving their approval. The NEDs should make sure that the governors are kept informed about the appointment process followed, ensuring that the governors are satisfied with the various stages of the process such as use of advertisements, the criteria for selection and how selection was carried out.

To give their approval, the council of governors needs to be confident that the appointment process has identified a candidate with sufficient experience to fulfil all essential aspects of the job description and that the process has been fair, open and transparent. The council of governors should receive a report setting out that due law and process has been followed and how the proposed candidate's skills and experience meet the agreed role and person specification. The primary responsibility for the appointment lies with the non-executives and the council of governors should only withhold its approval with good cause.

If approval is withheld, the council of governors must set out their reasons to the chair and the other NEDs. The reasons for withholding approval must be justifiable as there are likely to be financial consequences.

The process, the decision and the reasons for the decision should be set out in the foundation trust's annual report, whatever the outcome.

Appointment and removal of the auditor

The board of directors' audit committee should make recommendations to the council of governors about the appointment, re-appointment and removal of the external auditor and the approval of the remuneration and terms of engagement of the external auditor. Again, the council of governors may delegate the work involved to an auditor appointments committee, which is made up of governors and chaired by the chair of the audit committee before making its recommendation to the council of governors for decision.

If the council of governors does not accept the recommendation, it should include in the annual report a statement from the audit committee explaining the recommendation and should set out reasons why the council of governors has taken a different position.

5.3 Forward planning

As part of Monitor's *Compliance Framework* each foundation trust is required to submit an annual plan, which includes forecast financial performance, details of any major risks to compliance with their terms of authorisation and how the foundation trust intends to address these. The information provided in the annual plan must also include:

- commentary on the strategic overview for the foundation trust, changes to previous forecasts, risk analysis and membership plans
- a membership report
- board statements on risk, service performance, clinical quality, compliance with the terms of authorisation and board roles, structure and capacity
- financial projections
- updates in relation to Schedules 2 (mandatory goods and services) and 3 (mandatory education and training) of the foundation trust's terms of authorisation.

The *FT Code of Governance* states that governors can 'expect to be consulted on the development of forward plans for the trust and any significant changes to the delivery of the trust's business plan'. The role of the governors is to ensure that the interests of the trust's members are considered when establishing the strategic direction for the foundation trust.

5.4 Re-election of governors

All elected governors should be submitted for re-election at regular intervals.

The *FT Code of Governance* states that:

> 'Elected governors must be subject to re-election by the members of their constituency at regular intervals not exceeding three years. The names of governors submitted for election or re-election should be accompanied by sufficient biographical details and any other relevant information to enable members to take an informed decision on their election. This should include prior performance information such as attendance records at governor meetings and other relevant events organised by the NHS foundation trust for governors.'

Appointed governors may be re-appointed by their organisation for a further three-year period. The maximum term for all members of the board of governors is six years under the *FT Code of Governance*.

5.5 The future role of governors

The HSC Act 2012 changes fundamentally the way foundation trusts are governed and managed. One of the most important changes is that the council of governors will be given express statutory duties to hold the NEDs individually and collectively to account for the performance of the board and to represent the interests of the foundation trust's members and the public as whole.

As previously set out in this text, governors have a statutory duty to appoint the chair and NEDs of a foundation trust. The new duty to hold non-executives to account will mean governors will have to consider how they use their existing powers to performance manage non-executives. The appraisal and line management of NEDs has previously been the responsibility of the chair and so this will again highlight the potential conflict for the chairman in his dual role of chair of both the council of governors and board of directors. To support governors in this role, they will be able to require directors to attend a meeting to obtain information about their organisation's performance and that of its directors. Under the existing powers they could, if they were dissatisfied with performance, remove the NEDs.

In addition, as Monitor will no longer be reviewing significant or material transactions, then a role for the council of governors has been introduced. Foundation trusts may define some types of transaction as 'significant' in the terms of their constitution; if they do so then the foundation trust will need the consent of more than half of the council of governors to proceed with the transaction. However, the consent of more than half of the governors will always be required for any merger, acquisition or separation of the foundation trust. Unlike 'significant transactions', this is not an optional requirement and this means that, in practice, responsibility for signing off any merger or acquisition moves jointly to the directors and governors.

This extended role for governors raises interesting questions around their capacity and capability and many governors are likely to require significant training to understand and be able to discharge their duties.

To support governors in this role Monitor will establish an independent panel to give 'authoritative' advice to governors in response to governors' concerns about constitutional and governance issues. To refer a matter to the panel would require the approval of more than half of the governors' council so that referrals would be limited to material areas of concern. This might mean that the foundation trust will need to provide much more by way of ongoing support and advice to its council of governors.

The ICSA in its memorandum to Parliament states that:

'Significant resources will have to be made available to governors in order to hold the board of directors to account and understand the competitive market when asked to vote on significant transactions. The requirements on governors are going to be onerous, and councils of governors will require at least some, if not all, of their number to have the financial and commercial skills to evaluate foundation trust proposals in relation to mergers, acquisitions and other significant transactions . . . There is also concern as to how governors can reconcile their role as representatives of the membership and play a significant part in the strategic decision making process.'

TEST YOUR KNOWLEDGE 6.3

a What are the three possible constituencies of membership?
b What is the makeup of the council of governors?
c What are the statutory duties of the council of governors
d In what circumstances would Monitor make direct contact with the lead governor?
e What are the key proposed changes to the role of governor and what impact will these changes have?

6 Elections

Foundation trusts are required to include the DH's model election rules as part of their constitution. The rules make provision for both first-past-the-post and single transferable voting but not electronic voting. The requirement to declare membership of a political party is a requirement of the Model Election Rules.

The Model Election Rules set out a clear and strict timetable for the election proceedings that must be adhered to.

Section 60 of the NHS Act 2006 requires persons standing for and voting in the elections to make a declaration setting out the particulars of their qualification to vote or stand as a member of the constituency (or class/area) for which the election is being held. The constitution of each trust sets out the criteria for disqualification for standing as a governor, e.g. a person cannot be a governor of a foundation trust if they are bankrupt or have served a prison sentence of three months or more during the last five years.

Other grounds include:

- in the case of an elected governor, they cease to be a member of the constituency they represent
- in the case of an appointed governor, the sponsoring organisation withdraws their sponsorship of them
- they have previously served as a governor of the trust for a total of six years (whether such years were served consecutively or not)
- they have within the preceding two years been dismissed, otherwise than by reason of redundancy or ill health, from any paid employment with a Health Service Body
- their tenure of office as the chairman or as a member or director of a Health Service Body has been terminated on the grounds that their appointment is not in the interest of the health service
- they are a director of the trust, or a governor, executive director, NED, chairman, CEO of another Health Service Body (unless they are appointed by a Partnership Organisation that is a Health Service Body), or a body corporate whose business involves the provision of healthcare services, including for the avoidance of doubt those who have a commercial interest in the affairs of the trust
- they have been a director of the trust in the preceding five years prior to the date of their nomination to stand for election as an elected governor, or in the case of an appointed governor, the date of their appointment
- they have had their name removed from a list maintained under regulations pursuant to sections 91, 106, 123, or 146 of the 2006 Act, or the equivalent lists maintained by Local Health Boards in Wales under the National Health Service (Wales) Act 2006, and they have not subsequently had their name included in such a list
- they are a member of a Local Involvement Network
- they are incapable by reason of mental disorder, illness or injury of managing and administering their property and affairs
- they have refused without reasonable cause to undertake any training that the trust and/or council of governors requires all governors to undertake
- they are a member of a local authority Health Overview and Scrutiny Committee
- they are the subject of a Sex Offenders Order and/or their name is included in the Sex Offenders Register
- they are an immediate family member of a governor or director of the trust
- they have failed to repay (without good cause) any amount of monies properly owed to the trust
- they have failed to sign and deliver to the Secretary a statement in the form required by the trust confirming acceptance of the Governor's Code of Conduct
- they are a person who by reference to information revealed by a Criminal Records Bureau check is considered by the trust to be inappropriate on the grounds that their appointment might adversely affect public confidence in the trust or otherwise bring the trust into disrepute
- they have failed to make, or have falsely made, any declaration as required by the constitution
- they are a person who is a subject of a disqualification order made under the Company Directors' Disqualification Act 1986
- they have received a written warning from the trust for verbal and/or physical abuse towards trust staff
- the relevant Partnership Organisation that they represent ceases to exist.

7 Foundation Trust Network

The Foundation Trust Network (FTN) represents the views and promotes the common interests of NHS foundation trusts and those aspiring to foundation trust status.

The FTN was set up in June 2004 and currently has over 200 NHS organisations in membership – including nearly all of the authorised foundation trusts and most of the NHS trusts, mental health and ambulance trusts and, more recently, community services providers preparing for foundation trust status.

The FTN is led by a board of trustees, who are chairs and chief executives elected by our members. The FTN is an incorporated charity.

In June 2011 the FTN became an independent organisation, having previously been part of the NHS Confederation. Membership of the FTN is open to all FTs and trusts applying to become FTs; members are no longer required to be members of the NHS Confederation.

The FTN has established a track record as the national voice for the foundation trust movement. It has an extensive programme of influencing, networking and learning events for members with a variety of member benefits and opportunities to get involved in their work, including:

- **Influencing policy**: members benefit from a programme of policy work on topics ranging from regulation and finance to legal and insurance issues. This policy work is based on regular member consultations to ensure FT views are effectively represented to key decision makers.
- **Networks**: meetings are held three times a year for chairs and chief executives and mental health members and quarterly meetings for communications leads, HR directors, finance directors, clinical leaders, company secretaries and directors with commercial development responsibilities. Members benefit from sharing learning and emerging good practice and shape the work programme.
- **www.foundationtrustnetwork.org**: members have access to the 'members only' area of this website. Facilities include a range of online discussion forums for members.
- **Newsletters**: the regular e-bulletin, *In Touch*, highlights key issues, developments in the work programme and forthcoming events.
- **Seminars, conferences and dinners**: a major programme of seminars and conferences for members and host dinners for chairs and chief executives to discuss current issues affecting the foundation trust movement with key opinion formers.
- **Providing guidance and sharing information**: guidance and acting as a conduit between members to allow them to share information and good practice.
- **Board training and development**: members have access to practical support for FT boards, including research on effective approaches to board evaluation and appraisal.
- **Publications**: a regular publishing programme to share emerging learning, both within the FT movement and with the wider NHS.

8 The future for foundation trusts

As this chapter has already highlighted, the HSC Act 2012 changes the way foundation trusts are governed and managed significantly, as board members and governors take responsibility for the direction and transactions of their foundation trust. Foundation trusts will still be led by a unitary board, which is responsible for leadership and setting strategy, supervising management and influencing culture; however, the changes are intended to facilitate the board of directors being held to account without Monitor acting as a safety net in the same way.

The key changes to the governance of foundation trusts can be summarised as follows:

The role of governors – this will be expanded so that governors represent more fully the membership of the foundation trust. Governors will have:

- a statutory duty to hold the board of directors to account and specifically, to hold NEDs collectively and individually to account
- a specific duty to represent the interests of members as a whole and the interests of the public
- a role in approving constitutional change
- a role in the approval of mergers, acquisitions and significant transactions (these are to be defined in the constitution)
- a right to call some or all directors to a meeting to answer questions.

The council of governors – these now have to be called 'Councils', and not 'boards' to avoid confusion with boards of directors. The Council will have:

- no ongoing requirement to appoint commissioners as governors
- new powers to appoint governors to ensure the right balance of capacity and capability within the governor body
- a majority of elected public governors.

According to the ICSA in their memorandum to Parliament:

> 'Greater clarification is required to inform governors of their role, and potential liability, in those situations where a foundation trust may be heading towards insolvency. Governors will also need to be aware of the powers they have available to prevent a course of action by directors they believe to be financially threatening to the long term existence of the foundation trust, which does not sit within the definition of a 'significant transaction.'
>
> (HS134 – March 2011)

The role of directors – this will be expanded so that directors will have individual responsibility to promote the success of the foundation trust to maximise the benefits for the members as a whole, and the public. In addition directors will have:

- a role alongside governors in approving constitutional changes
- a duty to equip governors with the skills they need to do their job
- a duty to provide governors with board minutes and agendas
- to move away from the collective responsibility of boards and recognise that each board member will have individual duties
- an express duty to avoid conflicts of interest. Importantly, this is relaxed if the particular type of conflict has been authorised according to the constitution so it will be necessary to make sure that constitutions are written to take advantage of this provision.

In their memorandum to Parliament on the Bill the ICSA welcomed these new duties

> 'as it makes explicit the step change from being a senior manager to being an executive director, and brings the duties of foundation trust directors in line with the private sector.'
>
> (HS134 – March 2011)

The implications of these changes will require additional training and development for governors in their new role and a much more effective working relationship between the board of directors and council of governors. Care will also be required in the definition of 'significant transactions' otherwise foundation trusts will find they regularly have to seek governor approval on more minor or less significant proposals and judgement will have to be exercised where a number of minor transactions could in fact warrant the attention of the council of governors as collectively they represent a 'significant transaction'.

9 The governance challenge

In a memorandum to Parliament in response to the HSC Act 2012 the ICSA have commented as follows:

> 'Regardless of the freedoms proposed in the Bill, foundation trusts still have to operate a governance framework unique within the UK economy and one that presents its own challenges and costs. The additional layer of governance inherent within the dynamic between the council of governors and the board of directors will impact on financial and non-financial resources. The dual nature of the decision-making process on specific areas of business development disadvantages foundation trusts as their governance and accountability framework is more cumbersome operating an almost two-tier board approach.'
>
> (HS134 – March 2011)

The **two-tier** governance structure of NHS Foundation Trusts referred to above does not mean the two-tier board structure common in Germany as outlined in Chapter 7, rather it refers to the oversight of the council of governors alongside the unitary role of the board of directors, which is unusual in British public services. The evidence below demonstrates that the structure has led to confusion and conflict but that there has also been a huge amount of development work in clarifying the role and powers of the board and the council, and how they relate to one another.

9.1 The evidence

In 2005 the Healthcare Commission published *The Healthcare Commission's Review of NHS Foundation Trusts*. It was the most comprehensive review of the early experiences of foundation trusts and stated that:

- few foundation trusts took action to involve traditionally poorly represented groups of the population;
- the roles of governors were unclear beyond their statutory duties; opportunities for training, support and development were variable, as were the perceived legitimacy and influence of the governors
- the dual role of the chair of the board and the governors could cause conflict;
- there was an overlap of functions between the council of governors and public and patient involvement forums, with both seeking to represent the public and patients, which caused confusion;
- there was also overlap with OSCs and concerns about excessive local scrutiny; and
- there was low engagement of staff, as initiatives such as Agenda for Change were considered to have more effect on their working lives.

The FTN also carried out their review of governance in foundation trusts during 2005. Their publication *New Voices New Accountabilities: a guide to wider governance in foundation trusts* was based on case studies from the first wave of foundation trusts, and examined their success in recruiting and involving members and working with their new council of governors. The FTN review set out that there were already clear benefits of the new governance structure and the opportunity for it to deliver further improvements in the longer term.

A further review in March 2008 by Professor Chris Ham (University of Birmingham) and Peter Hunt (Mutuo) was undertaken for the DH to explore the governance in NHS foundation trusts. Remember, the original intention for foundation trusts was to establish public accountability for the healthcare services provided through a membership body and a two board structure. The findings of the review suggested that:

- the hybrid governance model adopted for foundation trusts was working increasingly effectively and that as the model developed, there was greater clarity about the role of the council of governors and how the knowledge and skills of governors can be used to best advantage
- the statutory powers of governors helped to ensure that they were taken seriously and not treated as rubber stamps
- there was less clarity on the role of the membership community and the most effective way of governors relating to members, however, members and governors were making a difference to how foundation trusts carry out their responsibilities
- further thought was required as to whether foundation trusts should be expected to make the same use of patient and public involvement mechanisms as other NHS organisations, or should relate to patients and the public mainly through members and governors.

This is in stark contrast to the findings of Lewis and Hinton (2005) in their review *Citizen and Staff Involvement in Health Service Decision-making: have National Health Service foundation trusts in England given stakeholders a louder voice?*. This review was based on a study at Homerton University Hospital NHS Foundation Trust in 2004/2005 and they found that governors and directors found the new role of foundation trust governor ambiguous and difficult to define. This lack of clarity impeded the development of the new governance function and governors' perception was that they had made little impact on the decisions of the trust during the year of study. They did, however, report evidence of an increased involvement of governors and the public in the activities of the trust.

The most recent review to be completed was the survey of NHS foundation trust governors conducted by Monitor between December 2010 and January 2011. The aims of the survey were to:

- determine to what extent governors thought they were holding foundation trust boards of directors to account, representing local interests and exercising their statutory powers and duties

- compare the results to those obtained from Monitor's 2007 survey of governors, in order to assess what progress has been made
- ask specific questions relating to some anecdotal beliefs about the governor role.

The survey findings demonstrate that there is a greater clarity around the role of the governor and that there are tangible achievements regarding representation of patients and members. Governors were also clearer about the trust's strategy and appropriately representing the views of their stakeholders.

9.2 The issues

There are a number of governance issues that arise for foundation trusts and they particularly highlight the challenges that arise in health service governance, which have been referred to earlier in this text.

Returning to basics again for the moment, remember that health service governance is concerned with the practices and procedures for trying to ensure that the individual parts of the NHS are run in such a way that they achieve their objectives and are in line with public sector values such as VFM and providing universal and free healthcare benefits to all those in need. This provides an interesting contrast to the objectives of a company in the private sector where a company's aim is to maximise the wealth of its owners (the shareholders), subject to various guidelines and constraints and with regard to other groups or individuals with an interest in what the company does.

The resulting key question relates to ownership and therefore who sets the objectives for the organisation, i.e. who owns the NHS organisation and the healthcare services it provides? The governance structure of foundation trusts has attempted to articulate the answer to this question. The foundation trust is accountable to its members and therefore should be governed according to their interests.

The implications of the changes proposed by the HSC Act 2012 drive this perspective forward by further empowering the role of governors, i.e. the representatives of the members. This accentuates the largest health service governance issue for foundation trusts, namely, how to establish an effective relationship between the members and their elected representatives – the governors.

It is not appropriate to liken the members of a foundation trust to the shareholders of a listed company as this does not reflect the complexity and breadth of the diversity of interests that are represented by foundation trust members, although there are limited grounds for viewing the governors as proxy shareholders. In other words, the member is authorising the governor to speak and act for them in respect of the business of the foundation trust. The challenge for foundation trusts has therefore been how to ensure that governors are aware of and informed by the healthcare concerns of their respective constituencies and the members they represent.

The other challenge in this respect relates to the considerable number of other arrangements that already exist to provide patient and public involvement and scrutiny of NHS decision making, such as LINk's and local government overview and scrutiny. How do these work alongside the membership and board of governors?

The mutual sector (explored in Section 9.3 below) has a long and wide experience of membership engagement and ongoing discussions continue to explore how foundation trusts can develop their governance structures to fully achieve the goal of being a membership organisation.

Other governance issues faced by foundation trusts include:

- **Governor capability**: the growing role for governors raises concerns about the training and development programmes available for governors. The increased responsibilities may also reduce or limit the number of people who are willing to fill the role.
- **Accountability**: governors must be accountable to their constituencies. If a governor is not representing the interests of the members who elected him then there must be clear procedures about how such a governor might be removed. The constitution currently sets out grounds for disqualification but these do not include failure to act in the interests of the members.
- **Dual role of the chair**: chairing both the board of directors and the council of governors will expose the chairman to ongoing conflicts of interest. With the increasing power of the council

of governors the chairman's role will be crucial and it will require high levels of interpersonal and listening skills.
- **Role of the company secretary**: a fundamental support for the chairman in this role is the company secretary or foundation trust secretary who will require 'a sophisticated understanding of the political dynamics at play within the governance structure'. Equally, the secretary will be the senior manager to whom the governors and members relate. They will be a useful player in helping to manage the relationships between stakeholders, and act as an early warning for the chair when issues arise.

9.3 Exploring other models

Mutuals

A mutual organisation, or **mutual society** is an organisation (which is often, but not always, a company or business) based on the principle of mutuality. A mutual organisation or society is often simply referred to as a mutual. A mutual exists with the purpose of raising funds from its membership or customers (collectively called its members), which can then be used to provide common services to all members of the organisation or society. A mutual is therefore owned by, and run for the benefit of, its members – it has no external shareholders to pay dividends to, and as such does not usually seek to maximise and make large profits or capital gains. Mutuals exist for the members to benefit from the services they provide. Profits made will usually be re-invested in the mutual for the benefit of the members, although some profit may also be necessary in the case of mutuals for internal financing to sustain or grow the organisation, and to make sure it remains safe and secure.

All mutuals share an important common bond – they are owned by, and run for the benefit of, their current and future members. Members might be consumers, service users, employees or stakeholders from the whole community.

Cliff Mills in *Public Services: made mutual* explains this clearly:

> 'A mutual society was "owned" by its members. The modern western mind generally has a narrow understanding of 'ownership', denoting a right over something which can be sold for money. The ownership of a traditional mutual society was not something which could be sold for money. The members owned their society, in the sense that ultimate constitutional control belonged to them: it was for them to agree any change to the constitution, to what their society was permitted to do (objects) or how it was governed. Nobody else "owned" their society – there was no other group, such as investor shareholders behind the scenes. But they could not sell their membership for money. Indeed the very act of doing so would be a destruction of the mutual covenant between the members, what we have come to call "demutualisation".'

The governance arrangements for mutuals is very different from corporate governance. As Cliff Mills goes on to describe:

> 'Ownership by members resulted in very different governance arrangements from those of traditional business. All members were treated equally, and every member had one vote, in spite of varying amounts of capital contribution and varying amounts of trade. Members elected representatives from among their number to form a board or committee to have responsibility for overseeing the affairs of the society on behalf of its members. Similar in many respects to the board of directors of a company, that board commonly had the power to appoint and employ a manager to run the day to day affairs of the society. Such a manager, who may become the chief officer of a substantial workforce in a successful society, was not a member of the board or committee: lacking any electoral mandate from the members, a manager remained the servant of the elected committee.'

Co-operatives

Co-operatives are a form of mutual organisation, which are fully or majority owned by their members – who may be employees, consumers, others in the community or a mix of these. Co-operatives work on one member, one vote – rather than one share, one vote – and sign up to an agreed set of values and principles and help to shape the decisions the co-operative makes.

Hybrid organisations

Sue Slipman, CEO of the FTN, presented a further model at the FTN's annual governance conference in October 2011. Based on the preliminary work of the Commission of Ownership she set out the possibility of foundation trusts becoming hybrid organisations that combine the best of the commercial sector (efficiency, delivery and 'consumer' focused) with the values of the public sector.

The question of defining the 'Ownership' structure of foundation trusts is challenging as it is not possible to privatise the £28 billion of public assets that foundation trusts are responsible for. Foundation trusts have a complex 'ownership' model with a single unitary board acting as 'the steward' accountable to:

- nationally to regulator and/or in future a PDC investment agency acting as a bank, and
- locally to members with governors as proxy shareholders.

Citing the examples of National Employment Savings Trust and the Probation Service, Sue Slipman set out the main characteristics of hybrid organisations:

- Social purpose that needs the delivery skills more usually associated with private sector.
- Part of wider agenda of social change.
- Not for profit organisations.
- Freed up to innovate and operate entrepreneurially.
- Ensure services available to people markets might not otherwise serve.
- Public assets locked in.

The move to self-regulation for foundation trusts promoted by the HSC Act will require a development of the concept of a hybrid organisation. In conclusion Sue Slipman argued that:

> 'The biggest guarantor of the independence of foundation trusts and their continued freedom to operate will be the development of the role of the governors and the relationships between the board and the governors.'

TEST YOUR KNOWLEDGE 6.4

a What the key changes will be introduced to Foundation Trusts and to Monitor by the HSC Act 2012?

b Why has the governance structure of foundation trusts led to confusion and conflict?

STOP AND THINK 6.1

How might the experiences of other types of organisations such as mutuals, co-operatives and hybrids help address some of the governance issues faced by foundation trusts?

CHAPTER SUMMARY

- NHS foundation trusts were a new type of NHS trust in England set up in 2006 and were part of the government's plan for creating a patient-led NHS.
- Although run locally, NHS Foundation Trusts remain fully part of the NHS. They have been set up in law as legally independent organisations called Public Benefit Corporations.
- Foundation trusts have significantly greater freedoms over the way they conduct their finances and are able to build up operational surpluses, retain proceeds from asset sales, raise capital in the public and/or private sectors and manage their organisations and their resources free from central government control.

- The functions of each foundation trust, according to the relevant provisions of the National Health Service Act 2006, are set out in its terms of authorisation as granted by Monitor.
- Foundation trusts are accountable to their local communities, their commissioners, Parliament, the CQC and Monitor.
- Monitor was established in January 2004 to authorise and regulate NHS foundation trusts and is independent of central government and directly accountable to Parliament.
- Monitor have also recommended that the council of governors appoint a Lead Governor who would lead the council of governors where it is not considered appropriate for the chair or another one of the NEDs to do so.
- The statutory duties of foundation trust governors are set out in The National Health Service Act 2006 and expanded further in the Monitor guidance: *Your Statutory Duties: a reference guide for NHS foundation trust governors*.
- Every authorised foundation trust will have a constitution that has been approved by Monitor, which will set out the governance arrangements for the foundation trust.
- The basic governance structure of all NHS foundation trusts includes the membership, the board of governors and the board of directors.
- The council of governors should hold the board of directors to account for the performance of the trust, including ensuring the board of directors acts so that the foundation trust does not breach the terms of its authorisation.
- The eligibility for membership of a foundation trust is open to local residents, patients and carers and staff employed by the trust, in the terms provided in each Trust's constitution.
- The model constitution sets out that a foundation trust membership will consist of two main constituencies, namely staff and public members. In addition a third may be included to represent patient members.
- The maximum term for all members of the council of governors is six years under the *FT Code of Governance*.
- Foundation trusts are required to include the DH's model election rules as part of their constitution.
- The HSC Act 2012 brings significant changes to the way foundation trusts are governed and managed and will require major changes as board members and governors take responsibility for the direction and transactions of their foundation trust.
- Other governance issues faced by foundation trusts include governor capability, accountability, the dual role of the chair and the importance of the role of the company secretary.
- The experiences of other types of organisations such as mutuals, co-operatives and hybrids may help to address some of the governance issues faced by foundation trusts.

CASE QUESTION 2.1

Review again the case study outlined at the beginning of Part Two. Having read the content of Part Two, how would you advise Helen Wrightford as company secretary on the governance best practice issues that have been identified from the board evaluation process?

PART **THREE**

Health service governance in practice

■ LIST OF CHAPTERS

7 The board of directors
8 Governance and boardroom practice
9 Remuneration issues
10 Reporting and the role of audit

■ OVERVIEW

The third part of this study text looks at the practical application of principles and provisions of best practice in health service governance.

Chapter 7 starts from the premise that an efficient and effective board is a key requirement of good governance. The board should have a clear idea of its responsibilities, and should fulfil these to the best of its abilities. There should be a suitable balance of skills and experience, and also power, on the board. This chapter considers the role and composition of a board and the duties and responsibilities of directors and committees. By the end of the chapter, you should have an understanding of what is needed to achieve an effective board, and how a weak board structure is a threat to good governance.

Chapter 8 deals with a variety of governance issues relating to the board of directors. The chapter explores the characteristics of effective boards and how the actual practice of boards compares with these characteristics. The effectiveness of a board is often damaged by poor boardroom behaviours, and the chapter sets out the guidelines on boardroom behaviours that are available. There are also important governance issues relating to the identification and appointment of new directors, and the induction and continuing professional development of board directors. Board evaluation is also a crucial part of developing appropriate boardroom practice.

Chapter 9 looks at the role of the remuneration committee, the problems with negotiating a satisfactory remuneration package for senior executives, and what the elements of that package should be. It explains why the remuneration of directors and senior executives has been a major corporate governance issue and the impact of these issues on NHS senior manager pay.

Chapter 10 considers the role of audit in ensuring accurate reporting for good health service governance. The key principles for health service governance of openness and transparency must therefore be underpinned by accurate and timely reporting. It examines the range of reporting requirements that are imposed on NHS organisations, as unlike in corporate governance where the annual report and accounts is seen as the most important communication between a company and its shareholders, this is not the case for health service governance. While significant, the annual report and accounts is not the sole means of communication for NHS organisations and there is a wide variety of reporting requirements, which are primarily to the regulators but which provide information to NHS stakeholders.

■ LEARNING OUTCOMES

Part Three should enable you to:

- advise on the structure and composition of the board to maximise effectiveness and meet regulatory requirements
- understand, interpret and apply the principles of the *FT Code of Governance* in relation to boardroom practice and behaviour and how the principles apply across the NHS
- identify key board behaviours that lead to effective boards
- understand the role and responsibilities of the key board committees
- identify the role of the remuneration committee in respect of NHS senior managers' remuneration
- understand the principles of Fair Pay and the need for control of severance payments in cases of poor performance
- explain the combined role of internal and external audit in NHS reporting to stakeholders
- identify the range of reporting requirements that NHS organisations are subject to
- identify the key mechanisms for communications with stakeholders.

PART 3 CASE STUDY

Internal audit has identified that Miranda Tabnorth's husband is a self-employed consultant who has been advising the trust on their Organisational Development strategy. The original contract for the services that he supplied was approved by Miranda and a competitive quote process was not utilised. While he was acting as their consultant he was also working for a training company who were tendering for the delivery of the trust's mandatory training package.

After three months of providing consultancy services to the HR team, the board is asked to approve his appointment as Director of HR and OD. This is not a board level appointment and the NEDs have not been involved in his appointment. The appointment process had been conducted by the Director of Finance and the Medical Director. As Director of HR and OD he will be reporting directly to Miranda, his wife.

The board of directors

CONTENTS

1. Governance responsibilities of the board
2. Board structures
3. The powers of directors
4. The duties of directors to their organisation
5. The statutory duties of directors
6. Liability of directors
7. NHS Code of Conduct and Accountability
8. Matters reserved for the board
9. The roles of chairman and chief executive officer (CEO)
10. Size and composition of the board
11. Non-executive directors (NEDs)
12. Senior independent directors (SIDs)
13. Board committees and non-executive directors (NEDs)
14. Effectiveness of non-executive directors (NEDs)

INTRODUCTION

An efficient and effective board is a key requirement of good governance. The board should have a clear idea of its responsibilities, and should fulfil these to the best of its abilities. There should be a suitable balance of skills and experience, and also power, on the board.

This chapter considers the role and composition of a board and the duties and responsibilities of directors and committees. By the end of the chapter, you should have an understanding of what is needed to achieve an effective board, and how a weak board structure is a threat to good governance.

This chapter (and the following chapter) will make a number of references to principles and provisions of the *UK Corporate Governance Code*. There will also be references to the FRC *Guidance on Board Effectiveness*, published in 2011, which broadly replaces the previous Higgs Guidance. The purpose of this guidance is to help the board of directors with implementing Sections A and B of the *UK Corporate Governance Code*. Specific references will also be made, where appropriate, to the voluntary codes for health service governance set out in Chapter 5, such as the *FT Code of Governance* and the *NHS Code of Conduct and Accountability*.

1 Governance responsibilities of the board

1.1 Responsibilities under the *UK Code*

The board of directors is the key decision-making body in an organisation. An organisation should have an effective board of directors dedicated to ensuring that the organisation achieves its objectives. The *UK Corporate Governance Code* states as one of its main principles:

> 'Every company should be headed by an effective board, which is collectively responsible for the long-term success of the organisation.'

The 2010 Code introduced the phrase 'long term' into this principle. This recognises that the board should not focus on short-term achievements, if these are inconsistent with longer-term success.

The *UK Code* also states that the role of the board should be to:

- provide entrepreneurial leadership for the company within a framework of prudent and effective risk management
- set the company's strategic aims
- make sure that the necessary financial and human resources are in place for the company to meet its objectives
- review management performance
- set the company's values and standards
- make sure that the company's obligations to its shareholders are understood and met.

The FRC *Guidance on Board Effectiveness* states that an effective board is one that:

- provides direction for management
- demonstrates ethical leadership, displaying and promoting throughout the company behaviours consistent with the culture and values it has defined for the organisation
- creates a performance culture that drives value creation without exposing the company to excessive risk of value destruction
- makes well informed and high quality decisions based on a clear line of sight into the business
- creates the right framework for helping directors meet their statutory duties under the Companies Act 2006, and/or other relevant statutory and regulatory regimes
- is accountable, particularly to those that provide the company's capital
- thinks carefully about its governance arrangements and embraces evaluation of their effectiveness.

The guidance adds that a board that demonstrates that it has suitable governance policies and systems in place is much more likely to generate trust and support among its shareholders and other stakeholders.

Except for its monitoring role, the board should not get involved with operational matters, for which the responsibility is delegated to executive management. The code also states that all directors must act in what they consider to be the best interests of the company, without specifying what those 'best interests' are or might be. *King III* identifies other responsibilities for the board, including responsibility for:

- ethical conduct and sustainability of the business
- compliance with laws, regulations and codes
- governing the relationships between the company and its stakeholders.

1.2 NHS trust boards

According to the DH, a NHS trust board has six key functions, for which it is held accountable by the Department on behalf of the Secretary of State. These are:

- to set the strategic direction of the organisation within the overall policies and priorities of the government and the NHS, define its annual and longer term objectives and agree plans to achieve them
- to oversee the delivery of planned results by monitoring performance against objectives and ensuring corrective action is taken when necessary
- to ensure effective financial stewardship through value for money, financial control and financial planning and strategy
- to ensure that high standards of health service governance and personal behaviour are maintained in the conduct of the business of the whole organisation
- to appoint, appraise and remunerate senior executives, and
- to ensure that there is effective dialogue between the organisation and the local community on its plans and performance and that these are responsive to the community's needs.

The *Healthy NHS Board* states that 'in unitary NHS boards, all directors are collectively and corporately accountable for organisational performance. A key strength of unitary boards is the opportunity provided for the exchange of views between executives and non-executives, drawing on and pooling their experiences and capabilities'.

The *FT Code of Governance* states that 'NHS foundation trust directors are ultimately and collectively responsible as a board for all aspects of the performance of the foundation trust. Therefore, they need to be able to deliver more focused strategic leadership and more effective scrutiny of the trust's operations.'

1.3 Decision-making

Decision-making is an important board activity. The board should have clear policies about what matters need a board decision or approval, and the processes required for each type of decision. Good decision-making can be improved by giving directors sufficient time to prepare for meetings, allowing sufficient time for issues to be discussed at board meetings, and making clear to executives what action they must take to implement board decisions.

The FRC Guidance recognises that even with suitable policies and procedures, the quality of decision-making by the board can be impaired by:

- a dominant personality or group of directors on the board, which can inhibit contribution from other directors
- insufficient attention to risk, and treating risk as a compliance issue rather than as part of the decision-making process
- failure to recognise the value implications of running the business on the basis of self interest and other poor ethical standards
- a reluctance to involve NEDs, or of matters being brought to the board for sign-off rather than debate
- complacent or intransigent attitudes
- a weak organisational culture
- inadequate information or analysis.

The guidance suggests that boards may wish to consider extra measures to reduce the risk of flawed decisions, such as:

- describing in board papers the process that has been used to arrive at and challenge the proposal prior to presenting it to the board, thereby allowing directors not involved in the project to assess the appropriateness of the process as a precursor to assessing the merits of the project itself; or
- where appropriate, putting in place additional safeguards to reduce the risk of distorted judgements by, for example, commissioning an independent report, seeking advice from an expert, introducing a devil's advocate to provide challenge, establishing a sole purpose sub-committee, or convening additional meetings. Some chairmen favour separate discussions for important decisions; for example, concept, proposal for discussion, proposal for decision. This gives executive directors more opportunity to put the case at the earlier stages, and all directors the opportunity to share concerns or challenge assumptions well in advance of the point of decision.

TEST YOUR KNOWLEDGE 7.1

a According to the *UK Code of Corporate Governance*, what are the governance responsibilities of a board of directors?
b How does the DH define the responsibilities of the board?
c According to the FRC *Guidance on Board Effectiveness*, what are the characteristics of an effective board?

2 Board structures

2.1 Unitary boards

Organisations in most countries have **unitary boards**, consisting of both executive and non-executive (NEDs) directors under the leadership of the chairman. A unitary board makes collective decisions and is accountable to the shareholders or major stakeholders. It is commonly accepted governance practice that the NEDs in a listed organisation should be independent, although this is not a legal requirement. In the NHS, the concept of a unitary board has not always been well understood or implemented. The dangers of not being a unitary board were reinforced by the *Integrated Governance Handbook* in 2006:

> 'To date, NHS Boards have performed in a diverse manner by separating out the roles of the various directors, i.e. finance, medical, nursing etc, and the non-executive director/lay individual input. The result of this is that, if the Board takes a decision, it is often deemed to be the decision of, say, the finance director or HR director, rather than being a corporate decision. Board corporacy is paramount. Each decision or agreement entered into in the boardroom is a fully accepted corporate decision. If a decision around finance is taken and the information brought to the Board clarifies the debate, if there are implications say, one month after the decision, the responsibility is of the corporate whole, rather than just the finance director.'

The concept of the unitary board is emphasised within the governance structure of the NHS foundation trust. While there may appear to be a two board structure with a Council of Governors and a Board of Directors, the Model Constitution and *FT Code of Governance* make it clear that the concept of the unitary board refers to the fact that within the board of directors the NEDs and the executive directors share the same liability. All directors, executive and non-executive, have responsibility to constructively challenge the decisions of the board and help develop proposals on priorities, risk mitigation, values, standards and strategy.

The *FT Code* is clear that 'every NHS foundation trust should be headed by an effective board of directors, since the board is collectively responsible for the exercise of the powers and the performance of the NHS foundation trust' (Principle A.1). To deliver this collective responsibility, the board of directors should meet sufficiently regularly to discharge its duties effectively and have a formal schedule of matters specifically reserved for decision by the board of directors. This should be complemented with a clear statement detailing the roles and responsibilities of the Council of Governors. These are set out in detail in Chapter 6.

There should also be a statement explaining how any disagreements between the Council of Governors and the Board of Directors will be resolved. The annual report should include a statement of how the board of directors and the council of governors operate, including a high-level statement of which types of decisions are to be taken by each of the boards and which decisions are to be delegated to the executive management by the board of directors.

The concept of a unitary board is now common practice within the NHS and continues to be the subject of a considerable amount of board development.

2.2 Two-tier boards

Some countries, including Germany and Austria, have **two-tier boards**. With a two-tier structure, there is a **supervisory board** and a **management board**.

The management board is responsible for managing the organisation. It is led by the chairman of the managing board, who is the CEO; its members are appointed by the supervisory board. It develops strategy for the organisation, in cooperation with the supervisory board, and is responsible for implementing the agreed strategy. It also has responsibility for risk management and for the preparation of the annual financial statements (which are examined by the auditors and the supervisory board.

The supervisory board is responsible for general oversight of the organisation and of the management board. Its members are elected by the shareholders, except that in public companies with more than 500 employees, a minimum proportion of the supervisory board must consist of representatives of the employees. The supervisory board is led by the chairman. It advises the management board and must be involved in decision-making on all fundamental matters affecting the organisation; these include 'decisions or measures which fundamentally change the asset, financial or earnings situations of the enterprise' (German *Corporate Governance Code*). The audit committee consists entirely of supervisory board members.

In a two-tier structure, there has to be a functional relationship between the management board and the supervisory board, and the chairman of the supervisory board plays a key role. He is responsible for making sure that the two boards work well together, and the most powerful individuals in the organisation are the chairman of the supervisory board and the CEO who is in charge of the management board. The CEO reports to the supervisory board chairman. If the relationship between these two works well, the chairman will effectively speak for the management at meetings of the supervisory board.

The management board consists entirely of executive directors. The supervisory board consists entirely of NEDs. In Germany, supervisory board members include:

- representatives of trade unions and/or the organisation's employees
- representatives of major shareholders
- former executives of the organisation.

The supervisory board NEDs are therefore not necessarily independent, particularly employee representatives. It can therefore be difficult to reconcile the differing views of employee representatives and representatives of major shareholders, without antagonising the executives on the management board. On the other hand, where there is a large number of former executives on the supervisory board, there is a risk that the supervisory board could take a lenient and easy-going view of what management are doing. In addition, some independent supervisory board directors might well be senior managers of other companies, where they are management board members. These individuals might therefore sympathise with the views of the management board.

The success of corporate governance depends on a good working relationship between the supervisory board and the management board, and in particular a good working relationship between the organisation chairman and the head of the management board. The German code states that 'the Management Board and Supervisory Board co-operate closely to the benefit of the enterprise' and the management board should discuss the implementation of strategy regularly with the supervisory board.

2.3 Criticisms of the two-tier board structure

The main concerns are as follows:

- Supervisory boards are too big, having up to 20 members. German supervisory boards include a large number of employee representatives, and large numbers can result in inefficient meetings.
- It has been common to appoint retired former managers of the organisation to the supervisory board, and these individuals might be tempted to retain some influence over the actions and operational decisions of their successors. This is not the purpose of a supervisory board. On the other hand, if former managers are appointed to the supervisory board, the supervisory board will benefit from their knowledge and experience of the business. In Germany former managers are now prohibited from 'moving upstairs' to the supervisory board for at least two years, unless the move receives the support of at least 25% of shareholders, because it is thought that for the first two years after retiring, a former executive will not be sufficiently independent.
- Companies with more than 500 employees are required to have workers' representatives or trade union representatives on the supervisory board. (Companies with more than 2,000 employees are required to have an even greater percentage of employee representatives on the supervisory board.) This requirement is an enforcement of the principle of 'co-determination', embodied in German law, that the workers as well as the management and owners should determine the future of their companies. Unfortunately, workers' representatives often lack the competence to consider strategic issues or are not independent

from the organisation. In some instances, worker members of a supervisory board opposing planned initiatives by the organisation have been accused of leaking confidential information to the press.
- Concerns about information leaks can damage communications between supervisory and management boards.

The German *Corporate Governance Code* suggests that in practice, the unitary board system and two-tier board system are becoming much more similar 'because of the intensive interaction between the Management Board and the Supervisory Board'. The German Code also suggests that the two types of board structure are 'equally successful'.

Developments in some German companies in recent years also suggest that the supervisory boards of large German companies are becoming more responsive to the interests of their shareholders.

CASE EXAMPLE 7.1

There was a bribery scandal at German engineering group Siemens in 2005, with allegations that senior managers had paid €1.3 billion in bribes worldwide to secure contracts. The supervisory board took legal action against the managers concerned, including the former CEO and chairman of the organisation. Its members believed that they had no choice other than to take legal action to obtain compensation, since shareholders would otherwise sue them. In December 2009 it was announced that settlements had been reached with nine former Siemens executives, who each agreed to pay compensation to the organisation.

The **Walker Report** in the UK (2009) on corporate governance in banks considered whether unitary boards contributed to the scale of the financial crisis in 2007–2009, and whether a two-tier board structure might be more suitable for large banks. Its conclusions were fairly critical of the two-tier structure:

'In practice, two-tier structures do not appear to assure members of the supervisory board of access to the quality and timeliness of management information flow that would generally be regarded as essential for non-executives on a unitary board. Moreover, since, in a two-tier structure, members of the supervisory and executive boards meet separately and do not share the same responsibilities, the two-tier model would not provide opportunity for the interactive exchange of views between executives and NEDs, drawing on and pooling their respective experience and capabilities in the way that takes place in a well-functioning unitary board.'

TEST YOUR KNOWLEDGE 7.2

a What is a unitary board? What are the benefits of a unitary board?
b What are the respective roles of a management board and a supervisory board in a two-tier board structure in Germany?
c What are the criticisms of a two-tier board structure?

3 The powers of directors

3.1 The general powers of directors – private sector

The powers of the board of directors are set out in an organisation's constitution. In UK companies, formed under the UK Companies Acts, this means the articles of association. UK company legislation provides a standard form of articles of association (known as **model**

articles of association). For companies formed under the Companies Act 1985 this means the 1985 Table A articles, which most companies have used as a model for their own articles. The Companies Act 2006 revised the model articles and introduced different model articles for public and private companies for new companies formed on or after October 2009. The powers of directors are broadly comparable, however, in all the model articles.

Article 3 of the new model articles for public companies states: 'Subject to the articles, the directors are responsible for the management of the company's business, for which purpose they may exercise all the powers of the company.' The shareholders may instruct the directors what they should do (or should not do) but only by passing a special resolution in general meeting, and a special resolution of the shareholders cannot invalidate what the directors have already done.

Article 5 of the new model articles for public companies allows the directors to delegate any of the powers conferred on them under the articles to any person (e.g. the CEO) or committee (e.g. to an audit committee), as they think fit. Standard articles of association in the UK, therefore, provide for the board collectively to be the main power centre in the organisation, but with delegation of powers to **board committees** and executive directors.

A distinction should be made between the powers and duties of executive directors as members of the board, and their responsibilities as managers of the organisation. Under the articles of association, managers have neither powers nor duties. The relationship they have with the organisation (including their authority and responsibilities) is established by their contract of employment and by the law of agency.

In health service governance the powers of the board of directors are set out in their governing document, e.g. foundation trusts have a written constitution, which has to be approved by Monitor. This is then further defined by the Schedule of Matters Reserved for the Board, the Scheme of Delegation, Standing Orders and Standing Financial Instructions, which will be covered in more detail later in this chapter.

4 The duties of directors to their organisation

The directors act as agents of their organisation. They have certain duties, which are to the organisation itself, but not to its shareholders, its employees or any person external to the organisation, such as the general public. Although an organisation is a legal person in law, it is not human. Since the relationship between directors and the organisation is by its very nature impersonal, it might be wondered just what 'duty' means.

The concept of duty is not easy to understand, and it is helpful to make a comparison with the duties owed by other individuals or groups.

Examples of individuals owing a duty to something inanimate are not common, although personnel in the armed forces have a duty to their country. It is more usual to show loyalty to something inanimate than to have a duty. For example, individuals might be expected to show loyalty to their country, and they might voluntarily show loyalty to their sports team or group of friends or work colleagues. Arguably, solicitors have a duty to their profession to act ethically, although the solicitors' practice rules in the UK specify that solicitors owe a duty of care to their clients. Similarly, doctors have a duty to act ethically, but their duty is to their patients. Duty is normally owed to individuals or a group of people. It might therefore be supposed that directors should owe a duty to their shareholders and possibly to the organisation's employees, but this is not the case.

- Accountability and responsibility should not be confused with duty.
- Directors have a responsibility to use their powers in ways that seem best for the organisation and its shareholders or major stakeholders.
- They should be accountable to the owners of the organisation, for the ways in which they have exercised their powers and/or the performance of the organisation.
- They have duties to the organisation.

If a person is guilty of a breach of duty, there should be a process for calling him to account. There might be an established disciplinary procedure, for example, in a court or before a judicial panel, with a recognised set of punishments for misbehaviour.

4.1 Common law duties and statutory duties of directors

Until the Companies Act 2006, the main legal duties of directors to their organisation were duties in common law – a **fiduciary duty** and **duty of skill and care** to the organisation. The Companies Act 2006 has now written the common law duties of directors into statute law. It states that these general duties 'are based on certain common law rules and equitable principles as they apply to directors, and have effect in place of those rules and principles as regards the duties owed to an organisation by a director' (Companies Act 2006, section 170). The Act goes on to state that the statutory general duties should be interpreted in the same way as the common law rules and equitable principles.

As far as the legislation is concerned, a 'company' means a company formed and registered under the companies legislation, and, therefore, NHS organisations that are not registered companies but organisations created by statutory instrument are not bound by this legislation. Good practice, however, would require an understanding of the general principles of the companies legislation and the nature of the original common law duties.

4.2 Fiduciary duty of directors

'Fiduciary' means given in trust, and the concept of a trustee (as established in US and UK law) is applicable. The directors hold a position of trust because they make contracts on behalf of the organisation and also control the organisation's property. Since this is similar being a trustee of the organisation, a director has a fiduciary duty to the organisation (not its shareholders).

If a director were to act in breach of his fiduciary duty, legal action could be brought against him by the organisation. In such a situation, 'the organisation' might be represented by a majority of the board of directors, or a majority of the shareholders, or a single controlling shareholder.

A director would be in breach of his fiduciary duty in carrying out a particular transaction or series of transactions in any of the following circumstances:

- The transaction is not in any way incidental to the business of the organisation. For example, the CEO of a building construction organisation might decide to trade in diamonds and lose large amounts of money in these diamond trading transactions.
- The transaction is not carried out **bona fide**, which means in good faith, with honesty and sincerity.
- The transaction has not been made for the benefit of the organisation but for the personal benefit of the director or an associate. A director has a fiduciary duty to avoid a conflict of interest between him or herself personally and the organisation, and must not obtain any personal benefit or profit from a transaction without the consent of the organisation. In other words, it would be a breach of fiduciary duty for a director to make a **secret profit** from a transaction by the organisation in which he has a personal interest.

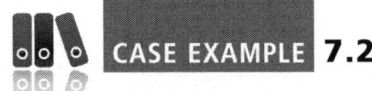 **CASE EXAMPLE 7.2**

An organisation wishes to buy some land and has identified a property for which it would be prepared to pay a large sum of money. The CEO secretly sets up a private organisation of his own to buy the property, and then sells this on to the organisation of which he is CEO, making a large profit in the process. The actions of the CEO are breach of fiduciary duty, because his actions have not been bona fide and he has made a secret profit at the expense of the organisation. Under the Companies Act 2006 these actions of the CEO would now be a breach of statutory duty.

4.3 A director's duty of skill and care

Directors are also subject to a duty of skill and care to the organisation. This was a common law duty that became a statutory duty with the Companies Act 2006. A director should not act negligently in carrying out his duties, and could be personally liable for losses suffered by the organisation as a consequence of such negligence.

The standard of skill and care expected of a director is the higher of the skill that he has or the skill that would objectively be expected of a director of the particular organisation. In the case *Re D'Jan of London [1993] Case law 7.2*, the judge ruled that the common law duty of care was the equivalent to the statutory test applied by section 214 of the Insolvency Act 1986. This statutory test refers to what would be expected of 'a reasonably diligent person having both:

- the general knowledge, skill and experience that may reasonably be expected of a person carrying out the same functions as are carried out by that director in relation to the organisation
- the general knowledge, skill and experience that that director has.

A director is expected to show the technical skills that would reasonably be expected from someone of his experience and expertise. If the finance director of a scientific research organisation is a qualified accountant, he would not be expected to possess the technical skills of a scientist, but would be expected to possess some technical skill as an accountant.

However, the duty of skill and care does not extend to spending time in the organisation. A director should attend board meetings if possible, but at other times is not required to be concerned with the affairs of the organisation. This requirement is perhaps best understood with NEDs, who might visit the organisation only for board or committee meetings. The duties of a director are intermittent in nature and arise from time to time only, such as when the board meets. If a director holds an executive position in the organisation, a different situation arises, because he is an employee of the organisation with a contract of service. This contract might call for full-time attendance at the organisation or on its business. However, this requirement arises out of his job as a manager, not out of his position as a director.

It is also not a part of the duty of skill and care to watch closely over the activities of the organisation's management. Unless there are particular grounds for suspecting dishonesty or incompetence, a director is entitled to leave the routine conduct of the organisation's affairs to the management. If the management appears honest, the directors may rely on the information they provide. It is not part of their duty of skill and care to question whether the information is reliable, or whether important information is being withheld.

A board of directors might make a decision that appears ill-judged or careless. However, the courts in the UK are generally reluctant to condemn business decisions made by the board that appear, in hindsight, to show errors of judgement. Directors can exercise reasonable skill and care, but still make bad decisions.

For a legal action against a director to succeed, an organisation would have to prove that serious negligence had occurred. It would not be enough to demonstrate that some loss could have been avoided if the director had been a bit more careful.

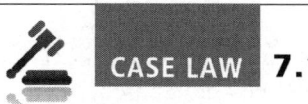

CASE LAW 7.1

Dorchester Finance Co. Ltd v Stebbing [1989]

In the UK legal case *Dorchester Finance Co. Ltd v Stebbing [1989]*, a company brought an action against its three directors for alleged negligence and misappropriation of the company's property. The company (Dorchester Finance) was in the money-lending business and it had three directors, S, H and P. Only S was involved full-time with the company; H and P were non-executives who made only rare appearances. There were no board meetings. S and P were qualified accountants and H, although not an accountant, had considerable accountancy experience. S arranged for the company to make some loans to persons with whom he appears to have had dealings. In the loan-making process he had persuaded P and H to sign blank cheques that were subsequently used to make the loans. The loans did not comply with the Moneylenders Acts and they were inadequately secured. When the loans turned out to be irrecoverable, the company brought its action against the directors.

It was held that all three directors were liable to damages. S, as an executive director, was held to be grossly negligent. P and H, as non-executives, were held to have failed to show the necessary level of skill and care in performing their duties as non-executives, even though it was accepted that they had acted in good faith at all times.

4.4 Wrongful trading and the standard of duty and care

The standard of duty and care required from a director has been partly defined in a number of UK legal cases relating to **wrongful trading**. Under the Insolvency Act 1986, directors may be liable for wrongful trading by the organisation, when they allowed the organisation to continue trading, but knew (or should have known) that it would be unable to avoid an insolvent liquidation. When such a situation arises and an organisation goes into liquidation, the liquidator can apply to the court for the director to be held personally liable for negligence. The duty of a director under the Insolvency Act was used in the case of Re D'Jan of London [1993] to illustrate a director's general duty of skill and care.

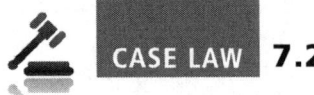

CASE LAW 7.2

Re D'Jan of London [1993]

An insurance broker completed a fire insurance proposal form with an incorrect answer, but a director of the company (Re D'Jan) applying for the insurance policy signed the form. The company premises burned down, and the insurance company, on discovering the mistake on the proposal form, repudiated all liability under the policy. The company went into insolvent liquidation. The liquidator brought an action against the director who had signed the proposal form, alleging a failure to exercise reasonable care to the company. The court found that although it would be unreasonable to expect a director to read every word of every document that he signed, in this case the form consisted of a few simple questions that the director was the best person to answer. The director was therefore guilty of a breach of duty of care, although, in this particular case, the director was exonerated on other grounds.

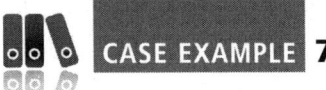

CASE EXAMPLE 7.3

Andrew Tuckey, former deputy chairman of Barings bank, was responsible for the supervision of Nick Leeson, the derivatives trader whose unauthorised speculative trading notoriously brought the bank to collapse in 1995. In a case concerning the disqualification of Tuckey as a director, it was alleged that he had failed to exercise his duty of care to the company. The situation was summarised as follows by the judge in the case, Mr Justice Parker:

- Directors, both individually and collectively, have a duty to acquire and maintain sufficient understanding of the organisation's business to enable them to discharge their duties properly.
- Subject to the articles of association, directors are allowed to delegate particular functions to individuals beneath them in the management chain. Within reason, they are also entitled to have trust in the competence and integrity of these individuals. However, delegation of authority does not remove from the director a duty to supervise the exercise of that delegated authority by the subordinate.
- There is no universal rule for establishing whether a director is in breach of his duty to supervise the discharge of delegated functions by subordinates. The extent of the duty, and whether it has been properly discharged, should be decided on the facts of each case.

When there is a question about the extent of the director's duties and responsibilities, a significant factor could be the level of reward that the director was entitled to receive from the company. Prima facie, the higher the rewards, the greater the responsibilities should be expected.

In the Barings case, Mr Justice Parker concluded that Tuckey had failed in his duties because he did not have a sufficient knowledge and understanding of the nature of the derivatives markets and the risks involved in derivatives dealing (which led to the collapse of Barings). He was therefore unable to consider properly matters referred to the committee of which he was chairman.

4.5 Duties of directors and delegation

Since directors owe a duty of skill and care to their organisation, it could be asked how much time and attention a director should give to the organisation's affairs, and to what extent a director can delegate responsibilities to another person without being in breach of his duty.

TEST YOUR KNOWLEDGE 7.3

a Why are the common law duties relevant for NHS organisations?
b What is the fiduciary duty of a director?

5 The statutory duties of directors

Although NHS organisations are not registered companies but organisations created by statutory instrument, they are not bound by the Companies Act 2006. Good practice, however, would require an understanding of the general principles of the Act, which are set out here.

The duties of directors in common law and equity to their organisation were introduced into UK statute law by the Companies Act 2006 (sections 171–177). These consist of a duty to:

- act within powers
- promote the success of the organisation
- exercise independent judgement
- exercise reasonable care, skill and diligence
- avoid conflicts of interest
- not to accept benefits from third parties
- declare any interest in a proposed transaction or arrangement.

5.1 Duty to act within powers

A director must act within his powers in accordance with the organisation's constitution, and should only exercise these powers for the purpose for which they were granted. If a director acts outside his powers to make a contractual agreement with a third party, the organisation is still liable for any obligation to the third party, provided that the third party has acted in good faith.

Directors should also ensure that they comply with the organisation's constitution. For example, when a group of directors meets, it must be clear whether the meeting is a full board meeting, a meeting of a board committee or an unofficial meeting of directors. Unless the meeting is a formal board meeting, the directors would be acting outside their powers if they took a decision on a matter that is reserved for decision-making by the board.

5.2 Duty to promote the success of the organisation

A director, in good faith, must act in the way he considers would be most likely to 'promote the success of the organisation for the benefit of its members as a whole'. The Act does not define 'success', but the term is likely to be interpreted as meaning 'increasing value for shareholders'. However, in doing so, a director must also have regard, among other matters, to the:

- likely long-term consequences of any decision
- interests of the organisation's employees
- need to foster the organisation's relationships with its customers, suppliers and others
- impact of the organisation's operations on the community and the environment
- desirability of the organisation maintaining its reputation for high standards of business conduct
- need to act fairly as between members of the organisation.

The Act does not create a duty of directors to any stakeholders other than the shareholders (members), but it requires directors to consider the interests of other stakeholders in reaching their decisions. The Act specifically mentions employees, customers, suppliers and the community. It therefore appears, in a small way perhaps, to promote a form of enlightened shareholder approach to corporate governance.

5.3 Duty to exercise independent judgement

A director must exercise independent judgement. However, this requirement does not prevent a director from acting in a way authorised by the organisation's constitution (e.g. accepting resolutions passed by the shareholders in general meeting) or from acting in accordance with an agreement already entered into by the organisation that prevents the director from using discretion. The requirement for independent judgement does not prevent a director from taking advice and acting on it.

The ICSA *Guidance on Directors' General Duties* comments as follows on this duty:

- A director must not allow personal interests to affect his independent judgement. This means that if the board is considering a contract in which a director has a personal interest ideally he should leave the meeting while the matter is being discussed. (This is also relevant to the duty of directors to avoid any conflict of interest with the organisation.)
- An executive director should not attend a board meeting to 'promote a collective executive line'. He should attend the board meeting in his own right and give the board the benefit of his independent opinion.
- Similarly directors representing a particular interest should 'set any representative function aside and make final decisions on their own merits'. For example, a director who is a representative of a family interest in the organisation 'may consult his family but be clear that he will make the final decision'.

5.4 Duty to exercise reasonable care, skill and diligence

This is similar to the common law duty of care.

5.5 Duty to avoid conflicts of interest

A director has a duty to avoid conflicts of interest with the interests of the organisation. However, this duty is not breached if the director declares to the board his interest in a transaction and the interest is authorised/approved by the board.

In the commercial world, it is inevitable that many directors will have a potential conflict of interest, whether direct or indirect, with their organisation. For example, an organisation might be planning to trade with another organisation in which one of its directors is a shareholder. In such a situation, the director concerned is required to declare his interest in the proposed contract and must not make a secret profit.

A director or a **connected person** might have a material interest in a transaction undertaken by the organisation. For example, the organisation might award a contract to a firm of building contractors to rebuild or develop a property owned by the organisation, and the director or his/her spouse might own the building organisation.

A director might also have a direct or indirect interest in a contract (or proposed contract) with the organisation. For example, the director might be a member of another organisation with which the organisation is planning to sign a business contract. Such a contract is not illegal, although the organisation can choose to rescind it should it wish to do so.

If a director has an interest in a contract with the organisation and has failed to disclose it, and has received a payment under the contract, he will be regarded as holding the money in the capacity of constructive trustee for the organisation (and so is bound to repay the money).

The 2006 Act recognises three situations in which an actual or potential conflict of interests may arise:

- A conflict of interest may arise in a situation where the organisation is not a party to an arrangement or transaction, but where the director might be able to gain personally from 'the

exploitation of any property, information or opportunity'. For example, a director might pursue an opportunity for his personal benefit that the organisation might have pursued itself.
- A conflict of interest may arise about a proposed transaction or arrangement to which the organisation will be a party. If a director has a direct or indirect personal interest in any such transaction or arrangement, he must disclose his interest to the board of directors before it is entered into by the organisation. An example would be a proposal to acquire a target company in which a director owns shares.
- A third type of conflict of interest arises with existing transactions or arrangements in which the organisation is already a party. It can be a criminal offence for a director not to make or update his declaration of interest in an arrangement or transaction to which the organisation is a party.

5.6 Duty not to accept benefits from third parties

A director must not accept benefits from a third party unless they have been authorised by the shareholders or cannot reasonably be regarded as creating a potential conflict of interest. Clearly, accepting a bribe from a supplier in return for awarding a supply contract would be a breach of this duty. It would also be illegal to accept lunch or dinner from the same supplier or customer every week, accepting an all-expenses paid holiday or accepting frequent invitations to 'hospitality' events. On the other hand it should be within the law to accept an invitation to a day out to tennis at Wimbledon, or an invitation to dinner to celebrate the successful completion of a project.

In practice many listed companies already have strict policies on the acceptance of gifts and corporate hospitality, especially from other companies that are or might be about to tender for business with the organisation. A policy might include a requirement for a director to obtain clearance from another director before accepting any such benefits, and for all instances of gifts or hospitality to be recorded in a register.

The Bribery Act 2010 deals with acts of bribery and sets out that an organisation may be liable for failing to prevent a person from bribing on its behalf but only if that person performs business services for the organisation. It contains a full defence for an organisation that show it had adequate procedures in place to prevent bribery. It is important to note that guidance on the Act sets out specifically that while hospitality is not prohibited by the Act, facilitation payments are classed as bribes under the Act.

5.7 Duty to declare interests in proposed transactions with the organisation

This duty is linked to the duty relating to conflicts of interest. A director must declare the nature and extent of his interest to the other directors, who may then authorise it.

A director may have a personal interest in a proposed transaction with the organisation. For example, a director may own a building that the organisation wants to buy or rent; or a director may be a major shareholder in another organisation that is hoping to become a supplier or customer. Proposed transactions do not necessarily create a conflict of interests, but they must nevertheless be declared, and subject to approval by the rest of the board. If a conflict of interest would arise from the proposed transaction, the director must take measures to ensure that the conflict is avoided.

5.8 Other statutory duties

Directors' responsibilities to third parties

Although the duty of directors is to their organisation, a breach of that duty could also affect outsiders. When the directors make a contract with an outsider, the contract is binding on the organisation when it is according to its constitution (articles of association). However, the directors might exceed their powers in making the contract, for example, because they should have obtained shareholder approval first, but failed to do so. Contracts entered into without proper authority are known as 'irregular contracts', and might seem to be void.

The main provision of UK company law is that an irregular contract is binding on an organisation when an outsider, acting in good faith, enters into the contract and the contract has been approved by the board of directors. The directors will be liable to the organisation for any loss suffered. This rule means that irregular contracts do not affect third parties (outsiders). Instead, when they occur, they would be a corporate governance problem.

Related party transactions and the UK Disclosure and Transparency Rules for listed companies

In listed companies, the requirements of UK law are reinforced by the UK Disclosure and Transparency Rules, which include a section on **related party transactions**. In broad terms, a related party means a substantial shareholder of the organisation, a director of the organisation, a member of a director's family or an organisation in which a director or family member holds 30% or more of the shares. A related party transaction is a transaction between an organisation and a related party, other than in the normal course of business.

For most related party transactions above a minimum size, a listed organisation is required to:

- make an announcement to the stock market giving details of the transaction
- send a circular to shareholders giving more details
- obtain the prior approval of the shareholders for the transaction.

The effect of the rules should be to prevent directors or major shareholders of UK listed companies from obtaining a personal benefit from any non-business transaction with their organisation, unless the shareholders have given their approval.

5.9 Borrowing powers of directors

In the UK, there is no restriction in law on how much the directors can borrow on behalf of their organisation unless the constitution (articles of association) includes a specific restriction. As far as the law is concerned, the borrowing powers of companies are limited only by what lenders are prepared to make available to them. Conceivably, the directors could therefore put the investment of their shareholders at risk by borrowing more than the organisation can safely afford.

Foundation trusts are also free to borrow from banks and other private sector lenders to improve the facilities and equipment available to patients. They are, however, subject to statutory controls – unlike voluntary or private providers of healthcare – which give Monitor powers to set limits on the amount they can borrow.

TEST YOUR KNOWLEDGE 7.4

a What are the seven statutory duties of directors under the provisions of the UK Companies Act 2006?
b In what circumstances is it acceptable for a director to have an interest in a third party transaction with the organisation?
c What are the provisions of the UK Disclosure and Transparency Rules for listed companies with regard to related party transactions with the organisation?

6 Liability of directors

The starting point for considering the liabilities of individual directors is understanding the role of the board and the corporate nature of the trust, PCT or foundation trust (in this section collectively referred to as the trust). Any such trust will be a corporate entity in its own right and will take decisions as such. As noted earlier, this has implications for the role of directors, who are collectively responsible for all decisions. However, the corporate nature of the organisation will mean that, in most instances, even if a decision is open to criticism, individual directors will not be legally liable. There is specific statutory protection where they are acting in good faith (see Section 265 of the Public Health Act 1875). This section covers the circumstances where such personal liability can arise.

6.1 Criminal liability

An individual who, in the course of his or her activities as a director, commits a criminal offence will of course carry personal responsibility and liability. Perhaps more significantly a director can, in some circumstances, be held to have committed a criminal offence where the offence arises under statute that includes explicit provision to hold a director liable. Examples are health and safety legislation, the Environmental Protection Act and the Data Protection Act.

With regard to corporate manslaughter, the law remains that it is necessary to show that a 'controlling mind' within the organisation (usually a director) is also guilty of manslaughter, that is to say has been guilty of gross negligence that directly caused the fatality. In practice it has proved very difficult to convict either large corporations or their directors on this basis. Current proposals introduce an approach that would address the difficulty of convicting the corporation, but would not affect the test for manslaughter.

6.2 Civil liability to third parties

Civil liability, which generally relates to the payment of compensation, can arise in either contract or tort. Liability in contract will only occur if the contract is entered into in the personal name of the director rather than that of the trust, or where a contract entered into by the trust is found to be **ultra vires** and the director has given a personal warranty or representation that the trust has appropriate powers. Directors therefore need to be careful about what assurances they give about the powers of the organisation.

The more usual risks are for the individual to have a claim in tort made against them, most commonly in relation to either negligence or defamation. Negligence arises where an individual acts without due care towards a person to whom they owe a duty of care, and causes foreseeable loss. Usually, as with clinical negligence claims, the claim is pursued against the trust, not the individual, and the NHS Litigation Authority will provide cover. Indeed, the Liabilities to Third Parties Scheme includes cover for directors similar to that available in the commercial market by way of directors' and officers' liability insurance.

Defamation is a potential risk, and while some degree of protection is afforded where public officers are acting honestly and in the course of their business, there are risks if they step outside the strict parameters of the role.

A potential threat is misfeasance in public office, but in practice this is very rare, and requires the establishment of deliberate malice, targeting the individual or a limited class of people who has/have suffered loss.

6.3 Claims by the trust

A final area of risk is that of claims by the trust. All directors owe a duty of care and skill to the trust, and breaches could give rise to claims. In this area there is a material difference between the position of executive and NEDs. The latter are protected by the terms of the standard Treasury indemnity unless they have been reckless. However, executives could in theory be the subject of claims even if they have only been negligent.

Although there are some high profile corporate cases, such as Equitable Life, in practice claims against the directors for negligently carrying out their duties are rare. It does however underline the need for directors to use care and skills in carrying out their role. Where a matter is outside their competence, they may want to consider whether they need independent advice.

A further area of claim by the trust would be for breach of fiduciary duty or for repayment of benefits improperly received. This can arise in two main ways.

The first is where a director abuses his or her position to make private gain. This could occur where a director arranged for a contract with a company in which he or she had an interest, without declaring the relevant interest. In such circumstances the trust can call for an account of the proceeds.

Second, and perhaps more commonly, situations arise where the auditors call into question officers' remuneration or retirement packages. Irrespective of the propriety of the individual's conduct, if the award of an enhanced pension was outside the powers of the trust, or decided upon improperly, it can be clawed back.

6.4 Indemnity

As indicated above, there is a degree of protection for directors. Non-executives will typically have the benefit of the Treasury approved wording (HSG 1999/104):

> 'A chairman or non-executive member or director who has acted honestly and in good faith will not have to meet out of his or her own personal resources any personal civil liability that is incurred in the execution or purported execution of his or her board function. Save where the person has acted recklessly.'

This indemnity may be extended to members of those committees that have delegated powers to make decisions or take actions on behalf of NHS boards. This covers the director for acts carried out in good faith in the execution or purported execution of the functions of the trust, short of recklessness. It does not cover criminal liability, and no indemnity could do so. There is some doubt about the position where the director is in fact acting outside the powers of the trust, particularly where to enforce the indemnity would be to allow a collateral enforcement of an ultra vires obligation against the trust.

Executive directors will generally be indemnified in relation to claims against them arising from third parties, but difficult issues can arise when staff make allegations of harassment, and trusts will need to tread carefully in such cases.

TEST YOUR KNOWLEDGE 7.5

a In what circumstances can personal liability arise?
b What kind of indemnity is provided by HSG 1999/104?

7 NHS Code of Conduct and Accountability

Not surprisingly, the duty to avoid conflicts of interest, not to accept benefits from third parties and to declare any interest in a proposed transaction or arrangement are very clearly set out in the Business Code of Conduct for NHS organisations. Given the scale and magnitude of the procurement of contracts and services within the NHS, there is clearly a significant need to regulate the behaviour of both the board and NHS staff in regard to managing conflicts of interests.

The *NHS Appointment Commission's Code of Conduct and Accountability* are quite clear in that NHS boards should act in a way that protects the interest of the NHS in the way they undertake their business:

- 'Accountability: Everything done by those who work in the NHS must be able to stand the test of parliamentary scrutiny, public judgements on propriety and professional codes of conduct.'
- 'Probity: There should be an absolute standard of honesty in dealing with the assets of the NHS: integrity should be the hallmark of all personal conduct in decisions affecting patients, staff, and suppliers, and in the use of information acquired in the course of NHS duties.'
- 'Openness: There should be sufficient transparency about NHS activities to promote confidence between the NHS organisation and its staff, patients and the public.'
- 'Chairs and board directors should act impartially and should not be influenced by social or business relationships.'

Furthermore, *Governing the NHS* guidance states:

> 'NHS boards should conduct themselves and the business of the trust in an open and transparent way that commands public confidence.'

The *Healthy NHS Board: principles for good governance* reinforces the importance of NHS boards acting, and being seen to act, with integrity and in the best interests of the organisation:

> 'Probity requires that the board maintains an up-to-date register of board members' interests. Board agendas should include an opportunity for board members to declare conflicts of interests that may relate to specific agenda items so that they can be managed appropriately.'

For NHS foundation trusts there is also a requirement for the board of directors to adopt appropriate standards of conduct and to be open and transparent in their decision-making and the manner in which conflicts of interest are managed.

It is worth remembering that these duties (as in common law) apply to non-executive as well as to executive directors. The fiduciary duty and the statutory duties of directors are referred to in the *UK Corporate Governance Code*, which includes a supporting principle that: 'All directors are fiduciaries who must act objectively in the best interests of the organisation and in accordance with their statutory duties.'

The consequences for breach of these duties are most likely to be legal action taken in the name of the organisation (perhaps by shareholders). However, failure to declare an interest could result in a criminal prosecution of the director concerned.

8 Matters reserved for the board

The main decision-making powers belong to the board of directors. Although the board delegates many of the operational decision-making responsibilities to executive management, it should:

- retain the most significant decisions to itself
- monitor the performance of the executive management.

An aspect of governance is therefore the nature of the decisions the board reserves to itself (rather than delegating them to executive management).

The *UK Corporate Governance Code* does not specify which matters should be reserved by the board for its own decision-making, but states simply in a provision that: 'There should be formal schedule of matters reserved for its decision.' It then goes on to state that the annual report should include a statement of how the board operates and a high-level statement of the types of decision that it reserves for its own decisions and the types of decision that it delegates to executive management.

The ICSA's Guidance Note on matters that should be reserved for the board's own decision-making, is consistent with the provisions of the *UK Code*. The list of items in the Guidance Note is quite long, and includes decisions relating to matters such as:

- approval of strategy
- approval of annual operating and capital expenditure budgets
- oversight of operations (including accounting, planning and internal control systems)
- compliance with legal and regulatory requirements
- performance review
- changes in corporate or capital structure
- approving the annual report and accounts
- declaring an interim dividend and recommending a final dividend
- approval of formal communications with shareholders
- approval of major contracts and investments
- approval of policies on matters such as health and safety, CSR and the environment.

The company secretary may be given the task of preparing and maintaining the list of matters to be reserved for the board (for board approval), and reminding the board whenever necessary that certain decisions should not be delegated.

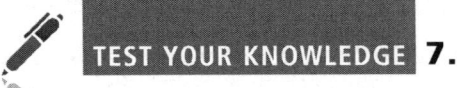

TEST YOUR KNOWLEDGE 7.6

List ten matters that should be reserved for decision-making by the board of directors.

9 The roles of chairman and chief executive officer (CEO)

9.1 The chief executive officer

The CEO leads the executive team, is responsible for the executive management of the organisation's operations and is the senior executive in charge of the management team and to whom all other executive managers report. Other executive managers might also be directors of the organisation, but the CEO is answerable to the board for the way the business is run and its performance.

In order to improve the standard of boardroom discussion, the CEO should also act as a spokesperson for the executive directors in board discussions and:

- explain the views of the executive directors to the rest of the board
- explain in a balanced way any differences of opinion within the executive team.

The CEO and the executive team also have certain corporate governance responsibilities. They have the primary responsibility for:

- communicating to employees the expectations of the board about the organisation's culture and values
- ensuring that appropriate standards of governance are applied at all levels within the organisation.

9.2 The chairman

Whereas the CEO is responsible for the executive management, the chairman's responsibilities relate primarily to managing the board of directors, and ensuring that the board functions effectively. To do this, he needs to ensure that the board discusses relevant issues in sufficient depth, with all the information needed to reach a decision, and with all the directors contributing to the discussions and decision-making. Key roles of a chairman are therefore to:

- set an appropriate agenda for board meetings
- ensure that relevant information is provided to the directors, in advance of the meeting
- encourage open discussions to board meetings, with constructive debate and discussion
- encourage all directors to contribute to discussions and decision-making.

The *UK Corporate Governance Code* states that 'The chairman is responsible for leadership of the board and ensuring its effectiveness on all aspects of its role.'

- 'The chairman is responsible for setting the board's agenda and ensuring that adequate time is available for discussion of all agenda items, in particular strategic issues.'
- 'The chairman should also promote a culture of openness and debate by facilitating the contribution of non-executives in particular and ensuring constructive relations between executive and non-executive directors.'
- 'The chairman should ensure that communications with shareholders are "effective".'

These principles emphasise the role of the chairman in trying to ensure that all directors, and in particular NEDs, contribute effectively to board discussions. There is always a risk that individuals who do not work full time for the organisation may have difficulty in challenging the views of full-time executive directors. The chairman should make sure that this does not happen.

The FRC Guidance states that: 'Good boards are created by good chairmen. The chairman creates the conditions for overall board and individual director effectiveness.' It emphasises that an effective chairman is a team-builder, developing a board whose members communicate effectively and enjoy good relationships with each other. He should develop a close relationship of trust with the CEO, giving support and advice while still respecting the CEO's responsibilities for executive matters. He should also ensure the effective implementation of board decisions, provide coherent leadership for the organisation and understand the views of the shareholders.

It also provides a detailed list of matters for which the chairman is responsible, which include:

- setting the board agenda, which is primarily focused on strategy, performance, value, creation and accountability, and ensuring that issues relevant to these areas are reserved for board decision
- making certain that the board determines the nature, and extent, of the significant risks the company is willing to embrace in the implementation of its strategy, and that there are no 'no go' areas that prevent directors from operating effective oversight in this area
- making certain that the board has effective decision-making processes and applies sufficient challenge to major proposals
- encouraging all board members to engage in board and committee meetings by drawing on their skills, experience, knowledge and, where appropriate, independence
- fostering relationships founded on mutual respect and open communication between the NEDs and the executive team
- developing productive working relationships with all executive directors, and the CEO in particular, providing support and advice while respecting executive responsibility
- taking the lead on issues of director development, including through induction programmes for new directors and regular reviews with all directors. Acting on the results of board evaluation
- ensuring effective communication with shareholders and other stakeholders and, in particular, that all directors are made aware of the views of those who provide the company's capital.

Table 7.1 (p. 142) sets out the key distinction in role for the chairman and CEO and is taken from the *NHS Healthy Board*.

More specifically, the *NHS Healthy Board* sets out some pointers for chairs and chief executives. The chair should *not*:

- be too operational, interfere with details of management
- exceed part-time hours
- take specific strategic decisions alone
- adopt bullying, macho 'hire and fire' culture.

Chief executives should *not*:

- be too controlling or autocratic towards the chair
- get too involved in NED role – e.g. no consultation on shaping board agendas
- break the fundamental rule of 'no surprises'
- be too entrenched in the organisation.

9.3 Independence of the chairman

As a general rule, the chairman should be independent when first appointed. This is a provision of the *UK Code* for listed companies and of the *FT Code of Governance* for foundation trusts.

It follows that the CEO of an organisation should not subsequently become the chairman; a former CEO will not be independent, although the *King III Code* states that a former CEO should not become chairman for at least three years after ceasing to be CEO, believing that this is sufficient time in which to become independent. If, exceptionally, it is proposed that the current CEO should become the chairman when the existing chairman retires, investors should be first consulted. The *UK Code* also states that the reasons for appointing a former CEO as chairman should be explained to shareholders both at the time of the appointment and in the next annual report and accounts.

A governance problem with 'promoting' the CEO to become the chairman is that the incoming CEO may find it difficult to run the organisation as he wishes because the former CEO is still on the board, monitoring what he/she is doing.

Table 7.1 Roles of chair and chief executive

	Chair	Chief executive
Formulate strategy	Ensures board develops vision, strategies and clear objectives to deliver organisational purpose	Leads strategy development process
Ensure accountability	Holds CE to account for delivery of strategy	Leads the organisation in the delivery of strategy
	Ensures board committees that support accountability are properly constituted	Establishes effective performance management arrangements and controls
		Acts as accountable officer
Shape culture	Provides visible leadership in developing a positive culture for the organisation, and ensures that this is reflected and modelled in their own and in the board's behaviour and decision making	Provides visible leadership in developing a positive culture for the organisation, and ensures that this is reflected in their own and the executive's behaviour and decision making
	Board culture: leads and supports a constructive dynamic within the board, enabling contributions from all directors	
Context	Ensures all board members are well briefed on external context	Ensures all board members are well briefed on external context
Intelligence	Ensures requirements for accurate, timely and clear information to board/ directors (and governors for FTs) are clear to executive	Ensures provision of accurate, timely and clear information to board/ directors (and governors for FTs)
Engagement	Plays key role as an ambassador, and in building strong partnerships with: – Patients and public – Members and governors (FTs) – Clinicians and staff – Key institutional stakeholders – Regulators	Plays key leadership role in effective communication and building strong partnerships with: – Patients and public – Members and governors (FTs) – Clinicians and staff – Key institutional stakeholders – Regulators

Even so, there have been several cases where a CEO has gone on to become chairman without any serious protest from shareholders or investor groups.

NAPF's *Corporate Governance Policy and Voting Guidelines* (2011) also recommend that if the chairman is not independent on appointment, the organisation should consult its investors and explain why it considers the appointment desirable. The shareholders should then consider the case on its merits.

9.4 Separating the roles of chairman and chief executive officer (CEO)

As leader of the management team and leader of the board of directors, the CEO and chairman are the most powerful positions on the board of directors.

It is important for the proper functioning of the organisation that the chairman and CEO work well together. Acting in alliance, the chairman and CEO can dominate the board and its decision-making, particularly if the chairman also has executive responsibilities in the organisation's management.

When the same person holds the position of both chairman and CEO, there is a possibility that he could become a dominant influence in decision-making in the organisation. As leader of the executive management team, a chairman-cum-CEO may be reluctant to encourage challenges from NEDs about the organisation's performance or to question management proposals about future business strategy.

In some countries (including the USA), it is common to find organisation leaders who are both chairman and CEO, although separation of the roles has become more common there. The *UK Code* states as a principle that the roles should be separated:

'There should be a clear division of responsibilities at the head of the organisation between the running of the board and the executive responsibility for the running of the organisation's business. No one individual should have unfettered powers of decision.'

The *UK Code* therefore states that the roles of chairman and CEO should not be performed by the same individual. In addition, the division of responsibilities between the chairman and CEO should be set out clearly in writing, to prevent one of them from encroaching on the area of responsibility of the other. The *FT Code of Governance* makes a similar statement.

When an individual holds the positions of chairman and CEO, he could exercise dominant power on the board, unless there are strong individuals on the board, such as a deputy chairman or a **SID**, to act as a counterweight. If the individual also has a domineering or bullying personality, the situation will be even worse, because a chairman-cum-CEO who acts in a bullying manner will not listen to advice from any board colleagues, and the board would not function as an effective body.

There is even a risk that the individual will run the organisation for his own personal benefit rather than in the interests of the shareholders and other stakeholders. The only way to prevent a chairman-cum-CEO from dominating an organisation is to have an influential group of directors capable of making their opinions heard. However, it is important to distinguish between:

- the position of 'unfettered power' that is created when the roles of chairman and CEO are combined and given to one individual
- acting in a dominant or tyrannical way, possibly out of self-interest.

Combining the two roles increases the risk that the organisation and its board will be dominated by a tyrannical individual, but this does not happen every time.

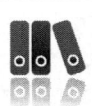

CASE EXAMPLE 7.4

The potential risk of an organisation and board being subjected to a dominant personality is illustrated by the case of the UK organisation Polly Peck International. Polly Peck, a FTSE 100 organisation during the 1980s, was effectively run by a single individual, Asil Nadir, who was both CEO and board chairman. The organisation collapsed without warning in October 1990. During the administration process, the system of internal controls at the organisation's London head office was found to be virtually non-existent. As a result, Nadir had been able to transfer large amounts of money from the organisation's UK bank accounts to personal accounts with a bank in Northern Cyprus, without any questions being asked. After the organisation collapsed, Nadir fled to Northern Cyprus, where he lives in exile.

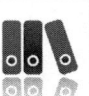

CASE EXAMPLE 7.5

In the UK, Mr Luc Vandevelde was appointed as chairman and CEO of Marks & Spencer some years ago, at a time when its business operations were in difficulty and the share price was falling sharply. This appointment attracted some criticism but appears to have been a successful short-term measure. By 2002, the organisation's fortunes had improved to the point where he relinquished the position of CEO and announced his intention to become part-time chairman. When, however, in 2008 the then CEO, Sir Stuart Rose, was also appointed as organisation chairman for a limited period until a successor to the role of CEO could be appointed this, given the previous appointment of Vandevelde, attracted strong criticism from institutional investors. Institutional investor Legal & General publicly criticised the decision by Marks & Spencer to appoint Sir Stuart Rose as executive chairman, saying it was an arrangement that made it difficult to appoint a successor to Sir Stuart as CEO. However, shareholders could not prevent the appointment of the new chairman because this was a decision of the board. Shareholders were able, however, to vote on the re-election of Sir Stuart Rose as director at the AGM in 2008, and 22% of shareholders either opposed his re-election or abstained in the vote.

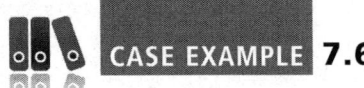 **CASE EXAMPLE 7.6**

Dr Bill Moyes headed up Monitor, the independent regulator for NHS foundation trusts, since it was established in January 2004 until January 2010 as its executive chairman. It was the board's view that the regulator's corporate governance principles, the stature and experience of the members of the board of directors, as well as a culture of open communication were conducive to board effectiveness with a combined chairman and CEO position. The board agreed separate objectives for the chairman and chief executive elements of his role and that he would be separately appraised on the chairman and chief executive aspects of his role by the deputy chair and the SID.

Following Dr Moyes' departure, the role was separated and Monitor was chaired by Steve Bundred and Dr David Bennett was appointed as an Interim CEO. Following the departure of Mr Bundred in March 2011, Dr Bennett was appointed as chairman while continuing as Interim CEO.

However, there might occasionally be situations where it is appropriate for the same person to be both chairman and CEO. When an organisation gets into business or financial difficulties, for example, there is an argument in favour of appointing a single, all-powerful individual to run the organisation until its fortune has been reversed. The combination of the roles of chairman and CEO might have been necessary in the short term to give an organisation strong leadership to get it through its difficulties.

9.5 The chairman's commitments

A problem with non-executive chairmen – as with NEDs generally – is that the individual may not have enough time to devote to the role of chairman because of a large number of other commitments. For example, the chairman of a large company may also be the chairman of another organisation so that he does not have enough time to fulfil all these roles adequately.

Chairmen need to be able to demonstrate that they have sufficient time to perform their role to the standards expected. NAPF's *Corporate Governance Policy and Voting Guidelines* state that where a chairman has 'multiple appointments', investors will require a 'compelling explanation' of how the chairman will be able to handle all the various appointments without any detriment to the organisation. The **Walker Report** suggested that the chairmen of large banks would need to spend about two-thirds of their time with the organisation.

The *UK Corporate Governance Code* is less specific on the amount of time that a chairman should commit to the organisation. However, a provision of the Code is that when a chairman is appointed, the **nomination committee** (see also Chapter 8) should prepare a job description, which should:

- include an assessment of the amount of time commitment that should be expected
- recognise the need for the chairman to make himself available in a time of crisis.

The chairman's other commitments should be disclosed to the board before his appointment and included in the next annual report and accounts. If there are changes to the time commitment required from or provided by the chairman, these should be disclosed to the board and reported in the next annual report and accounts.

 TEST YOUR KNOWLEDGE 7.7

a What is the role of a chairman? Why should this role not be combined with the role of CEO?
b What are the requirements of the *FT Code of Governance* with regard to the independence of the chairman?
c In what circumstances is it acceptable for an individual to be the chairman of more than one FTSE 100 companies at the same time?

The *FT Code of Governance* also sets out that the board of directors should not agree to a full-time executive director taking on more than one non-executive directorship of an NHS foundation trust or another organisation of comparable size and complexity, nor the chairmanship of such an organisation.

10 Size and composition of the board

The effectiveness of a board of directors depends on its size and composition.

10.1 The size of the board

The typical size of a board of directors varies with the size of the organisation and possibly also the industry or business sector in which it operates. In addition, the average size of boards in listed companies varies between different countries.

A board should not be larger than it needs to be. Large boards are more difficult to manage, because there are more individuals involved, and board meetings can be very long and time consuming. On the other hand, boards should be large enough for its members to collectively have the knowledge, skills and experience to make effective decisions.

The *UK Code* suggests that the board should be sufficiently large to avoid a situation in which it becomes over-reliant on one or two individuals, for example as chairmen of board committees (nominations, remuneration, audit and risk committees). It states:

> 'The board should be of sufficient size that the requirements of the business can be met and that changes to the board's composition and that of its committees can be managed without disruption, and should not be so large as to be unwieldy.'

The *Healthy NHS Board* suggests that:

> 'NHS boards should not be so large as to be unwieldy, but must be large enough to provide the balance of skills and experience that is appropriate for the organisation. The composition of the board should achieve a balance between continuity and renewal.'

STOP AND THINK 7.1

Select any NHS organisation that you know. Given the size and complexity of its business, make an estimate of how large its board of directors might be. Next, find the organisation's website and check the size and composition of its board. (If you have difficulty in finding this information, it should be contained in the directors' report in its report and accounts.) See how close your estimate was to being correct.

10.2 The composition of the board

The composition of a board of directors depends partly on its size. In the UK, the board of a large public company commonly consists of a:

- chairman
- possibly a deputy chairman
- CEO
- SID (who may also be the deputy chairman)
- executive directors
- NEDs.

In the NHS, the composition of the board is clearly dictated either by the model standing orders issued by the DH or, if a foundation trust, then by the Core Constitution required by Monitor.

Collectively, the members of the board should have sufficient skills and experience to provide effective leadership for the organisation. This suggests that they should have a variety of different backgrounds and expertise.

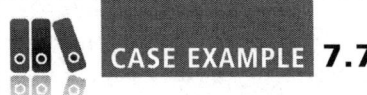

CASE EXAMPLE 7.7

Monitor Core Constitution (paragraph 20)

20.1 The trust is to have a Board of Directors, which shall comprise both executive and non-executive directors.
20.2 The Board of Directors is to comprise:
   20.2.1 a non-executive Chairman
   20.2.2 [*] other non-executive directors; and
   20.2.3 [*] executive directors.
20.3 One of the executive directors shall be the Chief Executive.
20.4 The Chief Executive shall be the Accounting Officer.
20.5 One of the executive directors shall be the finance director.
20.6 One of the executive directors is to be a registered medical practitioner or a registered dentist (within the meaning of the Dentists Act 1984).
20.7 One of the executive directors is to be a registered nurse or a registered midwife.

[*] denotes number to be inserted at the trust's discretion.

There should also be a suitable balance of power on the board, so that one individual or a small group of individuals is unable to dominate the board and its decision-making. In countries such as the UK, it is therefore considered appropriate to appoint independent NEDs to a board, because:

- they act as a counter-balance to executive directors, who may give priority to their own interests above those of the shareholders (and other stakeholders)
- they have skills and experience that executive directors do not have, because they come from a different background and so are able to contribute different ideas and views to board discussions and decision-making.

Because they do not have a strong personal financial interest in the organisation, NEDs are more easily able to represent the interests of the major stakeholders (e.g. shareholders) and to act (where required) as a restraint on executive management.

These principles relating to board composition are set out in the *UK Code* as follows:

'The board and its committees should have the appropriate balance of skills, experience, independence and knowledge of the company to enable them to discharge their respective duties and responsibilities effectively.'

'The board should include an appropriate combination of executive and non-executive directors (and in particular independent non-executive directors) such that no individual or small group of individuals can dominate the board's decision-taking.'

In the UK, a key principle of good corporate governance is that there should be sufficient independent NEDs on the board of directors to create a suitable balance of power and prevent the dominance of the board by one individual or by a small number of individuals. This is reflected in the *FT Code of Governance*. The *UK Code* sets out different requirements for large listed companies and for smaller companies. (Smaller companies are defined as companies outside the FTSE 350 for the whole of the year immediately prior to the reporting year.)

- Except for smaller companies, at least one half of the board, excluding the chairman, should be independent NEDs.
- For smaller companies, there should be at least two independent NEDs.

Guidelines about the composition of a unitary board differ between countries. The *King III Code*, for example, recommends that the majority of directors should be NEDs and the majority of NEDs should be independent, but also adds that there should be at least two executive directors on the board – the CEO and chief finance officer (finance director).

TEST YOUR KNOWLEDGE 7.8

a What would be the disadvantages of a large NHS organisation restricting the total size of its board to eight members?
b What are the provisions in the *UK Code* for the size and composition of the board of directors of a listed organisation in the FTSE350?

11 Non-executive directors (NEDs)

A NED is a member of the board of directors without executive responsibilities in the organisation. NEDs should be able to bring judgement and experience to the deliberations of the board that the executive directors on their own would lack.

To be effective, a NED has to understand the organisation's business, but there appears to be general consensus that the experience and qualities required of a NED can be obtained from working in other industries or in other aspects of commercial and public life. NEDs may therefore include individuals who:

- are executive directors in other public companies
- hold NED positions and chairmanship positions in other public companies
- have professional qualifications (e.g. partners in firms of solicitors)
- have experience in government, as politicians or former senior civil servants.

However, research has been carried out into identifying and recruiting suitable individuals as NEDs from a wider variety of sources and backgrounds (see below).

NEDs are expected not only to bring a wide range of skills and experience to the deliberations of the board, particularly in the area of strategy and business development, but also to ensure that there is a suitable balance of power on the board. A powerful chairman or CEO might be able to dominate other executive directors, but in theory at least, independent NEDs should be able to bring different views and independent thinking to board deliberations. Decisions taken by the board should therefore be better and more in keeping with the aims of good corporate governance.

CASE EXAMPLE 7.8

The Bristol Royal Infirmary Enquiry, July 2001 stated that:

> 'In our view, non-executive directors have a crucial role to play in representing the public interest in the conduct of the Trust's affairs. They must be people with a high level of ability and experience in the leadership and management of organisations . . . they should have a commitment to public service.'

Lessons for non-executive directors that resulted from the Bristol Enquiry were as follows:

- Non-executive directors can be prevented from exerting their authority by 'not being let in on issues' at senior executive level.
- Lack of sound knowledge about trust activity can lead to an inability to challenge chief executives' or executive directors' views.
- Role objectives may not be clarified and communicated. There was:
  - a variation in the roles played by non-executives on the Board
  - variation in what was expected of non-executives
  - a lack of clarity and direction for the role.

11.1 The *UK Corporate Governance Code* on non-executive directors (NEDs)

The *UK Code* has largely incorporated the recommendations from the Higgs Report on the role and effectiveness of NEDs. Key among them are:

- NEDs should 'constructively challenge and help develop proposals on strategy'
- NEDs should also scrutinise the performance of management in meeting agreed goals or targets of performance, and they should monitor the reporting of performance (to ensure that this is honest and not misleading)
- NEDs should satisfy themselves about the integrity of the financial information produced by the organisation, and that the financial controls and systems of risk management are 'robust and defensible'
- they should be responsible for deciding the remuneration of executive directors
- they should have a significant role in the appointment (and where necessary removal) of executive directors and in succession planning for the major positions on the board.

The *UK Code* recognises there are matters that the NEDs should discuss without executive directors being present, and a provision of the *UK Code* is that:

- the chairman should hold meetings with the NEDs without executive directors being present
- without the chairman and led by the SID (see Section 10 'Senior independent directors'), the NEDs should meet at least once a year to discuss the performance of the chairman. They should also meet on other occasions if this is considered necessary or appropriate.

All of these principles have been adopted by the *FT Code of Governance*.

11.2 FRC Guidance on the role of NEDs

The guidance makes the following recommendations on the role of NEDs:

- A NED should, on appointment, devote time to a comprehensive, formal and tailored induction and should devote time to developing and refreshing their knowledge and skills.
- NEDs need to make sufficient time available to discharge their responsibilities effectively.
- Their letter of appointment should state the minimum time that the NED will be required to spend on the company's business, and indicate the possibility of additional time commitment when the company is undergoing a period of particularly increased activity, such as an acquisition or takeover, or as a result of some major difficulty with one or more of its operations.
- NEDs should insist on receiving high-quality information sufficiently in advance so that there can be thorough consideration of the issues prior to, and informed debate and challenge at, board meetings. High-quality information is that which is appropriate for making decisions on the issue at hand – it should be accurate, clear, comprehensive, up-to-date and timely; contain a summary of the contents of any paper; and inform the director of what is expected of him or her on that issue.

11.3 The Walker Report on the role of NEDS in banks

The Walker Report suggested that the role of NEDs is crucial to the effectiveness of a board in formulating and implementing business strategy. The report included the following comments:

- Shareholders have a right to expect that in a unitary board there should be a material input from the NEDs to decisions on strategy and oversight of strategy implementation. It should also be expected that when there is such shared decision-taking between executive and NEDs, the organisation should perform better in general and over time than if strategy were determined exclusively by the executive management. This expectation appeared to have been justified by the banking crisis in the USA and Europe.
- NEDs should provide a 'disciplined but rigorous challenge on substantive issues'. This should be seen as the norm, not an exception, and if any NED has insufficient strength of character to participate in providing a challenge, his continued suitability to remain as a board member should be thrown into question.

'This does not, of course, mean open season for challenge to the executive team. Appropriate balance will only be achieved where the executive expects to be challenged, but where the board debate surrounding such challenge is conducted in a way that leaves the executive team with a sense of having drawn benefit from it.'

11.4 Independence of non-executive directors (NEDs)

NEDs are either independent or non-independent. A NED is not independent if his opinions are likely to be influenced, in particular by the senior executive management of the organisation or by a major stakeholder.

Independent NEDs are supposed to bring an independent view to the deliberations of the board. However, they are in a difficult position as they are legally liable in the same way as executive directors. For example, they have the same fiduciary duties to the organisation, and the duty of skill and care. As fellow directors, they might also be reluctant to blow the whistle on their executive colleagues. If they have been selected and appointed by the chairman or the CEO, they will be less likely to ask tough questions about the way the organisation is being run.

The *UK Code* does not suggest that all NEDs should be independent. Non-independent NEDs are permissible, although the majority of the total board should consist of independent NEDs. If there are NEDs on the board who are not considered to be independent, this could create problems with the size and composition of the board and it may be considered necessary to appoint independent NEDs to act as a counterbalance to the NEDs who are not independent.

The *FT Code of Governance* states that:

'The board of directors should identify in the annual report each non-executive director it considers to be independent. The board should determine whether the director is independent in character and judgement and whether there are relationships or circumstances which are likely to affect, or could appear to affect, the director's judgement. The board of directors should state its reasons if it determines that a director is independent notwithstanding the existence of relationships or circumstances which may appear relevant to its determination . . .'

So what is meant by 'independent'? It is easier to answer this question by specifying what is 'not independent'. A NED is *not* independent if his opinions are likely to be influenced by someone else, in particular by the senior executive management or by a major stakeholder. The independence of an NED could be challenged, for example, if the individual concerned:

- has a family connection with the CEO – a problem in some family controlled public companies
- until recently used to be an executive director in the organisation
- until recently used to work for the organisation in a professional capacity (e.g. as its auditor or corporate lawyer)
- receives payments from the organisation in addition to their fees as an NED.

A person cannot be independent if he personally stands to gain or otherwise benefit substantially from:

- income from the organisation, in addition to his fee as a NED
- the company's reported profitability and movements in the organisation's share price.

A NED cannot be properly independent, for example, if he accepts a fee from the organisation for consultancy work. Consultancy involves the individual in the operational aspects of the organisation, and by implication puts him on the side of the executives. Nor can an individual be independent if he has been awarded a large number of share options by the company. Holding share options gives the individual a direct interest in the share price of the company around the time the options can be exercised. He might therefore favour decisions that improve the reported profitability of the company at this time, because good financial results are likely to be good for the share price.

Occasionally, NEDs are appointed to represent the opinions of a major stakeholder (e.g. in NHS teaching hospitals the appointment of a NED from the related University or Dental school). In such cases, the individual can be expected to voice the wishes of the stakeholder, and so could not be regarded as independent.

To ensure that NEDs should not rely for their tenure in office on one or two individuals, the *UK Code* recommends that they should be selected through a formal process.

Executive directors cannot be independent. Not only are they involved in the running of the organisation's operations and report (and are accountable) to the CEO for this aspect of their work, they also rely on the organisation for most (if not all) of their remuneration.

11.5 Criteria for judging independence

The *UK Corporate Governance Code*, and as quoted above, the *FT Code*, both require the board to identify in the annual report each NED it considers to be independent. Although this is a matter for the board's judgement, both codes set out the circumstances in which independence would usually be questionable:

- The director has been an employee of the organisation within the last five years.
- The director has a material business relationship with the organisation (or has had such a relationship within the last three years). This relationship might be as a partner, shareholder, director or employee in another organisation that has a material business relationship with the organisation.
- The director receives (or has received) additional remuneration from the organisation other than a director's fee, or is a member of the organisation's pension scheme, or participates in the organisation's share option scheme or a performance-related pay scheme.
- The director has close family ties with any of the organisation's advisers, directors or senior employees.
- The director has cross-directorships or has significant links with other directors through involvement in other companies or organisations. A cross-directorship exists when an individual is a NED on the board of Organisation X and an executive director on the board of Organisation Y, when another individual is an executive director of Organisation X and an NED on the board of Organisation Y.
- The director represents a significant shareholder or stakeholder.
- The director has served on the board for more than nine years since the date of his first election (six in the case of the *FT Code*).

These criteria of independence should be applied to the chairman (on appointment) as well as other NEDs. Circumstances may change, and the independence of NEDs should be kept under review.

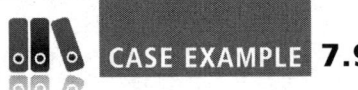

CASE EXAMPLE 7.9

A chairman of an NHS trust had served a three-year term of office and was one year into her second three-year term when the trust was authorised as a foundation trust. At the date of authorisation the chairman was offered the remaining two years of her term of office which she accepted.

At the end of that second term of office the Council of Governors agreed that while they would be happy to appoint the chairman for a further term of three years the appointment had to be subject to open competition. The role was advertised, candidates interviewed, and the chairman was reappointed for a further three-year term.

At the end of the third term of three years, the company secretary advised that since the *FT Code of Governance* now set out a six-year term of office any further terms of office would be for one year and would have to be subject to open competition.

The chairman refused to accept this, claiming that her previous term of office before the trust became an FT did not count and that she had only served five years. The chairman was advised similarly by the trust's lawyers and the Governor's Nominations Committee was advised accordingly.

When the position was made clear the chairman refused to stand for a further term of office and resigned.

11.6 Independence of serving directors

There is a general view that the independence of a NED is likely to diminish over time, as the NED becomes more familiar with the organisation and executive colleagues. The risk is that the NED will take more of the views of executive colleagues on trust and will be less rigorous in his questioning. This is noted in the *UK Code*, the *King III Code* and the *FT Code*.

However there will be circumstances where NEDs, having served their full terms, may exceptionally remain on the board and the *UK Code* is pragmatic in its approach to the nine-year rule. If the board considers that a director is still independent even after nine years' service, he may still be considered 'independent' for the purposes of the corporate governance provisions.

The *FT Code of Governance* takes a similar approach stating that:

'Any term beyond six years (e.g. two three year terms) for a NED should be subject to particularly rigorous review, and should take into account the need for progressive refreshing of the board.

'NEDs may in exceptional circumstances serve longer than six years (e.g. two three year terms following authorisation of the NHS foundation trust), but subject to annual re-appointment. Serving more than six years could be relevant to the determination of a NED's independence.'

11.7 Protecting the independence and effectiveness of board committees

As a way of protecting the independence and improving the effectiveness of board committees, the *UK Code* includes the following supporting principles:

- When deciding the chairmanship and membership of board committees, consideration should be given to the benefits of ensuring that committee membership is refreshed (i.e. membership rotation) and that undue reliance is not placed on particular individuals.
- The only individuals who are entitled to attend meetings of the nomination, remuneration and audit committees are the chairman and members of the committee, although other individuals may attend at the invitation of the committee.

11.8 Comparison of executive and non-executive directors (NEDs)

Unlike NEDs, executive directors are full-time employees of the organisation, with executive management responsibilities as well their responsibilities as directors. For the executive directors, there is a tension between:

- their role as members of the board, 'one step down from the shareholders'
- their role as senior operational directors, 'one step up from management'.

Executive directors, led by their CEO, may often want to present a united front to the rest of the board, to justify what the management team has done and achieved, or what it would like to do. However, if the executive directors come together with a united opinion, this will question their ability to fulfil the role of all directors to provide effective challenge in discussions on strategy. In comparison, independent NEDs do not have this problem, which is why they should be more effective in providing effective challenge in board discussions, encouraged by the chairman.

The problems for executive directors are therefore that:

- they may be inclined to support the views of the CEO on all matters, including strategy
- they may mistrust the NEDs as 'outsiders' who do not know much about the organisation and its business.

In recognition of this problem, the FRC Guidance suggests that executive directors should see themselves as representatives of the shareholders rather than as executive managers who are responsible and accountable to the CEO. The chairman should encourage this attitude among the executive directors, partly through ensuring that they receive appropriate induction and training for their role as organisation director.

Executive directors should have a very detailed knowledge of the organisation and its business, and should apply this knowledge when making judgements about organisation strategy. However, they should also recognise that constructive challenge from NEDs is an essential part of good governance, and they should welcome and encourage such challenges. For an effective board, the executive directors and NEDs must work constructively together.

> **TEST YOUR KNOWLEDGE 7.9**
>
> a What are the intended functions of independent NEDs?
> b According to Higgs, what are the four broad roles of NEDs?
> c According to the *UK Code* of Corporate Governance, what are the roles of NEDs?
> d List six circumstances in which a NED would not normally be considered independent.
> e Why does the *FT Code of Governance* stipulate no more than two three-year terms of office for NEDs?

12 Senior independent directors (SIDs)

In anticipation of the potential for problems arising between shareholders and the chairman and CEO, the *UK Corporate Governance Code* requires that the board of directors of large companies should nominate an independent NED as the SID, whom shareholders could approach to discuss problems and issues when the normal communication route through the chairman has broken down. In addition, if the chairman fails to pass on the views of the institutional shareholders to the NEDs, there should be another channel of communication that could be used instead.

The role of the SID has also been taken up by the *FT Code of Governance* for foundation trusts. The FT board of directors appoints one of the independent NEDs to be the SID, in consultation with the council of governors. The SID is then available to members and governors if they have concerns, which contact through the normal channels of chairman, chief executive or finance director have failed to resolve or for which such contact is inappropriate. The code states that the SID may also be the deputy chairman.

The FRC Guidance makes a distinction between the role of the SID in 'normal times' and when the board is undergoing 'a period of stress'.

At normal times, the role of the SID is to:

- provide support for the chairman
- ensure that the views of other directors, particularly the other NEDs, are conveyed to the chairman
- ensure that the views of the shareholders, particularly matters that concern them, are conveyed to the rest of the board
- ensure that the chairman is giving sufficient attention to succession planning
- carry out the annual review of the performance of the chairman, in conjunction with the other NEDs (see Chapter 5).

At times of stress for the board, the role of the SID should be to take the initiative to resolve the problem, working with the other directors and stakeholders and/or the chairman, as appropriate. Examples of problems where intervention by the SID may be appropriate include situations where:

- there is a dispute between the chairman and the CEO
- shareholders or the NEDs have expressed serious concerns that are not being addressed by the chairman or CEO
- the strategy pursued by the chairman or CEO is not supported by the rest of the board
- there is a very close relationship between the chairman and the CEO
- decisions are being taken without the approval of the board
- succession planning is being ignored.

Issues where intervention may be required should be considered when defining the responsibilities of the SID and should be set out in writing.

Critics of the SID concept argue that the chairman should be able to resolve difficulties between an organisation and its shareholders/stakeholders, and the position of SID should therefore be superfluous. Opening up the possibility of an additional channel of communication for shareholders/stakeholders is perhaps more likely to undermine organisation–shareholder relationships than improve them.

However, the *ICGN Global Corporate Governance Principles* put forward reasons why a 'lead independent director' or independent deputy chairman is necessary:

- If the chairman is the CEO or former CEO, or was for another reason not independent when first appointed, the SID should provide independent leadership for the board, and should have a key role in setting the agenda for board meetings and acting as spokesman for the independent members of the board.
- Even when the chairman was independent when first appointed, his role inevitably brings him closer than the NEDs over time to the views of the CEO and executive management.
- The SID should provide leadership to the independent members of the board when this situation creates a problem.
- The ICGN Principles also recognise the role of the lead independent director as an alternative conduit for communication with the shareholders.

13 Board committees and non-executive directors (NEDs)

An aspect of best practice in governance is that for some issues that the board should decide, the executive directors should be excluded from the decision-making or monitoring responsibilities. This is achieved by delegating certain responsibilities to committees of the board. A board committee might consist entirely or mostly of NEDs, and have the responsibility for dealing with particular issues and making recommendations to the full board. The full board is then usually expected to accept and endorse the recommendations of the relevant board committee.

In the UK, three committees are recommended by the *UK Corporate Governance Code*:

- a nomination committee
- an audit committee
- a remuneration committee.

In the UK there is no statutory requirement for a nomination committee or a remuneration committee, but, following the implementation of the EU Statutory Audit Directive in 2008, quoted companies are required to have an audit committee. The roles of these committees are explained in subsequent chapters.

Some boards might establish other committees. For example, an organisation might have an environment committee if its business activities are likely to have important consequences for the environment, involving government regulation, the law and public opinion. However, there is no requirement for these committees to consist wholly or mainly of NEDs.

In the NHS, the model standing orders and core constitution require all NHS trusts to have the same three committees.

Table 7.2 (p. 154) summarises the *UK Code*'s recommendations about membership of board committees.

14 Effectiveness of non-executive directors (NEDs)

There are differing views about the effectiveness of NEDs. The accepted view is that NEDs bring experience and judgement to the deliberations of the board that the executive directors on their own would lack. An alternative view is that the effectiveness of NEDs can be undermined by:

- lack of knowledge about the business operations of the organisation
- insufficient time spent with the organisation
- the weight of opinion of the executive directors on the board
- delays in decision-making.

Table 7.2 Summary of the *UK Code*'s recommendations regarding membership of board committees

Nominations committee	Audit committee	Remuneration committee
Chairman should be the chairman of the board or an independent NED	Composition: all independent NEDs – in large companies, at least three, in smaller companies two	Composition: all independent NEDs – in large companies, at least three, in smaller companies two
Composition: majority of members should be independent NEDs	In smaller companies, the chairman of the board may also be a member of the audit committee (but not chairman of the committee), in addition to the independent NEDs – but only if he was independent on appointment to the chairmanship	The chairman of the board may also be a member of the audit committee (but not chairman of the committee), but only if he was independent on appointment to the chairmanship
If the board chairman is the company chairman, he should not act as chair when the committee is considering a successor for the chairmanship	At least one member of the committee should have 'recent and relevant financial experience'	

14.1 Insufficient knowledge

The quality of decision-making depends largely on the quality of information available to the decision-maker. The *UK Code* states that the board as a whole should be 'supplied in a timely manner with information in a form and of a quality appropriate to enable it to discharge its duties'. However, the senior executives in an organisation control the information systems, and so control the flow of information to the board. It is quite conceivable, for example, that the CEO and other executive directors might have access to management information that is withheld from the board as a whole, or that is presented to the board in a distorted manner. Lacking the 'insider knowledge' of executive managers about the business operations, and having to rely on the integrity of the information supplied to them by management and executive directors, restricts the scope for NEDs to make a meaningful contribution to board decisions.

14.2 Insufficient time

NEDs often have executive positions in other companies and organisations, where most of their working time is spent. As a general rule, NEDs do not have an office at the organisation headquarters and may spend at most one or two days a month on the organisation's business. A further criticism of NEDs is that some individuals hold too many NED positions, with the result that they cannot possibly give sufficient time to any of the companies concerned. It could be argued, for example, that an individual cannot be an effective NED of an organisation if he is also the CEO of another public organisation and holds four or five other NED positions in other companies.

The *UK Code* states that all directors should be able to allocate sufficient time to the organisation to discharge their responsibilities effectively. Although this principle of the code applies to all directors, the main concern is with NEDs (since executive directors are usually full-time employees) and in particular the chairman. The *UK Code* requires that when a chairman is appointed, the nomination committee should prepare a job specification that includes an assessment of the expected time commitment and recognising the need for the chairman to be available to the organisation in times of crisis.

Similarly, when a NED is appointed (other than a chairman), the letter of appointment should set out the expected time commitment.

14.3 Overriding influence of executive directors

Yet another criticism of NEDs is that if a difference of opinion arises during a meeting of the board, the opinions of the executive directors are likely to carry greater weight, because they know more about the organisation. NEDs may be put under pressure to accept the views of their executive director colleagues. This potential problem provides an argument for the role of a strong SID, to ensure that the opinions of the independent NEDs are properly considered.

14.4 Delays in decision-making

It may be argued that NEDs delay decision-making within an organisation. Major decisions should be reserved for the board; therefore, to implement an important new strategy initiative it may be necessary to call a board meeting. The time required to hold the meeting, giving the NEDs sufficient time to reach a well-informed opinion about the matter, may delay the implementation of the proposed strategy. It has also been argued that NEDs may be conservative in outlook, whereas the board of directors needs to be 'entrepreneurial'.

One counter-argument is that when a major new strategy or initiative is proposed, it should be given full and careful consideration before a decision is made. NEDs, with their range of skills and experience, can contribute positively to this decision-making process.

14.5 Myners Report and criticisms of non-executive directors (NEDs)

Weaknesses in the system of appointing NEDs has been recognised for many years and criticisms made in 2002 are probably still valid today. In February 2002 Paul (later Lord) Myners issued a UK government-backed report into pension fund investment. He accused boards of directors of public companies of being a 'self-perpetuating oligarchy', which failed to stand up for shareholders' rights against over-powerful executives. He condemned NEDs as the 'missing link' in the chain of good corporate governance. In particular, he criticised the way NED appointments were made and the number of NED positions that some individuals held.

The law makes no distinction between executive and non-executive directors. In principle, the NEDs could be equally liable with the executive directors for negligence and failure of duty. Arguably, this threat of criminal or civil liability could make NEDs more likely to support their executive colleagues.

TEST YOUR KNOWLEDGE 7.10

What are the main criticisms that have been made about NEDs?

CHAPTER SUMMARY

- Every organisation should be headed by an effective board, which has the collective responsibility for the long-term success of the organisation. Various corporate governance codes have identified the responsibilities of the board.
- According to the DH a NHS trust board has six key functions, for which it is held accountable by the Department on behalf of the Secretary of State.
- In most countries, there is a unitary board structure. In a few countries, notably Germany, there is a two-tier board structure with a supervisory board of NEDs led by the organisation chairman and a management board of executives led by the CEO. The two boards need to interact closely and constructively, even though one has a supervisory role over the other.
- In the NHS, the concept of a unitary board has not always been well understood or implemented. The dangers of not being a unitary board were reinforced by the *Integrated Governance Handbook* in 2006:
- Directors, and not shareholders/stakeholders, may exercise all the powers of the organisation. These powers are defined in the organisation's constitution (or articles of association) but are subject to some restraints in provisions of company law.
- In health service governance the powers of the NHS board of directors are set out in their governing document, e.g. foundation trusts have a written constitution that has to be approved by their

- regulator Monitor. This is then further defined by the Schedule of Matters Reserved for the Board, the Scheme of Delegation, Standing Orders and Standing Financial Instructions.
- In the NHS, the composition of the board is dictated either by the model standing orders issued by the DH or, if a foundation trust, then by the Core Constitution required by Monitor.
- In UK common law, directors have a fiduciary duty and a duty of skill and care to the organisation. This duty is owed to the organisation, not the shareholders/stakeholders. The common law duties of directors have now effectively been included in UK statute law, with the inclusion of a number of statutory general duties of directors in the Companies Act 2006.
- These statutory duties are the duties to act within their powers, promote the success of the organisation, exercise independent judgement, exercise responsible care, skill and diligence, avoid conflicts of interest, not accept benefits from third parties and declare any interest in a proposed transaction.
- The chairman is the leader of the board and the CEO is the leader of the executive management team.
- The *UK Code* states that the chairman should be independent on first appointment. It is therefore inappropriate to appoint a former CEO as chairman.
- The *UK Code* also states that the roles of chairman and CEO should not be combined and given to one individual, because this would create a position of 'unfettered power' on the board and would disturb the balance of the board and the ability of NEDs to challenge the executive management.
- A board should not be so large that it is unwieldy nor too small so that it lacks sufficient skills and experience. The *UK Code* recommends that at least 50% of the board (excluding the chairman) should be independent NEDs, except for smaller companies (listed companies outside the FTSE350) where there should be at least two independent NEDs.
- NEDs fulfil various roles: they contribute to discussions and decision-making by the board on strategy, they review the performance of executive management, they have a responsibility to ensure the integrity of financial information issued by the organisation and the effectiveness of risk management and internal control, and they are involved in the appointment of new directors and the remuneration of executive directors and other senior executives.
- 'Independence' of a NED is defined by the *UK Code* in terms of circumstances where a NED would normally be considered 'not independent'.
- The *UK Code* recommends that one of the independent NEDs should be nominated as the SID.
- The *UK Code* (and other national governance codes) calls for the establishment of board committees with governance responsibilities. The remuneration committee and the audit committee should consist entirely of independent NEDs and the nominations committee should have a majority of independent NEDs.
- There have been criticisms of NEDs. These include the argument that they are ineffective because they devote insufficient time to the organisation or have insufficient knowledge of the organisation's business.

Governance and boardroom practice

■ CONTENTS

1. Good boardroom practice
2. Board behaviour
3. Appointments to the board
4. Nomination committees
5. Succession planning
6. Refreshing board membership
7. Induction and training of directors
8. Performance evaluation of the board
9. Conflicts of interest
10. Hospitality policy and registers

■ INTRODUCTION

This chapter deals with governance issues relating to the board of directors. Board performance and operation was highlighted by the NHS Confederation in 2005 in their publication *Effective Boards in the NHS?* and in the NHS Leadership Council's *The Healthy NHS Board*. In particular *Effective Boards in the NHS?* outlined research, carried out by the NHS Confederation and the NHS Clinical Governance Support Team, which examined what board members believed were the characteristics of effective boards and how the actual practice of their boards compared with these views. In 2009, the ICSA also issued *Boardroom Behaviours*, suggesting that the effectiveness of a board is often damaged by poor boardroom behaviours, and recommending that guidelines on boardroom behaviours should be produced. There are also important governance issues relating to the identification and appointment of new directors, such as diversity, and the **induction** and continuing professional development of board directors. Board evaluation is a crucial part of developing appropriate boardroom practice. The DH has recently produced a Board Governance Assurance Framework, which assists aspirant foundation trust boards through a combination of self and independent assessment processes to ensure that they are appropriately skilled, and prepared to achieve FT authorisation. This will no doubt be a benchmark for NHS board evaluation in the future.

1 Good boardroom practice

1.1 Boardroom practice

Boardroom practice describes the way in which a board conducts its procedures and reaches its decisions.

The FRC *Guidance on Board Effectiveness*, issued in 2011, states that:

'An effective board develops and promotes its collective vision of the company's purpose, its culture, its values and the behaviours it wishes to promote in conducting its business. In particular it:

- provides direction for management;
- demonstrates ethical leadership, displaying – and promoting throughout the company – behaviours consistent with the culture and values it has defined for the organisation;

- creates a performance culture that drives value creation without exposing the company to excessive risk of value destruction;
- makes well informed and high quality decisions based on a clear line of sight into the business;
- creates the right framework for helping directors meet their statutory duties under the Companies Act 2006, and/or other relevant statutory and regulatory regimes;
- is accountable, particularly to those that provide the company's capital; and
- thinks carefully about its governance arrangements and embraces evaluation of their effectiveness.'

'An effective board should not necessarily be a comfortable place. Challenge, as well as teamwork, is an essential feature. Diversity in board composition is an important driver of a board's effectiveness, creating a breadth of perspective among directors, and breaking down a tendency towards "group think".'

The FRC *Guidance on Board Effectiveness* goes on to say that:

'Well-informed and high-quality decision making is a critical requirement for a board to be effective and does not happen by accident . . . Boards can minimise the risk of poor decisions by investing time in the design of their decision-making policies and processes, including the contribution of committees.'

'Good decision-making capability can be facilitated by:
- high quality board documentation;
- obtaining expert opinions when necessary;
- allowing time for debate and challenge, especially for complex, contentious or business critical issues;
- achieving timely closure; and
- providing clarity on the actions required, and timescales and responsibilities.'

1.2 Frequency of board meetings

A basic requirement of an effective board is that there should be regular board meetings. The *UK Corporate Governance Code* states simply that the board should meet sufficiently regularly to discharge its duties effectively, and there should be a formal schedule of matters reserved for the board.

1.3 The agenda

The agenda for board meetings is a governance issue in the sense that the chairman decides what the board will discuss when he sets the agenda. Although directors can raise matters as 'any other business', most of the time at board meetings is spent in discussion of the items listed by the chairman on the agenda.

It is therefore important that the agenda should include all matters reserved for board decision, whenever they arise. The company secretary can assist the chairman by providing advice and reminders.

1.4 Information

To enable them to contribute effectively to board discussions, directors must be provided with relevant information. They should receive relevant documents in advance of a board meeting, so that they have time to read them and think about the issues they deal with. The *UK Code* states that:

'The board should be supplied in a timely manner with information in a form and of a quality sufficient to enable it to discharge its duties.'

The chairman has the responsibility for ensuring that directors receive the information that they need in sufficient time. The code states that management has an obligation to provide the required information, but that the directors should ask for clarification or additional information if required.

The *Intelligent Board Report* states that 'every member of the board needs sufficient information at a high enough level to be confident that the organisation is well run, but not so much information that it becomes difficult to tell what is important' and that 'good governance is underpinned by intelligent information'.

Such information enables the board to:

- set an appropriately challenging, but achievable, strategic direction
- identify the strategic issues that require discussion or decision, and distinguish these issues from operational detail
- provide constructive challenge
- make sure that tax payers are receiving VFM
- identify trends in performance
- enable comparisons with the performance of similar organisations
- understand the needs, views and experiences of users and non-users from all backgrounds and communities
- make sure that users are receiving a high-quality service
- anticipate the potential impact of key policy, technological and socioeconomic developments
- assure themselves that the organisation is complying with standards and other regulatory requirements.

All information should:

- be clearly and simply presented, including graphic overviews as well as brief commentary
- be updated in a timely manner
- direct the board's attention to significant risks, issues and exceptions
- provide a level of detail appropriate to the board's role.

Information flows should be both formal and informal. Information is provided formally in documents or files, but this is supplemented by informal communication by e-mail, telephone or face-to-face conversation. Whether providing information formally or informally, the company secretary should ensure that there are good information flows between the board and its committees, between committees, and between executive managers and NEDs.

1.5 Support

As well as receiving relevant and timely information, directors should be given access to independent professional advice, at the organisation's expense, when they consider this necessary in order to fulfil their duties as director. For example, a director might ask to consult a lawyer for advice on a matter where the legal position is not clear.

NEDs and possibly also executive directors may also need administrative support or advice on routine matters, and board committees should be provided with sufficient resources to carry out their duties, and all directors should have access to the advice and assistance of the company secretary.

2 Board behaviour

There is a general consensus among recently published reports and reviews in both corporate and health service sectors that the quality of governance depends ultimately on the culture and behaviour of individuals, and consequently the ability of procedures and regulation to provide good governance is limited.

The **Walker Report** argued that both character and culture of the board members are important for an effective board. It commented that:

> 'Board conformity with laid-down procedures ... will not alone provide better corporate governance overall if the chairman is weak, if the composition and dynamic of the board is inadequate and if there is unsatisfactory ... engagement with its owners.'

The report went on to argue that the main weaknesses in the boards of banks had been caused by behavioural factors and a failure to challenge.

> 'The sequence in board discussion on major issues should be: presentation by the executive, a disciplined process of challenge, decision on the policy or strategy to be adopted and then full empowerment of the executive to implement. The essential 'challenge' step in the sequence appears to have been missed in many board situations and needs to be ... clearly recognised and embedded for the future.'

Effective Boards in the NHS? identified the behaviour and culture of a board as key determinants of the board's performance. From the interviews, the research identified four characteristics of effective boards:

- a focus on strategic decision-making
- board members who trust each other and act cohesively/behave corporately
- constructive challenge by board members of each other
- effective chairs who ensure meetings have clear and effective processes.

Some boards appeared to be too trusting, with little constructive challenge or debate about strategic issues. Reasons for this lack of challenge included the desire to present a united public face in public meetings. The perceived differences between non-executive and executive roles needs to be addressed as challenge should not be seen as the preserve of non-executives scrutinising the executive team.

The report concluded that a culture that enables board business to be conducted in a sharp and focused manner is required at board level, making clear what decisions are required of the board and what action will follow as a result of the decisions.

As far back as 2002, Jeffrey Sonnenfeld argued in the *Harvard Business Review* ('What makes boards great', *Harvard Business Review*, September 2002) that the behaviour of individual board members rather than the structures of the board were key determinants of organisational performance. Sonnenfeld argued that good board governance cannot be legislated but can be built over time. The 'best bets' for success are:

- a climate of trust and candour in which important information is shared with all board members and provided early enough for them to digest and understand it
- a climate in which dissent is not seen as disloyalty and in which mavericks and dissenters are not punished
- a fluid portfolio of roles for directors so individuals are not typecast into rigid positions on the board
- individual accountability with directors given tasks that require them to inform the rest of the board about issues facing the organisation
- regular evaluation of board performance.

The *Healthy Boards Report* identified boards as 'social systems' and summarised the techniques and practices that support and hinder the effectiveness of these social systems in Table 8.1.

2.1 ICSA report: *Boardroom Behaviours*

In 2009, the ICSA submitted a report to Sir David Walker who was reviewing the corporate governance issues that may have contributed to the 2007–2009 banking crisis in the UK. The ICSA report suggested that the corporate governance problem was partly attributable to inappropriate 'boardroom behaviours'.

Behavioural problems were only a part of the problem of ineffective governance, the report suggested, but insufficient attention had been given to the problem, and there should be better guidance to directors on how to improve board behaviours.

The report suggested that best practice in boardroom behaviour is characterised by:

- a clear understanding of the role of the board
- the appropriate deployment of knowledge, skills, experience and judgement
- independent thinking
- the questioning of assumptions and established orthodoxy
- challenge, which is constructive, confident, principled and proportionate
- rigorous debate
- a supportive decision-making environment
- a common vision
- the achievement of closure on individual items of board business.

Table 8.1 Techniques and practices that support and hinder boards

Ways of working that support good social processes	Ways of working that obstruct good social processes
Building a crystal clear understanding of the roles of the board and individual board members	Board members behaving in a way that suggests a 'master-servant' relationship between non-executive and executive
Actively working to develop and protect a climate of trust and candour	Executive directors only contributing in their functional leadership area rather than actively participating across the breadth of the board agenda
Building cohesion by taking steps to know and understand each other's backgrounds, skills and perspectives	Demonstrating an unwillingness to consider points of view that are different from individual directors' starting positions
Encouraging all board members to offer constructive challenges	Challenge primarily coming from non-executive directors, rather than all directors feeling empowered to challenge one another in board meetings
Sharing corporate responsibility and collective decision-making	Challenging in a way that is unnecessarily antagonistic and not appropriately balanced with appreciation, encouragement and support
Ensuring that neither chair nor chief executive power and dominance act to stifle appropriate participation in board debate	Working in ways that don't demonstrate overall confidence in the executive and that feed individual anxiety and insecurity about capability

The report commented that:

> 'Despite the importance of these . . . considerations, it is remarkable that there is practically no guidance in the Code on the main drivers of, and factors affecting, boardroom behaviours . . . To improve on existing standards of behaviour in the boardroom, directors need to develop a greater awareness of, and commitment to, "fit for purpose" governance as the means by which the board can collectively agree the business objectives of the company and a strategy for their implementation by executive management.'

Directors need to see best practice in governance as a 'business facilitator' and not a 'business killer'. The pursuit of best practice in governance should be seen as a way of achieving competitive advantage, because it strengthens the process and quality of decision-making by the board. Directors also need to be aware that failure to perform at a satisfactory level can have negative consequences, and directors need to be aware of their duties and potential liabilities. Failure to provide best practice in governance, and failure to perform at a satisfactory level, creates a risk to the reputation of boards of directors and individual directors.

2.2 Mapping the Gap

The ICSA research project – Mapping the Gap: highlighting the disconnect between governance best practice and reality in the NHS (July 2011) – was initiated to examine the degree to which trust boards in the NHS understood issues of governance, and the extent to which actual boardroom behaviour reflected guidance on best practice. The resulting report stated that respondents rated constructive challenge in the top three contributors to sound decision-making, but that the boardroom behaviours observed suggests that more challenge was required to improve discussions and decisions. The project further identified that on average respondents saw board trust and collective behaviours as a minimal contributory factor in an effective board. However, in the meetings observed there were a number of behaviours that did not suggest that all board members were fully engaging with the business to be transacted as can be seen in the table below. Examples of poor boardroom behaviour included using electronic devices, conversing with colleagues, interrupting, reading non-board papers, arriving late, fidgeting, exchanging knowing looks/raising eyebrows/rolling eyes.

2.3 Guidance on boardroom behaviours

The **ICSA report: Boardroom Behaviours** provided an outline of the guidance that might be useful to directors about boardroom behaviours:

- All directors, including executive directors, need to improve their performance in these important areas of boardroom behaviours. The process of achieving this for NEDs can be made more effective by giving them greater exposure to the organisation's operations.
- A knowledgeable board is a function of board balance, and there may be insufficient balance if the board is shrunk to just two executive directors (CEO and finance director) in order to achieve a majority of NEDs without making the board too big.
- Diversity of board membership is necessary to provide sufficient independent challenge.
- High standards of performance evaluation are needed to increase the effectiveness of a board.
- At the moment the remuneration of executive directors appears to focus on maximising short-term 'value' rather than pursuing the goal of a sustainable business. Remuneration arrangements should give more emphasis to the behaviours of directors in the boardroom, working in the long-term interests of the organisation.
- In terms of developing a wider perspective of the business, directors should look 'forward and out, as well as backwards and in'.
- The board should lead by example, 'evidenced by high levels of visibility and integrity, strong communications, and demanding expectations'.
- Practical issues, such as the timely circulation of board papers, 'can have a disproportionate effect on the quality of decision-making'.

TEST YOUR KNOWLEDGE 8.1

a List the techniques and practices that support and hinder the effectiveness of a healthy board.
b According to the *UK Code of Corporate Governance*, how often should a board of directors meet?
c How does the agenda for board meetings contribute to good governance?
d What are the characteristics of best practice in boardroom behaviour, as identified by the ICSA (2009)?
e Explain the meaning of the statement that directors should look on best practice in governance as a 'business facilitator', not a 'business killer'.

3 Appointments to the board

3.1 Board size and composition

The membership of a board of directors changes regularly, as some individuals resign or retire and new appointments are made. Generally in the private sector there are no regulations on the overall size of the board but NHS organisations have a provision about the composition of the board in their Standing Orders. These are set out by the DH in the NHS trust model standing orders, reservation and delegation of powers and standing financial instructions (March 2006). Foundation trusts will have a provision about board size within their constitutions.

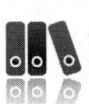

CASE EXAMPLE 8.1

The model standing orders for NHS trusts set out the composition of the Trust Board, which must be in accordance with the Membership, Procedure and Administration Arrangements Regulations, as follows:

- The Chairman of the Trust (Appointed by the NHS Appointments Commission).
- Up to five non-officer members (appointed by the NHS Appointments Commission).
- Up to five officer members (but not exceeding the number of non-officer members) including:
  - the chief executive; and
  - the Director of Finance.

The trust shall have not more than 11 and not less than eight members (unless otherwise determined by the Secretary of State for Health and set out in the Trust's Establishment Order or such other communication from the Secretary of State).

Similar model standing orders exist for SHAs and PCTs.

3.2 Board appointments in the NHS

In the NHS, the appointment of the chairman and NEDs has been generally overseen by the NHS Appointments Commission; however, foundation trust chairmen, are appointed by the Council of Governors and foundation trust NEDs are appointed by the Council of Governors.

The NHS Appointments Commission has the responsibility for ensuring that NHS organisations have chairs and non-executives who are capable, trained and supported to fulfil the function of governance. The NHS Trust Development Agency will be taking over this role as the HSC Act comes into force

The main functions of the NHS Appointments Commission have been to:

- appoint, re-appoint and, where necessary, to terminate the appointment of chairs and non-executives of SHAs, PCTs, NHS trusts and special health authorities
- ensure chairs and non-executives receive relevant and appropriate training
- ensure through annual performance review that chairs and non-executives are supported and developed in their role and feel valued
- ensure chairs and non-executives receive all necessary support through mentoring programmes
- ensure that overall NHS boards add value to the NHS locally and more widely.

The Commission follows the Commissioner for Public Appointment's Code of Practice, which guarantees that NHS and other regulated public appointments follow a fair, open and transparent appointments process, which commands public confidence, with appointment based on the principle of merit. The Code of Practice (August 2009), which is mandatory, sets out the regulatory framework for public appointments processes within the Commissioner's remit.

The code sets out the following principles:

- **Merit**. All public appointments must be governed by the overriding principle of selection based on merit, by the well-informed choice of individuals who through their abilities, experience and qualities match the need of the public body in question.
- **Independent scrutiny**. No appointment must take place without first being scrutinised by an independent panel or by a group including membership independent of the department filling the post.
- **Equal opportunities**. Departments should sustain programmes to deliver equal opportunities principles.
- **Probity**. Members of public bodies must be committed to the principles and values of public service and perform their duties with integrity.
- **Openness and transparency**. The principles of open government must be applied to the appointments process, its working must be transparent and information provided about the appointments made.
- **Proportionality**. The appointments procedures should be subject to the principle of proportionality, that is, they should be appropriate for the nature of the post and the size and weight of its responsibilities.

NEDs hold a statutory office under the National Health Service Act (2006) and their appointment does not create any contract of service or contract for services between the individual and the NHS trust.

At present, the Appointments Commission engage and support NHS trusts throughout the entire recruitment and selection process. It works with the trust's Nomination Committee (see Section 3) to conduct a full campaign, including developing a job description and person specification, advertising the post and supporting the interview process. The Commission's Health and Social Care Appointments Committee makes the final appointment decision based on the recommendation of the selection panel that assesses the merit of each application received.

Anyone currently employed by the NHS is disqualified from chair and non-executive appointments within the NHS. If existing chairs or non-executives subsequently take up NHS employment they would automatically be disqualified and required to resign. The purpose of creating non-executives is to ensure independent representation, i.e. non-staff members, on public bodies and counterbalance the executive team. People who work for the NHS would not be regarded as 'independent' by the general public.

The Appointments Commission ensures that all appointments of chairs and non-executives to NHS boards throughout England are made in a way that is open, transparent and fair to all applicants. All appointments are made in accordance with the Commissioner for Public Appointments. The Commission values and promotes diversity and is committed to equality of opportunity for all and appointments made on merit. It positively encourages applications from people from all sections of the community, from all backgrounds and with a broad range of experience. All decisions made are based on merit and the ability to meet the candidate specification.

The appointment process for foundation trust chairman and NEDs has already been set out in detail in Chapter 6.

3.3 Appointments in the corporate sector

Corporate governance is less specific than health service governance in this regard, although it is an accepted principle of good corporate governance that the power over board appointments should rest with the whole board. Under UK corporate governance, new appointments are made to the board at any time during the year, but each newly appointed director must offer himself for re-election at the next AGM. (The chairman of the company and the chairmen of the board committees are appointed by the board, and chairmanship appointments are not subject to shareholder approval at the next AGM.)

Recommendations about new appointments should not belong exclusively to the chairman and/or the CEO. Appointments should be made on merit and against objective criteria; however, in practice, criticism has been expressed about the way in which most appointments are made, particularly appointments of NEDs. This criticism centres on the fact that most NED appointments come from a fairly small circle of successful businessmen, many of whom know each other, whereas the net should be cast much wider and individuals from more diverse backgrounds should be chosen.

While the *UK Corporate Governance Code* remains a voluntary code, it states that there should be 'a formal, rigorous and transparent procedure for the appointment of new directors to the board'. The procedure of identifying candidates for a directorship should be rigorous, and candidates should be investigated thoroughly before the directorship is offered. The *UK Code* states that appointments should be made on 'merit' and 'against objective criteria'. However, it does not specify what these 'objective criteria' should be.

The procedure should be transparent so that shareholders and other stakeholders are able to see what is happening (what type of person the company is looking for and why a particular individual has been appointed). A formal procedure involves the nomination committee.

The Davies Review

Perhaps somewhat controversially, the code also states that appointments to the board should be made 'with due regard to the benefits of diversity on the board, including gender'. This reflect the widely expressed concern that the boards of major UK companies are dominated by middle-aged to older white males with a commercial or financial background, and that there are not enough directors with different attributes, talents and experience to provide boards with an appropriate balance. The relative shortage of female board directors has been well-publicised in the **Davies' Review** 'Women on Boards' (February 2011).

The review made a strong case for greater diversity on boards, and recommended in particular that there should be a greater proportion of women on the boards of FTSE350 companies. Its general argument in favour of greater diversity was that diverse and balanced boards: 'are more likely to be effective boards, better able to understand their customers and stakeholders, and to benefit fresh perspectives, vigorous challenge and broad experience. These in turn lead to better decision-making.'

The report rejected the view, for example, that directors (and particularly NEDs) should have had experience of financial responsibilities before their appointment. 'Although there is a real need for financial literacy, financial responsibility . . . can be taught and should not be a prerequisite for appointments.'

The review made ten recommendations, which can be summarised as follows:

- FTSE 100 companies should aim to have a minimum of 25% female representation on their board by 2015.
- All FTSE 350 chairmen should set out their target for the percentage of board members who are women by 2013 and 2015.
- Quoted companies should be required to disclose each year the proportion of women on the board, in senior executive positions and in the whole organisation. The *UK Corporate Governance Code* should require listed companies to establish a policy for boardroom diversity including measurable policy objectives. They should also disclose each year a summary of this policy and report on the progress towards achieving the policy objectives.
- The *UK Code* requires the nomination committee to report on its work in the annual report. In line with this requirement, companies should disclose 'meaningful information' about its appointment process and how it addresses the issue of diversity (including a description of the nomination and selection process).
- When searching for a new board appointee, companies should occasionally advertise the position because this may result in greater diversity among applicants.
- Executive search consultants should draw up a voluntary code of conduct for their 'industry' that addresses gender diversity and best practice with regard to research criteria and nomination processes for appointments to boards in FTSE350 companies.

The changes required will be incorporated in an updated version of the code to be published in 2012. These changes will require the inclusion of a description of the board's policy on diversity, including gender in the annual report and that the evaluation of the board should consider the balance of skills, experience, independence and knowledge of the company on the board, its diversity, including gender.

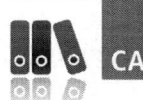

CASE EXAMPLE 8.2

A Canadian study 'Not just the right thing, but the bright thing', looking at public, not-for-profit and private boards, found that boards with three or more women on them showed very different governance behaviours to those with all-male boards. The more gender-balanced boards were more likely to identify criteria for measuring strategy, monitor its implementation, follow conflict of interest guidelines and adhere to a code of conduct. They were more likely to ensure better communication and focus on additional non-financial performance measures, such as employee and customer satisfaction, diversity and CSR. They were also more likely to have new director induction programmes and closer monitoring of board accountability and authority.

4 Nomination committees

The guidance for the NHS can be found in the DH guidance *The Intelligent Board*, which recommends that all NHS trusts should have a nomination committee, audit committee and remuneration (and terms of service) committee as part of their governance arrangements, reporting to the board of directors.

The nomination committee membership is appointed by the board of directors and is usually made up of at least three members, including the chairman of the NHS trust and the majority of whom shall be independent NEDs, and free of any conflict of interest. Only members of the committee have the right to attend committee meetings and other individuals such as the chief executive, the head of human resources and external advisers may be invited to attend for all, or part of, any meeting, as and when appropriate. The committee chairman shall be the chair or vice-chairman of the board of directors or an independent NED. Members conflicted on any aspect of an agenda presented to the committee, such as succession planning for an executive director vacancy, are required to declare their conflict and withdraw from discussions. Please refer back to Chapter 6 for the role of nomination committees in foundation trusts.

- This is very similar to the detailed corporate governance guidelines on the role of the nomination committee, in the *UK Code* that sets out a similar recommended framework: the search for new directors should be carried out by a nomination committee of the board, to which the full board delegates the responsibility
- the nomination committee should make recommendations to the board
- the board should consider the recommendations of the committee, and in normal circumstances should be expected to accept the recommendation.

It is important to note that a nomination committee does not have the authority to make new appointments; it simply carries out the search and makes the recommendation. Appointing new directors is a matter for the board, and decisions should therefore be made by the whole board.

It is also important to note that the need for a new board appointment, or a replacement for an existing board member (**succession planning**), is not necessarily decided by the nomination committee. The chairman has responsibility for ensuring that the composition of the board is appropriate. The need for a new NED may also emerge from the annual review of board performance, if an existing NED has not been performing as well as expected, or if a gap is identified in the range of skills and experience that the board needs. The chairman is also responsible for ensuring that there is succession planning for board positions, and may therefore ask the nomination committee to identify potential successors.

The *UK Code* similarly recommends that a nomination committee should be made up of a majority of independent NEDs and that the committee chairman should be either the board chairman or an independent NED. If the board chairman is the chairman of the nomination committee, he should not chair the committee when it is dealing with the succession to the chairmanship.

The existence of a majority of NEDs should ensure that the appointments process is not dominated by the chairman and CEO. The committee should consider new appointments to the board and make recommendations to the full board. The full board should then reach a decision about offering a position to the individual concerned so that final responsibility for board appointments remains with the board as a whole.

4.1 The main duties of the nomination committee

In the NHS the main role of the nomination committee is to:

- regularly review the structure, size and composition (including the skills, knowledge and experience) required of executive directors of the board compared, to its current position and make recommendations to the board with regard to any changes
- give full consideration to succession planning for all executive directors in the course of its work, taking into account the challenges and opportunities facing the trust, and what skills and expertise are therefore needed on the board of directors in the future
- before any appointment is made by the board of directors, evaluate the balance of skills, knowledge and experience on the board, and, in the light of this evaluation prepare a description of the role and capabilities required for a particular executive appointment. In identifying suitable candidates the committee shall:
    - use open advertising or the services of external advisers to facilitate the search
    - consider candidates from a wide range of backgrounds
    - consider candidates on merit and against objective criteria, taking care that appointees have enough time available to devote to the position
- review the job descriptions of the executive director role as required

- keep under review the leadership needs of the organisation, with a view to ensuring the continued ability of the organisation to deliver services effectively
- keep up to date and fully informed about strategic issues and commercial changes affecting the trust and the environment in which it operates
- review annually the performance evaluation process for executive directors ensuring it is fit for purpose.

The committee shall also make recommendations to the board of directors concerning:

- formulating plans for succession for executive directors
- membership of the audit and remuneration committees, in consultation with the chairmen of those committees
- any matters relating to the continuation in office of any executive director at any time including the suspension or termination of service.

The committee also ensures that the full range of eligibility checks have been performed and references taken and found to be satisfactory.

This is based on the principal duties of the nomination committee which were summarised in the Higgs *Suggestions for Good Practice* and which have been adopted in the NHS. See also the ICSA Guidance notes 'NHS Primary Care Trust Executive Directors Nomination Committee' and 'NHS Foundation Trust Non-Executive Directors Nomination Committee'.

The *UK Code* requires that a separate section of the annual report should describe the work of the nomination committee, including the process it used in relation to appointments that were made during the year. An explanation should be given if neither the services of an external search consultancy ('headhunters') nor advertising were used in making the appointment of chairman or NED. (If advertising the vacancy or a headhunter was not used, this would suggest that the appointment was made of a person that the nomination committee already knew or who was recommended privately: this would be contrary to the requirement for a formal, rigorous and transparent appointment procedure.) Executive directors may be appointed from within the company, so the requirement applies only to the appointment of a chairman or NED.

This is mirrored in the provisions of the *FT Code of Governance*.

4.2 Criteria for appointment

The *UK Code* includes several provisions about criteria for appointment to the board that are reflected in the health service governance for NHS organisations.

- The committee 'should evaluate the balance of skills, experience, independence and knowledge and experience of the board, and, in the light of this evaluation, prepare a description of the role and capabilities required for the particular appointment' (and (see above) from 2012 the code will also require gender diversity in this evaluation).
- On initial appointment, the chairman should meet the criteria for independence.
- For the appointment of a chairman, the nomination committee should prepare a job specification, including an assessment of the time required and recognising the need for the chairman's availability in times of crisis.
- The departing chairman should not chair the nomination committee when it is meeting to consider the appointment of the successor to the chairmanship.
- A proposed new chairman's other significant commitments should be disclosed to the board and council (FTs only) before an appointment is made, and included in the annual report. (Subsequent changes should also be disclosed and reported.)

4.3 Practical aspects of board appointments: time commitment

In practice, a nomination committee is likely to carry out its responsibilities by:

- using a firm of headhunters to find individuals outside the firm who might be suitable for appointment (as NED, CEO, finance director, and so on)
- vetting the candidates put forward by the headhunters
- making a selection and recommendation to the full board or council.

When an individual is appointed to the board, the appointment may be for a fixed term. This is usually the case with NEDs; in the UK, NEDs are typically appointed on a fixed three-year contract, which may then be renewed at the end of each three-year term. Executive directors are commonly appointed for an indeterminate length of time, subject to a minimum notice period (typically six months in the NHS).

'All directors must be able to allocate sufficient time to the company to discharge their responsibilities effectively' (*UK Code*). Executive directors are full-time appointments, so the problem of time commitment is not usually significant for them (unless the executive is also appointed as NED for another company). The main problem is ensuring that the chairman and NEDs give sufficient time to the company. More time will probably be required from the chairman than from a NED, and some NEDs (e.g. the chairman of the audit committee) will be expected to commit more time than other NEDs.

When the nomination committee prepares a job description for the position, this should include an estimate of the time commitment expected. A NED should undertake that he will have sufficient time to meet what is expected of them. This undertaking could be written into the NED's letter of appointment.

Governing the NHS (June 2003) said this:

'In our view a [NHS] non-executive serving on a board, which is properly focused on its governance responsibilities and which is properly supported by papers and information from the executive team, should be able to fulfil the role in 2½ days. This may be regarded as the minimum acceptable commitment. Clearly some individuals will be able to give more time to the organisation and where this is helpful we are not suggesting that it should be discouraged. However, these additional duties should not be regarded as an extension or part of their board role or cross the boundaries set out above.'

NED posts currently being advertised on the Appointment Commission website still show a minimum time commitment of 2½ days per month. The commitment for a NHS chair is commonly around 3½ days per week.

If an individual who is proposed to the board as chairman or NED has significant time commitments outside the organisation, this should be disclosed to the board (and council) before the appointment is made.

An organisation should also protect itself against the risk that an executive director is unable to commit sufficient time to the company because of NED appointments with other companies. The *UK Code* states that the board should not allow one of its own executive directors to take on:

- more than one NED post in a FTSE 100 company, or
- the chairmanship of a FTSE 100 company.

4.4 The talent pool for new directors

Following publication of the Higgs Report in 2003, the government set up a taskforce under the chairmanship of Laura Tyson, then Dean of the London Business School, to look into the recruitment and development of NEDs. The *Tyson Report on the Recruitment and Development of Non-Executive Directors* was published in June 2003. The report argued that a range of different experiences and backgrounds among board members could enhance the effectiveness of the board, and suggested how a broader range of NEDs could be identified and recruited. The Report criticised the practice (current at that time) of appointing individuals without a formal interview. This method of recruitment tended to overlook a number of potentially rich sources of NEDs.

Although elements of the Tyson Report remain valid, the Davies 'Women on Boards Review' has taken the issue of diversity considerably further as we have seen earlier in the chapter.

In the NHS, the requirement to openly advertise all NED appointments under the auspices of the Appointments Commission has gone some way to addresses these issues both in terms of ethnicity and gender. The Equality Act 2010 also imposes a duty on public bodies to achieve equal opportunities in the workplace and in wider society. The Act is supported by specific duties, which require public bodies to publish relevant, proportionate information demonstrating their compliance with the Equality Duty; and to set themselves specific, measurable equality objectives. NHS trusts must set objectives that eliminate unlawful discrimination, harassment and victimisation, advance equality of opportunity and foster good relations.

> **TEST YOUR KNOWLEDGE 8.2**
>
> a Explain the composition of an NHS trust board as outlined by DH's model standing orders.
> b What are the key principles that the Appointments Commission must follow in the appointment of NHS NEDs?
> c What are the responsibilities of a nomination committee?
> d What are the provisions in the *UK Corporate Governance Code* relating to nominations and appointments to the board?
> e How much time should NEDs be required to commit to the organisation, and should this be a contractual commitment?
> f What were the recommendations of the 2011 Davies Review?

4.5 Accepting an offer of appointment as a non-executive director (NED)

The formal procedures for appointing a new NED are the same for the appointment of an executive director. However, a NED will be less familiar with the organisation than a senior executive manager and he should not accept an appointment unless he is satisfied that there are no matters of concern.

An individual should only be willing to accept an appointment as NED if:

- the organisation does not use unethical business practices and has a good reputation
- the organisation is a going concern and is not in financial difficulties
- he can commit to the role the time that the organisation expects
- the individual believes that he can contribute positively to the effectiveness of the board
- there is no risk that the directors of the organisation could be held liable for any breach of duty, or that there is sufficient directors' and officers' liability insurance as protection against this risk
- the fee that the organisation has offered is adequate.

As the ICSA has commented:

> 'By making the right enquiries, asking the right questions and taking care to understand the replies, a prospective director can reduce the risk of nasty surprises and dramatically increase the likelihood of success.'

Guidance from the ICSA on the due diligence that a prospective NED should undertake recommends asking questions about:

- the business, e.g. its nature and size, and the organisation's market share, financial performance and financial position
- governance and stakeholder relations – who the major stakeholders are, and about the structure of the board of directors and its committees
- the role that the NED would be expected to perform, including membership of board committees. The prospective NED should be satisfied that he has the necessary qualities or experience to make an effective contribution to work of the organisation's board
- the organisation's risk management systems and controls
- ethical issues, and whether there are any ethical matters that might give cause for concern.

NHS NEDs might also want to ask questions about the impact of any health reform legislation.

Answers to many of these questions can be obtained from published documents that are available, in paper form or on a website, to the general public. These include the annual report and accounts of the organisation, the organisation's constitution, standing orders or articles of association, any **sustainability report** or social and environmental report that the organisation publishes, and press reports about the organisation.

Terms of engagement

If a prospective NED decides to accept the offer of the appointment, terms of engagement should be agreed with the organisation (either the board as a whole or its nomination committee). The terms that must be agreed are as follows:

- The initial period of tenure in office (normally three years).
- **Time commitment**. The organisation must indicate how much time the NED is expected to commit to the organisation, and the NED should make this commitment. This should be included in the formal letter of appointment.*
- **Remuneration**. The annual remuneration of the NED should be agreed. This is usually a fixed annual fee. It is generally considered inappropriate for NEDs, including the chairman, to be remunerated on the basis of incentive schemes linked to company performance, because this would undermine their independence.

* Typically, NEDs of listed companies are expected to commit between 15 and 30 days each year, and possibly more for a committee chairman. NHS NEDs are expected to commit a minimum of 30 days each year, with more for a committee chairman.

The terms of engagement should be set out in a formal letter of appointment. As well as including details of the role that the NED will be required to perform (including initial membership of board committees), the expected time commitment, the tenure and the remuneration, the letter of engagement should also:

- specify that the NED should treat all information received as a director as confidential to the company
- indicate the arrangements for induction
- give details of directors' and officers' liability insurance that will be available
- indicate the need for an annual performance review process for directors
- state what organisation resources will be made available to the NED (e.g. desk, computer terminal and telephone).

A sample letter of appointment for a NED can be found on the ICSA website.

TEST YOUR KNOWLEDGE 8.3

a What issues should an individual consider before accepting the offer of an appointment as independent NED of an NHS organisation?
b How much time should NEDs of an NHS organisation be required to commit and should this be a contractual commitment?

5 Succession planning

The key positions on the board of directors are the chairman of the board and the CEO. The individuals holding these positions will retire or resign at some time, e.g. because the individual has reached retirement age or has come to the end of a fixed-term contract.

The board of directors should try to ensure a smooth succession, with a replacement lined up to take the place of the departing individual. In the case of a departing CEO, the successor might be an existing executive manager who has been groomed for the role. In the case of a departing chairman, the successor might be an external appointment. A smooth succession is desirable to avoid disruptions to the organisation's decision-making processes or changes in policy or direction. The succession can also be planned well in advance, so that the newly appointed individuals will have an opportunity to learn about their new role before the actual succession occurs.

The FRC *Guidance on Board Effectiveness* states that while 'Executive directors may be recruited from external sources, companies should also develop internal talent and capability'. Initiatives might include middle management development programmes, facilitating engagement from time to time with NEDs, and partnering and mentoring schemes.

The positions of chairman and CEO (and finance director and CFO) are important and it is undesirable to have vacancies in these positions for more than a short time. Ideally, the successor should be in place for immediate appointment. This is why succession planning should be carried out in advance.

Succession planning should be delegated to the nomination committee. If the board of a listed company intends to breach the governance code by appointing the current CEO as the next chairman, it would be advisable for a suitable representative of the board (e.g. the chairman of the nomination committee or the SID) to discuss the reasons for their choice with major shareholders and representative bodies of the institutional shareholders. These discussions should take place well in advance of any final decision about the appointment.

There should also be succession planning for NEDs. As stated above, NEDs are typically appointed in the UK for a fixed period of three years, but, see below, it is now a requirement of the *UK Code* that directors of FTSE 350 companies should stand for re-election annually. The three year contract may be extended at the end of that time for another three years and so on. Over time, a NED may lose some of his independence. It was explained in the previous chapter that a NED is generally considered 'not independent' if he has been with the company for nine years or more.

The *FT Code of Governance* and the *UK Code* both include a provision that any term beyond six years for a NED should be subject to particularly rigorous review. The board should be continually refreshed, and this is achieved by appointing a new NED when the three-year term of an existing NED reaches its end or in the case of a FTSE350 company where a NED has performed poorly, nor supporting his or her annual re-election.

The nominations committee may recommend the re-appointment of a NED at the end of his first year term, but should be more inclined to terminate the appointment after six years, when the second three-year term ends.

 STOP AND THINK 8.1

The chairman of a foundation trust who was facing a re-appointment process in order to continue as the chairman of the trust is insisting on chairing the governors nominations committee that would be carrying out the appointment process.

What is your advice to the nominations committee about the conflict of interest that would arise and how would you resolve it?

6 Refreshing board membership

The *FT Code of Governance* and the *UK Code* state that there should be 'progressive refreshing of the board'. Refreshing the board calls for succession planning as outlined above, and the nomination committee should be aware when a vacancy is expected to arise and should plan in advance to appoint the type of person it considers would improve the balance of skills and experience on the board.

However, in listed companies, the board is also refreshed through the re-election of directors by the shareholders at AGMs. The procedures for this are primarily a matter for the company's constitution (articles of association). However, it is widely accepted that directors should be subject to re-election by the shareholders at regular intervals.

In the UK, the corporate governance code until 2010 recommended that each director should be subject to election by the shareholders at the AGM following his appointment, and then subject to re-election every three years (until the director resigns, chooses not to stand for re-election or is removed from office).

The financial crisis in banking in 2007–2009 led to a re-assessment of this provision, when it was argued that some or all of the board should be subject to annual re-election. Annual re-election increases the accountability of the directors to the shareholders and also gives more power to the shareholders, who are able to threaten to vote against a director at the next AGM (instead of possibly having to wait up to three years before having the opportunity).

After extensive consultation by the FRC, the provisions included in the 2010 *UK Code* are:

- annual re-election of directors of FTSE 350 companies
- annual re-election of all NEDs who have served longer than nine years on the board
- the same recommendations as before for directors of other companies subject to the *UK Code*: all other directors to be subject to re-election at the first AGM following their appointment and re-election subsequently at intervals of no more than three years.

The *UK Code* also requires that when the board proposes a NED for election at an AGM, they should present reasons why the directors believe that the individual should be appointed. When a director is proposed for re-election, the chairman should confirm to the shareholders that following a formal performance evaluation of the individual, he has concluded that the individual's performance continues to be effective and the individual remains committed to the role.

The requirement for the board to ensure planned and progressive refreshing means that re-election of current directors, particularly NEDs, should not be an automatic process. As indicated earlier, plans to refresh the board with new NEDs should be a part of succession planning.

TEST YOUR KNOWLEDGE 8.4

a Why is it desirable to plan for **board succession**?
b How is the board of an NHS organisation regularly refreshed?
c What are the requirements in the *UK Corporate Governance Code* regarding the re-election of directors?

7 Induction and training of directors

7.1 Induction of new directors

The induction of directors is a process by which new directors familiarise themselves with the business, its products or services and how it operates. New directors need induction in order to become effective contributors to the board decision-making process. The need for induction is more important for NEDs than for internally appointed executive directors, who should be familiar with much of the business before their appointment to the board. However, newly appointed executive directors may not be familiar with all the responsibilities and duties of being a director, and may need induction to make them more aware of what will be expected of them in their new role.

In the NHS, the Appointments Commission has provided a structured induction to new NEDs with ongoing support around key issues. The induction is provided in partnership with the NHS and SHAs, and involves a year-long induction programme, which is planned to complement training received locally. The Appointments Commission induction programme has three key stages:

- On taking up the post an induction pack is issued, which includes terms and conditions, codes of conduct, roles and responsibilities, guidance on the appraisal process, and what to expect in the way of local training, together with a list of useful contacts.

- After three months, a two-day residential course is offered, which includes presentations on key topics, such as finance, legal issues and decision-making and interactive working sessions. It also provides opportunity to network with other newly appointed NEDs from around the country.
- Ongoing development is then offered through a number of online training opportunities that can be tailored to suit specific interests, skills and experience. Modules include governance, finance and strategic planning.

The *UK Code of Corporate Governance* states that **all** directors should receive **induction** on joining the board and that 'to function effectively all directors need appropriate knowledge of the organisation and access to its operations and staff'.

The chairman is responsible for ensuring that new directors receive 'full, formal and tailored' induction. Although there is no specific reference to the company secretary, the chairman will probably ask the company secretary to arrange for each director to receive a personalised induction programme. The aim should be to make the director an effective member of the board quickly, and an induction programme may therefore focus initially on providing essential information and familiarity with the organisation, such as visits to key sites, meetings with senior management and staff and providing copies of previous board meetings and copies of any current strategy documents. Over time, further induction may then be provided.

Reading is an effective way for an individual to absorb new information quickly, and the company secretary might therefore wish to give a new director a selection of documents as an induction pack.

FRC *Guidance on Board Effectiveness* provides useful guidance on induction.

A NED should, on appointment, devote time to a comprehensive, formal and tailored induction that should extend beyond the boardroom. Initiatives such as partnering a NED with an executive board member may speed up the process of him or her acquiring an understanding of the main areas of business activity, especially areas involving significant risk. The director should expect to visit, and talk with, senior and middle managers in these areas.

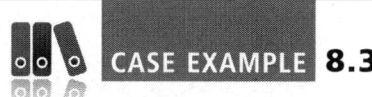 **CASE EXAMPLE 8.3**

NHS Board development

GatNet is a Practice Based Commissioning cluster of 34 practices, based in a former PCT locality, serving around 200,000 people. It is the biggest of six Consortia in NHS South of Tyne and Wear, formed from three former clusters. There is a strong sense of identity and shared history. The practices have collaborated in an out-of-hours cooperative and in a Community Based Care organisation (CBC).

GatNet created a clear, well-planned and facilitated development process. The PCT has supported the development programme, which has included:

- a development programme with the board and extended to other clinicians to secure succession planning
- 360-degree appraisal and psychometric tests were used to support clinical lead development
- commissioning skills – e.g. training in peer review of referrals for GPs and leaning of management skills for members of the clinical team;
- time out to work through the shape and function of the Commissioning Board
- regular time in/time out sessions (TITO) for clinicians and managers (influenced by their needs).

7.2 Induction of an executive manager as an executive director

The induction process described above is much more relevant to an individual joining as a director from outside the organisation. For an individual who is already an executive manager of the organisation and now appointed as executive director, the induction process needs a different focus. A senior executive of the organisation should already be familiar with many aspects of the organisation's operations (although his induction might include visits to parts of the organisation he has not worked with before).

An executive manager 'promoted' to the board is much more likely to lack knowledge and experience about being a director and governance. (However, some large companies try to give their senior executives experience as a director, by allowing them to take a position as a NED in another organisation.)

An induction programme for such an individual may therefore need to focus on matters such as:

- the role of the board, including matters reserved for the board and oversight of management
- the powers and duties of directors, and the rights of shareholders/stakeholders (the new director should be given a copy of the organisation's constitution (articles of association))
- the role of board committees
- the role of the board in monitoring risk and **internal control** (see also Chapter 12)
- membership of the board and its committees, how the board operates and the role of the company secretary
- frequency of board meetings
- what the new director will be expected to contribute
- who the major shareholders/stakeholders are and their relationship with the organisation
- compliance with governance requirements
- the potential liabilities of directors
- directors' liability insurance
- organisation policy on CSR
- arrangements for monitoring the performance of board members.

And for listed companies the law relating to fair dealing by directors (the law on insider dealing) and in the UK the Model Code on share dealing by directors should be set out.

This list is not exhaustive. However, in some cases it might be considered too long. The main point is that an executive manager appointed as a director needs to learn about the differences in the roles of manager and director, and that he has not been appointed as a director simply to be a 'high level' executive of the organisation.

7.3 Training and professional development

Directors should keep their knowledge and skills up to date, so that they can continue to perform effectively, and the organisation should ensure that this is provided. The appropriate training and personal development for each individual director will depend on the director's personal situation.

- All directors may need training or updating when there is a change in an important aspect of the law or when new regulations are introduced that affect the organisation's operations or its governance.
- Members of board committees may need to be updated or may need to acquire greater in-depth knowledge of matters affecting the work of their committee.
- Directors may need to be informed about an important new service or product or an important new acquisition for the organisation.

Reflecting as it does the *UK Code*, the *FT Code of Governance* states that:

> 'The chairman should ensure that the directors continually update their skills and the knowledge and familiarity with the company required to fulfil their role both on the board and on board committees. The company should provide the necessary resources for developing and updating its directors' knowledge and capabilities.'

FRC Guidance states:

> 'Non-executive directors should devote time to developing and refreshing their knowledge and skills, including those of communication, to ensure that they continue to make a positive contribution to the board. Being well-informed about the company, and having a strong command of the issues relevant to the business, will generate the respect of the other directors.'

The particular training and development needs for each individual director should be assessed by the chairman, but each director should be able to make suggestions about the type of training or development that might be suitable for him personally. The *UK Code* includes a provision that the chairman should agree a personalised approach to training and development with each director. This should be reviewed regularly. The obvious time to do this is during the annual performance review of the director.

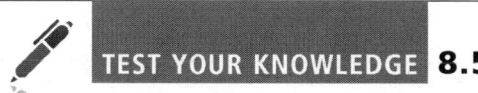 **TEST YOUR KNOWLEDGE 8.5**

What should the induction of a new director consist of?

8 Performance evaluation of the board

8.1 Requirement for annual evaluation

A possibly contentious issue in both corporate and health service governance is the extent to which the performance of directors should be monitored and assessed, and what form such assessments should take. In the UK, a requirement for company directors to undergo formal performance appraisals each year was introduced into the *UK Corporate Code* in 2003.

The *FT Code of Governance* and the *UK Code* states as a main principle that the board should undertake a 'formal and rigorous annual evaluation of its own performance and that of its committees and individual directors'.

Evaluation of individual directors should aim to show whether each director:

- continues to contribute effectively
- continues to demonstrate commitment to the role (e.g. in terms of time spent carrying out the director's duties, attendance at board and committee meetings, and on other duties).

The evaluation of performance is particularly important for NEDs. Executive directors commit all or most of their time to the organisation and should be fully familiar with the business and the organisation's operations. In contrast, NEDs spend only a part of their time with the organisation, even though they make up the membership of key board committees – the audit and remuneration committees in particular. There is a possibility that NEDs will lose some of their enthusiasm for the organisation, and may get into a habit of missing meetings and not spending as much time with the organisation as expected. In some cases, a director may fail to keep up to date with an important area of his supposed expertise. The FRC *Guidance on Board Effectiveness* states that 'evaluation should be bespoke in its formulation and delivery'.

Originally, the UK Code did not recommend how the performance evaluation of the board, its committees and individual directors should be carried out, or who should do it. It became established practice, however, that except for the performance review of the chairman himself, the chairman should organise the performance review process and should be closely involved in it.

One approach is for the chairman to carry out the reviews personally, possibly with advice and assistance from the company secretary. Alternatively, the chairman may be responsible for deciding on the process that should be used for the performance review, and should act on the findings of the review, but may hand the responsibility for conducting the review to the SID. Organisations may also use the services of specialist external consultants.

The NHS Appointments Commission has an established evaluation system in place for NHS NEDs, which sets out the key principles and minimum standards for a performance and development review process (appraisal) for chairs and NEDs. It provides a framework for:

- holding all chairs and NEDs to account for their performance
- setting appropriate objectives, consistent with the chair or NED role;
- identifying learning and development needs
- supporting succession planning and the management of the NED talent pool
- ensuring the process is proportionate to the chair/NED role, i.e. appropriate to the nature of the role and the size/weight of responsibilities.

Key principles:

- There should be, as a minimum, an annual performance and development review meeting for the chair and each NED, throughout the term of their appointment. This could be supplemented by interim review(s), where necessary and appropriate.
- Individuals should be made aware, on appointment, that they will be appraised, the standards against which they will be appraised, and have an opportunity to contribute to and approve their reports.
- The annual performance and development review meeting should be clearly recognised as such by the individual, i.e. it should not be an informal 'coffee shop' conversation or an 'add-on' to a different conversation.
- Performance Reviews should be evidence-based with relevant examples for conclusions drawn.
- Objectives for the chair/NED should reflect a link to the key objectives of the organisation, where possible.

All performance reviews must be formally recorded. This is a requirement of Office of the Commissioner of Public Appointments and is also vital in the event of any complaint requiring investigation. Evidence that a review has taken place and details of the performance assessment made must be recorded and sent to the Appointments Commission on completion of the review meeting.

The *FT Code of Governance* and the *UK Code* requires that the board should state in the organisation's annual report how the performance evaluation of the board, its committees and individual directors has been carried out. In addition the *FT Code of Governance* requires the outcomes of the evaluation of the executive directors to be reported to the board of directors and for the chief executive to take the lead on the evaluation of the executive directors.

8.2 Evaluation of the board

In the UK, the potential value of external consultants has been recognised, and the *UK Code* now states that for the evaluation of the board as a whole:

- the evaluation of the board of FTSE companies should be 'externally facilitated' at least every three years; in other words, the company should use specialist external consultants at least once every three years, and
- where the company uses external consultants, the company should make a statement of whether the consultants have any other connection with the company. (Independent consultants are more likely to provide better advice.)

This is echoed in the *FT Code of Governance*, which requires the statement in the annual report to explain why the NHS foundation trust adopted a particular method of performance evaluation, bearing in mind the desirability for independent assessment.

A FTSE 350 company might therefore use external consultants in one year, and then the chairman might use the lessons obtained from the consultants to carry out an internal performance evaluation for the next two years. In year four, external consultants might be used again as a way of learning new lessons or checking the quality of the internal evaluation process.

The possible reasons for an ineffective board may be any of the following.

- Insufficient information provided to the directors to enable them to make properly considered decisions.
- Directors not given sufficient time before a board meeting to read relevant papers, and so arrive at the meeting not properly briefed.
- Directors not bothering to take time before a board meeting to read relevant papers, and so arrive at the meeting not properly briefed.
- Individual directors failing to attend meetings of the board or meetings of board committees.
- Individual directors not being given enough opportunity to contribute to discussions in board meetings (this would arguably be a failing of the chairman rather than an indication of an ineffective board).
- The board failing to carry out its responsibilities in full.
- The board failing to take its annual performance evaluation seriously enough.
- The board making ill-considered (bad) strategic decisions.

To assess the performance of the board, a comparison should be made between what the board should be expected to achieve, and what it has actually achieved. One way of doing this may be to provide answers to a set of questions about performance, possibly through discussions at a special board meeting.

Questions that may provide a useful basis for assessment of board performance are set out below:

- Does the board have any specific performance objectives, e.g. in terms of business performance or dividend payments? How well has the board performed against any such targets?
- What has the board contributed to the development of strategy and what has the board done to oversee the implementation of strategy and achievement of strategy targets?
- What has the board contributed to ensuring that the company has a robust and effective risk management system?
- Is the board concerning itself with the appropriate issues? Is the list of matters reserved for the board suitable or should it be amended?
- Is the board an appropriate size and is the mix of members suitable (in terms of spread of experience, knowledge, skills and/or background)? Are changes needed?
- How well does the board communicate with management, employees, shareholders and other stakeholders?

Questions may also be asked about the effectiveness of boardroom practice:

- Do board members receive relevant and clear information in good time for board meetings and decision-making? Is the amount and quality of this information adequate?
- Have there been sufficient board meetings in the past year?
- Are the board meetings too short to be effective or too long?

The Board Governance Assurance Framework introduced by the DH in January 2012 for aspirant foundation trusts set out a clear benchmark as to what constitutes effective board room practice. The self-assessment, which is then followed up by an independent examination, would look at the following areas:

1 Board composition and commitment
    1.1 Board positions and size
    1.2 Balance and calibre of board members
    1.3 Board member commitment
2 Board evaluation, development and learning
    2.1 Effective board level evaluation
    2.2 Whole Board Development Programme
    2.3 Board induction, succession and contingency planning
    2.4 Board member appraisal and personal development
3 Board insight and foresight
    3.1 Board performance reporting
    3.2 Efficiency and Productivity

  3.3 Environmental and strategic focus
  3.4 Quality of board papers and timeliness of information
4 Board engagement and involvement
  4.1 External stakeholders
  4.2 Internal stakeholders
  4.3 Board profile and visibility
  4.4 Future engagement with FT Governors.

8.3 Evaluation of board committees

Board committees should be evaluated in a similar way to the board as a whole. For each committee, there should be a comparison between what the committee is responsible for doing and what it has actually done:

- Has the nomination committee been successful in identifying suitable individuals for board appointments?
- Have any individuals been appointed to the board who, in retrospect, were not as good as originally thought?
- Has the nomination committee done any succession planning and if so, how good have its plans been?
- Has the committee made clear recommendations to the board, and has the board acted on its recommendations?
- Is the committee an appropriate size and is the mix of members suitable? Are changes needed?
- Have there been enough committee meetings during the past year?

Similar questions can be asked about the remuneration committee and audit committee, whose work is described in later chapters.

8.4 Evaluation of individual board members

The performance of individual executive directors as executive managers is not dealt with by a governance code, because individual executive performance is not a governance issue. For governance purposes, the evaluation of performance relates to performance as a director.

 For an independent NED, key questions for evaluation include the following:

- How many board meetings has the director attended, and how many times has he been absent?
- How well prepared has the individual been for meetings, e.g. has he read the relevant papers in advance?
- What has been the quality of contributions of the individual to board meetings, e.g. on strategic development and risk management?
- Has the individual shown independence of character, or has he tended to go along with the opinions of certain other board members?
- How many board committee meetings has the director attended and how many has he missed?
- What has the individual contributed to committee meetings?
- Has the time commitment of the director been sufficient? Has the time commitment been as much as expected, or as much as stated in the director terms of appointment?
- Does the NED continue to show interest in and enthusiasm for the organisation?
- Are there reasons why the director may no longer be considered independent?
- Does the director communicate well with the other directors and with senior executives of the organisation?

The *UK Code* states that: 'Individual evaluation should aim to show whether each director continues to contribute effectively and to demonstrate commitment to the role (including commitment of time for board and committee meetings and any other duties).'

8.5 Evaluation of the chairman

The NHS Appointments Commission also plays a key role in the annual appraisal of NHS chairs. This is then used as part of the evaluation process, e.g. the SHA chairman will use the appraisals as part of their review of all of the chairs appointed in their regional area. NEDs of the respective trusts will also be consulted as part of that evaluation process. In foundation trusts, the evaluation of the chairman is undertaken by the governors assisted by the SID (see Chapter 6).

The *UK Code* states that the NEDs, led by the SID, should be responsible for the performance evaluation of the chairman, 'taking into account the views of executive directors'. However, the actual performance review of the chairman may be conducted for the NEDs by external consultants.

The chairman's performance should be assessed by comparing his responsibilities with his achievements, and asking whether he has been successful in providing the board leadership that should be expected of him.

This is reflected in the *FT Code of Governance* for the evaluation of a FT chairman and requires the input of the Council of Governors.

8.6 Using the results of a performance review

To obtain practical value from an annual evaluation of the board, its committees and its individual directors, the board should be prepared to act on its findings whenever performance is not considered to be as good as it should be. The chairman has the responsibility for acting to deal with poor performance.

The *UK Corporate Governance Code* makes the following provisions for how the performance review should be used:

> 'The chairman should act on the results of the performance evaluation by recognising both the strengths and weaknesses of the board and, where appropriate, proposing new members to be appointed to the board or seeking the resignation of directors.'

In the preface to the 2010 *UK Code*, the chairman of the FRC stated:

> 'Chairmen are encouraged to report personally in their annual statements how the principles relating to the role and effectiveness of the board have been applied.'

The recommendation is that the chairman of a company should recognise his personal responsibility for performance and effectiveness of the board, and a company should not simply disclose its procedures for assessing performance in a 'boiler plate' fashion.

The chairman may also consider the need for changes to the composition of board committees and may ask for the resignation of a committee chairman. Some improvements may be achieved by changing board procedures (e.g. holding meetings more frequently, or changing the dates of meetings to give management more time to prepare the information required).

Although the chairman has the primary responsibility for acting on the results of the annual performance review, the FRC guidance 'Improving Board Effectiveness' states that: 'The results of a board evaluation should be shared with the board as a whole and fed back, as appropriate, into the board's work on composition, the design of induction and development, and other relevant areas.'

8.7 Problems with performance reviews

The performance evaluation of the board and its directors is recognised in the UK as a valuable tool for the assessment of the effectiveness of the board, and institutional investors have shown an interest in obtaining information about the evaluation process. They want to know that an evaluation has taken place, but they also need assurance that the evaluation process is of a suitable quality standard and rigour. This is a reason why the *UK Code* introduced a requirement for external consultants to be used at least every three years.

Investors would also like to know more about the action that has been taken following an annual performance review, because they want assurance that the review is being used to improve the effectiveness of the board. However, it may be difficult to provide as much information about the performance review, especially the review of individual directors, without compromising the confidentiality of the exercise.

This has encouraged a similar approach in the NHS, as key stakeholders have expressed a similar concern about board performance.

TEST YOUR KNOWLEDGE 8.6

a What are the requirements in the *FT Code of Governance* and the *UK Code* for the performance evaluation of the board, its committees and its individual directors?
b What is the purpose of an annual performance evaluation of the board and its directors?
c How does the NHS Appointments Commission underpin the evaluation of board chairs and NEDS?
d What factors should be considered when reviewing the performance of a NED?
e How might a chairman arrange for the evaluation of the performance of the board and its directors?

9 Conflicts of interest

The board of directors of an NHS organisation has a legal obligation to act in the best interests of that organisation, in accordance with the governing document, and to avoid situations where there may be a potential conflict of interest. As such, there are requirements for board members to register personal financial interests that may be perceived as conflicting with that overriding duty.

The Appointment Commission's *Code of Conduct and Accountability* are quite clear in that NHS boards should act in a way that protects the interest of the NHS in the way they undertake their business.

Furthermore, *Governing the NHS* guidance states: 'NHS boards should conduct themselves and the business of the Trust in an open and transparent way that commands public confidence.'

The Healthy NHS Board: principles for good governance reinforces the importance of NHS boards acting, and being seen to act, with integrity and in the best interests of the organisation: 'Probity requires that the board maintains an up-to-date register of board members' interests. Board agendas should include an opportunity for board members to declare conflicts of interests that may relate to specific agenda items so that they can be managed appropriately.'

Boards in NHS foundation trusts are also required to adopt appropriate standards of conduct and to be open and transparent in their decision-making and the manner in which conflicts of interest are managed.

It is, therefore, essential that there are clear and robust systems in place for identifying and managing real and potential conflicts of interest of board members to protect the reputation and tangible assets of the NHS trust, as well as the reputation of individual board members.

As the *NHS Code of Conduct* states: 'Boards have a clear responsibility for corporate standards of conduct and acceptance of the Code (of Conduct) should inform and govern the decisions and conduct of all board directors.'

9.1 What are conflicts of interest?

Conflicts arise when the interests of directors, or 'connected persons', are incompatible or in competition with the interests of the trust. Such situations present a risk that directors may make decisions based on these external influences, rather than the best interests of the organisation:

a A 'connected person' to a director is defined in s252 (2) of the Companies Act 2006 as: members of the directors' family (s253 defines these as – spouse or civil partner; any other person with whom the director lives as a partner in an enduring family relationship, and that partners' children or step-children under 18 years of age; children or
b a body corporate with which the director is connected;
c a person acting in his capacity as a trustee of a trust – (i) the beneficiaries of which include the director or a person who by virtue of (a) or (b) is connected with him, or (ii) the terms of which confer a power on the trustees that may be exercised for the benefit of the director or any such person, other than a trust for the purposes of an employees' share scheme or pension scheme;

d a person acting in his capacity as a partner – (i) of the director, or (ii) of a person who by virtue of (a) to (c) is connected with that director;

e a firm that is a legal person under the law by which it is governed and in which – (i) the director is a partner, (ii) a partner is a person who by virtue of (a) to (c) is connected with the director, or (iii) a partner is a firm in which the director is a partner or in which there is a partner who by virtue of (a), (b) or (c) is connected with the director.

The most common types of conflicts of interest include:

- direct financial interest
- indirect financial interest
- non-financial or personal interests
- conflicts of loyalty.

Direct financial interest

The most easily recognisable form of conflict of interest arises when a director obtains a direct financial benefit over and above the agreed remuneration and terms of service package agreed by the nomination committee. Examples include:

- the award of a contract to a company or other business with which a director is involved, and
- the sale of assets at below market value to a director.

Indirect financial interest

This arises when a close relative of a director benefits from the trust. Directors will benefit indirectly if their financial affairs are bound with those of the relative in question through the legal concept of 'joint purse', as would be the case if the relative were the spouse, partner, dependent child of the director, or directly connected in some other way.

Non-financial or personal conflicts

These occur where directors receive no financial benefit, but are influenced by external factors. For instance:

- to gain some other intangible benefit or kudos, or
- awarding contracts to friends or personal business contacts.

Conflict of loyalties

Directors may have competing loyalties between the trust to which they owe a primary duty and some other person or entity. Conflicts of interest may present problems in the form of:

- inhibiting free discussion
- resulting in decisions or actions that are not in the interests of the trust, and
- risking the impression that the trust has acted improperly.

Decisions made under a conflict of interest may be legally challenged and could result in personal liability for the director. The aim of a conflict of interest policy, therefore, is to protect both the organisation and the individuals involved from any appearance of impropriety.

9.2 Declaration of interests

A conflict of interest policy should require the board chairman and board members to act impartially and not be influenced by social or business relationships. No one should use their public position to further their private interests. Where there is potential for private interests to be material and relevant to NHS business, the relevant interest should be declared and recorded in the Register maintained by the company secretary.

Any interest, that arises during the course of a meeting, should be declared immediately, and should be recorded in the relevant minutes. When a conflict of interest is established, the person should withdraw and play no part in the relevant discussion or decision. Interests which should be regarded as 'relevant and material' are:

- directorships, including non-executive directorships, held in private companies or PLCs (with the exception of those of dormant companies)
- ownership or part-ownership of private companies, businesses or consultancies likely or possibly seeking to do business with the NHS
- majority or controlling share holdings in organisations likely or possibly seeking to do business with the NHS
- a position of trust in a charity or voluntary organisation in the field of health and social care
- any connection with a voluntary or other organisation contracting for NHS services
- any other commercial interest relating to any relevant decision to be taken by the trust.

Any change in interests should be declared as soon as it is recognised, and should be declared, where appropriate, at the next board meeting following the change occurring.

The Register of Interests is maintained by the company secretary who formally records the declarations of interests made by members of the board. These details must be kept up-to-date by means of at least an annual review of the register in which any changes to interests declared during the preceding months will be incorporated.

The register is available to the public and to the trust's internal and external auditors and should be published on the trust's website, to ensure compliance with Information Commissioner's Office Publication Scheme. The details of the interests of board members will be published in the trust's annual report.

10 Hospitality policy and registers

The Hospitality Policy is intended to assist all employees of an NHS trust (and this includes all board members) in following the various NHS guidance and relevant legislation on the giving and receipt of hospitality or gifts. This covers both the receipt and delivery of hospitality and gifts. Any hospitality, gifts or benefits accepted should be entered on the hospitality register by means of a standardised form. Each employee has a personal responsibility to declare hospitality and gifts in accordance with the policy.

Under the Prevention of Corruption Acts, 1906 and 1916: it is an offence for employees corruptly to accept any gifts or consideration as an inducement or reward for; doing, or refraining from doing, anything in their official capacity; or showing favour or disfavour to any person in their official capacity. Under the 1916 Act, any money, gift or consideration received by an employee in public service from a person or organisation holding or seeking to obtain a contract will be deemed to have been received corruptly unless the employee proves to the contrary.

Under NHS Standing Orders and European Commission Directives on Public Purchasing for Works and Supplies, the requirement is for fair and open competition between prospective contractors or suppliers.

Circular HSG (93) 5 Standards of Business Conduct for NHS Staff (January 1993) provides guidelines for NHS employers and employees. This sets out that NHS employers are responsible for ensuring the guidelines are brought to the attention of all employees, and that machinery is put in place to ensure they are effectively implemented. A Hospitality Policy is intended to fulfil these requirements by providing clear guidance to employees and by establishing a hospitality register.

The NHS guidance also sets out that it is the responsibility of staff to ensure that they are not placed in a position which risks, or appears to risk, conflict between their private interests and their NHS duties. This applies to both staff who commit resources directly (e.g. ordering of goods or services) or indirectly (e.g. by policy development).

Examples of hospitality, gifts or benefits where a declaration may be necessary include the following:

- meals and drinks
- crate and bottles of wine or spirits
- tickets for sporting events/theatre, etc.
- events where the cost of your accommodation is paid for by a research company
- national and international seminars where your placement has been paid for by the company organising the seminar

- sponsored golf events
- lecture trips (national and international)
- site visits to prospective suppliers of goods and services where hospitality, gifts or benefit is provided or loaned.
- gifts of equipment by drug companies

The above list is not exhaustive, but it will give an indication of the types of items that may need to be declared. Most trusts set a financial threshold, e.g. if the item has a value of more than £50 then it must be declared.

10.1 Acceptable hospitality

Hospitality is generally defined as attendance at a social or leisure event or conference (or an occasion that could be perceived as such an event) where the attendance is being funded by a third party. NHS guidance provides that modest hospitality is an accepted courtesy of a business relationship. However, the recipient should not allow themselves to reach a position whereby he or she might be deemed by others to have been influenced in making a business decision as a consequence of accepting such hospitality. The frequency and scale of hospitality accepted should not be significantly greater than the recipient's employer would be likely to provide in return. Where an employee is offered and receives hospitality from any external body while at work or outside work when they are acting in the capacity of employee of the trust they are required to declare this. Again, most trusts set a financial threshold for the declaration.

As a general principle, all offers of hospitality received from commercial third parties should be refused. Attendance at relevant commercially sponsored conferences and courses is acceptable, but only where acceptance will not, and cannot be seen as compromising purchasing or other decisions in any way. Receipt or provision of such sponsorship should be recorded in the hospitality register.

Employees should pay particular attention to the circumstances in which hospitality is offered: the provision of hospitality by an individual or organisation during a tendering process or where a contract is shortly to end, or where performance of the contract is in question, or in any other circumstance where acceptance might compromise the position of the employee or of the trust, is not acceptable.

10.2 Acceptance of gifts

Employees should not accept gifts that may be capable of being construed as being able to influence a purchasing decision or cast doubt on the integrity of such decisions. Casual gifts offered by contractors or others, for example at Christmas time, should be declined except when they are of low intrinsic value, for example small stationery items such as:

- diaries
- calendars
- staplers
- pens.

NHS guidance provides that any gifts of higher value offered or received should be declined. Where it is not easy to decide whether a gift should be accepted or not, advice should be sought from the line manager. Where an employee is offered and receives gifts or benefits from any external body while they are at work or outside work when they are acting in the capacity of employee of the trust they are required to declare this. Again, most trusts set a financial threshold for the declaration.

The acceptance or giving of monetary gifts, including vouchers, is not acceptable in any circumstances.

10.3 The Bribery Act 2010

The Bribery Act 2010 came into force in July 2011 and made it a criminal offence for commercial organisations to fail to prevent bribes being paid on their behalf. NHS organisations are included within the definition of 'commercial' and therefore if any NHS organisation fails to take appropriate steps to avoid (or at least minimise) the risk of bribery taking place it could face large fines and even the imprisonment of the individuals involved and those who have turned a blind eye to the problem. The Act makes it a criminal offence:

- to give or offer a bribe, or to request, offer to receive or accept a bribe, whether in the UK or abroad (the measures cover bribery of a foreign public official), and
- for a director, manager or officer of a business to allow or turn a blind eye to bribery within the organisation.

The Act also introduces a corporate offence of failure to prevent bribery by persons working on behalf of a commercial organisation. However, organisations will have a defence against prosecution if they can show that they have adequate procedures in place to prevent bribery.

Guidance from the Ministry of Justice describes six guiding principles that set out the approach that organisations should take to prevent bribery occurring in their organisation. These are:

1 **Proportionate procedures**: designed to prevent bribery by anyone associated with the organisation and should be proportionate to the level of bribery risk to the organisation.
2 **Top level commitment**: senior management teams must show a commitment to preventing bribery, and promote a culture that does not tolerate acts of bribery.
3 **Risk assessment**: an assessment of both internal and external risks of bribery to the organisation should be carried out regularly and documented.
4 **Due diligence**: there must be effective due diligence procedures in place in respect of those involved in the organisation or carrying services out on behalf of the organisation.
5 **Communication**: the organisation's stance on bribery should be clearly communicated to all employees and all those carrying out services on behalf of the organisation. This should include appropriate training.
6 **Monitoring and review**: there should be an ongoing review process that regularly monitors the effectiveness of the procedures in place to prevent bribery.

These principles can be implemented by updating existing documentation. For example:

- Update policies and procedures by adding an anti-bribery statement to the organisation's employee handbook / intranet – this should be adequately communicated to all staff.
- Amend whistleblowing policies to make specific reference to bribery, and encourage disclosure of bribery offences.
- Training/a presentation to make employees aware of the strengthened legislation around 'bribery', particularly in relation to corporate hospitality and the organisation's policy on business conduct (or similar).
- Update/add a clause on bribery to the employment contract.
- Ensure all employees are under an express obligation to report any potential acts of bribery, including where an employee has personally committed an act of bribery.
- Ensure recruitment checks are robust.
- Add bribery to the matters covered by a disciplinary policy.
- Review remuneration structures so that they comply with the new law where applicable.

TEST YOUR KNOWLEDGE 8.7

a What are the most common types of conflicts of interest?
b What is the definition of a 'connected person'?
c What kind of gifts and hospitality are acceptable?
d What defence is available to an organisation under the Bribery Act 2011?

CHAPTER 8 Governance and boardroom practice

CHAPTER SUMMARY

- There are certain fundamental requirements for an effective and efficient board. These include: having directors of appropriate character, sufficiently frequent board meetings, and appropriate agendas for board meetings; providing timely and sufficient information to all directors (but particularly NEDs); providing administrative support and advice to directors; and, when required, access to professional advice for directors. The provision of administrative support and advice to NEDs is usually the responsibility of the company secretary.
- In the NHS, the appointment of the chairman and NEDs has been overseen by the NHS Appointments Commission (the exception being, foundation trusts, where they are appointed by the Council of Governors). The Commission is a Special Health Authority, which has the responsibility for ensuring that NHS organisations have chairs and non-executives who are capable, trained and supported to fulfil the function of governance.
- The board of directors may delegate to a nomination committee the task of recommending new appointees to the board. In the UK, the *FT Code of Governance* and the *UK Corporate Governance Code* recommends that a majority of the nominations committee should be independent NEDs and that its chairman should be either the chairman of the board or an independent director.
- The nomination committee should also be responsible for making recommendations for board succession and changes in the size and composition of the board. The committee should also consider the need to refresh the board with new NEDs, and should therefore also make recommendations about the re-appointment of NEDs who are reaching the end of their contract.
- Appointments to the board are made by the board as a whole, on the recommendation of the nomination committee, but directors of listed companies who have been appointed must (in the UK) stand for election by the shareholders at the following AGM.
- Before accepting the offer of appointment as NED, an individual should consider a range of issues. A NED is typically appointed with a three-year contract and is paid a fixed annual fee. Contracts may be renewed at the end of each three-year period, although the independence of a NED may be brought into question if he has held the position for nine years or more.
- In the past it has been usual practice in the UK for directors to stand for re-election every three years, at the AGM. A new requirement was introduced by the *UK Corporate Governance Code* in 2010. All directors of FTSE 350 companies and NEDs who have been board members for more than nine years should stand for re-election annually.
- There should also be suitable induction for new directors. This is the responsibility of the chairman, who may delegate the task to the company secretary. Directors should also receive further training throughout their term in office. The chairman is responsible for ensuring that appropriate training is provided.
- The *FT Code of Governance* and the *UK Code* states that there should be an annual performance review of the entire board, its committees and individual directors. This is the responsibility of the chairman, but at least every three years the performance evaluation process should be 'externally facilitated' by specialist consultants.
- The NEDs, led by the SID, should carry out the performance review of the chairman. The NHS Appointments Commission also plays a key role in the annual appraisal of NHS chairs, e.g. the SHA chairman will use the appraisals as part of their review of all of the chairs appointed in their regional area. NEDs of the respective trusts will also be consulted as part of that evaluation process. In foundation trusts, the evaluation of the chairman is undertaken by the governors assisted by the SID.
- The performance review of the board should assess its effectiveness. Guidelines have been issued about how the performance of the board, its committees and its individual directors (particularly the NEDs) may be assessed.
- The board of directors of an NHS trust has a legal obligation to act in the best interests of the organisation, in accordance with the trust's governing document, and to avoid situations where there may be a potential conflict of interest. As such, there are requirements for board members to register personal financial interests, which may be perceived as conflicting with that overriding duty.
- The Hospitality Policy is intended to assist all employees of an NHS trust (and this includes all board members) in following the various NHS guidance and relevant legislation on the giving and receipt of hospitality or gifts.

- NHS trusts are a corporate entity in their own right and the directors are collectively responsible for all decisions. The corporate nature of the organisation will mean that, in most instances, even if a decision is open to criticism, individual directors will not be legally liable. There is specific statutory protection where they are acting in good faith (see Section 265 of the Public Health Act 1875).
- There is a degree of protection for directors. Non-executives will typically have the benefit of the Treasury approved wording (HSG 1999/104). This covers the director for acts carried out in good faith in the execution or purported execution of the functions of the trust, short of recklessness.
- Under The Bribery Act 2012 it is an offence for commercial organisations (including NHS organisations) to fail to prevent bribes being paid on their behalf. The Act makes it clear that it is senior management's responsibility to demonstrate commitment to preventing bribery and ensure that it is communicated to all employees and those carrying out services on behalf of the organisation.

Remuneration issues

■ CONTENTS

1. Remuneration as a governance issue
2. Principles of senior executive remuneration
3. Elements of remuneration for executive directors and other senior executives
4. The design of performance-related remuneration
5. The remuneration committee
6. The remuneration of non-executive directors (NEDs)
7. Compensation for loss of office
8. Disclosure of directors' remuneration details
9. Further guidance

■ INTRODUCTION

The remuneration of executive directors and other senior executives in the corporate sector has been a contentious issue, partly because of the amounts paid to top executives in some companies and partly because remuneration for senior executives has risen by a much bigger percentage than increases in pay for other employees. While remuneration packages should be sufficient to attract and retain executives of a suitable calibre, they should not be excessive. Such packages should also reward executives for successful performance, in both the short term and the longer term, because pay incentives are expected to encourage executives to perform better.

A further area of concern to both the NHS and the corporate sector is the payment of large 'rewards for failure' and contracts of employment for senior executives should try to minimise the risk of these severance payments when a senior director fails to perform to a satisfactory standard and is dismissed.

This chapter looks at the role of the remuneration committee, the problems with negotiating a satisfactory remuneration package for senior executives, and what the elements of that package should be.

Shareholders and other stakeholders cannot decide the remuneration of executive directors and cannot vote to reject contracts of employment that have already been agreed. However, in the UK they have a legal right to be given information about directors' remuneration and to approve any new long-term incentive scheme for executives.

1 Remuneration as a governance issue

The case study below neatly sets out the dilemma around remuneration within the NHS. Moves to greater independence and local accountability offer a freedom on remuneration for NHS executive directors, and the increasing complexity of the organisations calls for the best candidates possible yet there is pressure on the government to ensure pay levels reflect the current economic climate.

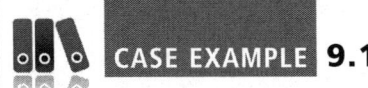

CASE EXAMPLE 9.1

In May 2011, research on boardroom pay in the health service by pay analysts Incomes Data Services (IDS) and reported in the *The Independent* newspaper revealed that the basic pay of NHS chief executives had jumped by 4.5%, with median earnings now more than £150,000. The research also found a widening wage gap between foundation and non-foundation bosses.

The report, which studied accounts for the year to March 2010, found that:

'around one in eight non-medical chiefs and seven out of 10 medical directors in England earned more than £150,000 last year, The basic salary of non-medical chief executives in the NHS increased by an average of 4.5%, three times higher than the DH's pay guidance rise of 1.5%.'

Steve Tatton of IDS was quoted as saying:

'For those wanting to see NHS directors' pay curbed, our latest pay findings may come as a disappointment. The government has stressed the importance of senior staff in the public sector showing leadership in the exercise of pay restraint in the current economic climate. With salary rises running at these levels, such restraint so far does not seem to have been a feature of boardroom pay deliberations, especially in foundation trusts. The government wants to bear down on senior executive pay in the public sector, yet it also wants to see decisions made locally without interference from central authorities. The issue for NHS organisations is will they be free to pay their senior executives what they decide is necessary or will they have to follow externally imposed pay restraints?'

'Median total earnings of chief executives in foundation trusts was £164,500 compared to £152,500 for those in non-foundation trusts, the report said. Foundation trusts have considerably more independence over the level of remuneration awarded to their executives, whereas others such as primary care and ambulance trusts are governed by prescribed guidelines determined by the Department of Health, IDS said.'

Taken from *The Independent*, Tuesday, 10 May 2011.

As the economic climate tightens the financial position for the NHS, attention will continue to focus on the level of pay to executive directors within the NHS and the lessons learnt from corporate governance will offer further insight to health service governance in this area. The remuneration levels that are on offer in the corporate sector will also influence the NHS remuneration levels as can be seen by the response of the NHS Confederation to the IDS report referred to above:

'NHS organisations are large and complex in nature and require the right managerial skills to be led effectively. A large city hospital could have a budget of between £500 million and £1 billion and employ as many as 10,000 staff – comparable to many FTSE 250 companies. Because of the challenging nature of a chief executive's role, NHS boards must consider a range of factors, including pay, to encourage the best candidates in to these positions. The NHS is looking to involve more clinical staff in top management positions. Given that a number of hospital doctors will be paid more than NHS chief executives, this factor must be taken into consideration when making a decision on pay.'

David Stout, Deputy CEO, NHS Confederation

The remuneration of executive directors and senior executives was not seen as a major problem of corporate governance until the 1990s in the UK and early 2000s in the USA. A sense that something might be wrong began when the general public, alerted by the media, criticised some top executives for being paid far more money than they were worth, and investment institutions criticised directors for receiving ever-increasing rewards even when their company performed badly.

In many listed companies in the UK during the 1980s and early 1990s, the CEOs and executive chairmen were involved in deciding their own remuneration package. Concern about remuneration has grown in other countries, particularly with regard to the banking crisis in

2007–2009 and the high rewards earned by senior bankers in spite of the large amounts of public funds provided to prevent banks from financial collapse.

Throughout the 2000s in the UK, the remuneration of top corporate sector executives has risen rapidly regardless of company performance, the effects of global recession, and at a faster annual rate than the remuneration of other company employees, whereas a principle of good corporate governance is that remuneration should be linked to some extent to company performance, so that a director will earn more if the company does well, but less if it does badly.

Within NHS organisations there is to a certain extent a greater level of regulation. All NHS organisations (except NHS foundation trusts) are required to follow either the VSM Pay Framework or Agenda for Change. The VSM Pay Framework is published by DH. VSM means chief executives, executive directors and others with board-level responsibility who report directly to the CEO. At present the VSM Framework applies to senior staff in PCTs, ambulance trusts, SHAs and special health authorities. The government has declared a pay freeze for 2011/2012 and 2012/2013.

The Agenda for Change system allocates posts to set pay-scales using a job evaluation scheme. Directors within acute and mental health trusts have their pay set within this system unless they are a foundation trusts. All foundation trusts have the freedom to use local terms and conditions when setting pay for all employees; however, in practice all but one (Southend University Hospital NHS Foundation Trust) has continued to be guided by VSM and to operate Agenda for Change for their staff.

1.1 Public attitudes

In corporate governance a general belief that directors pay themselves far too much can have a damaging effect on the stock market. Private investors may be reluctant to invest in companies that reward their leaders far more than they deserve. It can be particularly damaging to the capital markets when public anger is stirred against directors who continue to pay themselves more when their companies are performing badly. The problem emerged in the UK during the 1990s, largely as a result of the privatisation of state-owned industries such as water and electricity supply companies. The same individuals who had run the former state-owned enterprises were appointed as directors of newly established listed companies, with a much improved remuneration package. The popular press led a campaign against 'fat cat' directors, such as the leaders of British Gas and United Utilities.

Public attitudes about remuneration within the NHS are interesting, which was recognised, although not specifically, in the *Hutton Review of Fair Pay* in the public sector issued in March 2011:

> 'Success [of the public sector] would be a fundamental building block in supporting economic growth and social well-being, but it cannot be done without motivated, high calibre public servants, along with managers to lead them. But while the British public is very sympathetic to front line delivery staff, it is hostile to the public sector managers responsible and accountable for the effective deployment of resources – and even more hostile to their pay. In the eyes of some, they are the quintessential "burdens" on the rest of us.'
>
> Will Hutton

The review set out that some of this public reaction is quite reasonable since public sector managers have also benefited from the significant growth of the earnings for the top levels of remuneration, particularly in the last ten years. However, some balance is required here. As the Hutton Interim Report demonstrated, £1 of every £100 earned by the top 1% of earners in the UK is earned by public sector employees.

However, the perception remains that the public sector is no less awash with 'fat cats' than the private sector; indeed in one poll a quarter of respondents thought that public sector executives earned more than their private sector counterparts. Despite the inaccuracy, 'the public has the right to know that pay is deserved, fair, under control and designed to drive improving public sector performance'.

Rewards for failure

In the UK, during 2002–2003, there was institutional investor concern, supported by widespread media coverage, about large remuneration packages for senior corporate directors where the size of the reward did not seem sufficiently linked to performance, and large **severance payments** (payments on dismissal) to outgoing senior executives who had been ousted from their job following poor company performance. High severance payments to unsuccessful directors were seen as 'rewards for failure'. Following the global banking crisis of 2007–2009, there was also widespread criticism of remuneration in banks, whereby top executives and traders received large bonuses even though their bank may have been close to collapse or in need of government financial support to remain in business.

Similar problems of rewards for failure have been seen in the NHS and raises very clear issues of health service governance.

CASE LAW 9.1

In **Gibb v Maidstone and Tunbridge Wells NHS Trust**, G was employed as the trust's CEO with a basic annual salary of £150,000 and an entitlement to six months' notice. Following outbreaks of the 'super bug' *C. difficile* at hospitals managed by her, there were a significant number of deaths and widespread public anger and anxiety. G left the trust under a Compromise Agreement that agreed to pay her around £250,000 including around £75,000 pay in lieu of notice and a compensation payment of £175,000. The compensation payment, which had been agreed, was challenged by G's successor as being ultra vires, i.e. beyond the powers of the NHS trust to award. G issued proceedings against the trust to recover the £175,000. The High Court found that the £175,000, which had been agreed under the Compromise Agreement, was irrationally generous and was therefore outside of the Trust's powers to award. It held that G was not therefore entitled to recover the £175,000. The trust had failed to ensure that it did not reward for failure, and the £175,000 was over and above any contractual or statutory entitlement that G may have had. The Court also held that she was not entitled to any other lesser payment (such as compensation for unfair dismissal). While G could have claimed for unfair dismissal, she had not done so. G therefore failed to recover the £175,000, which had been an agreed payment under the Compromise Agreement. G was out of time to bring a claim for unfair dismissal, but if she had still been within time, she could have issued proceedings against the trust.

The NHS trust was a public body so it was clearly of relevance to those involved in the public sector. The trust had failed to follow specific guidance for NHS bodies in assessing compensation and had acted outside its authority.

The problem of inappropriate remuneration policies for senior executives is now well recognised both within the NHS and the corporate sector, but a satisfactory solution has not necessarily been found. However, a distinction should be made between the unethical 'corporate greed' of some senior executives, and a reasonable desire by senior executives to be well remunerated for what they do. Similarly, it important to make the distinction between high rewards that are justified by performance, and high rewards that are earned in spite of poor performance.

STOP AND THINK 9.1

From your general reading or awareness of the business and/or NHS news, can you name any other example of public anger or concern about remuneration for senior executives? Is there a difference between the corporate sector and the NHS?

Are you aware of any opposition by institutional investors or political involvement in the discussions about a director's remuneration package, and what their reasons for opposing it were?

1.2 Why is remuneration a governance issue?

Remuneration of senior executives is a governance issue for several reasons:

- Excessive remuneration for senior corporate executives that is not clearly linked to good performance can undermine confidence in the stock markets.
- Executives should not be rewarded for failure.
- Large organisations need to attract and retain talented professionals to provide them with effective leadership. Top executives are attracted and retained by the remuneration packages they are offered.
- Organisations need effective boards and senior executive management. Remuneration incentives can be used to motivate executives to perform better and to achieve better results, however, remuneration incentives should be designed carefully to align the interests of the organisation and executives as much as possible, in both the short term and the longer term.
- The remuneration of senior executives may antagonise employees (and employee representatives), when it appears that senior executives are paid excessive amounts in comparison with their own pay. A sense that benefits or rewards are unfairly distributed could lead to industrial unrest within the organisation.

A further reason that this is a governance issue relates to the stability and continuity of the board. The IDS study referred to in Case example 9.1 found that turnover in non-foundation trust boardrooms had increased from 17% to 24% in the year to March 2010 and from 14% to 21% for foundation trusts. In his review on fair pay Will Hutton identified that there were real concerns in the NHS, where the average tenure of NHS acute trust chief executives was just two years and four months, compared with the average tenure for FTSE 100 chief executives at 5.9 years. He went on:

> 'Such short tenures not only compare unfavourably with the private sector (average tenure for FTSE 100 chief executives is currently 5.9 years), but are also not conducive to successful management: business management research suggests that most chief executives need an average of 30 months to complete their learning curve upon taking up a new role.'

Accusations that the remuneration packages of senior executives has got out of hand are made harder to defend if there is no robust framework to justify top levels of pay. Remuneration as a governance issue can apply to senior executives below board level, as well as to directors, although the constraints of the VSM Framework do operate within the NHS to manage this issue. NHS senior managers whose pay falls within the national framework received no uplift to basic pay for the 2010/2011 financial year, and pay levels will be frozen for a further two years from April 2011.

STOP AND THINK 9.2

What are the potential problems for good governance when the annual remuneration of senior executives rises at a very much higher percentage rate than the salaries of other employees over a period of several years?

TEST YOUR KNOWLEDGE 9.1

For what reasons is the remuneration of senior executives considered a corporate governance issues in some countries?

1.3 *Hutton Review of Fair Pay* in the public sector

The *Hutton Review* was published in March 2011 and sets out a new Fair Pay Code for senior pay, to be adopted by all organisations delivering public services, on a 'comply or explain' basis based on:

- the principle of fairness as due desert, i.e. reward should be proportional to the weight of each role and each individual's performance
- pay levels being set according to a fair process
- recognition that an organisation's success derives from the collective efforts of the whole workforce.

The review also set out 12 recommendations to the government that together form the framework for fairness:

- **Using pay multiples to track executive pay against that of all employees**: the government should not cap pay across public services, but should require that from 2011–2012 all public service organisations publish their top to median pay multiples each year to allow the public to hold them to account.
- **Informing the public debate through annual Fair Pay Reports**: to support citizen accountability, the government should commission the Senior Salaries Review Body to publish annual Fair Pay Reports, starting from 2011–2012.
- **Re-calibrating the pay of Non-Departmental Public Body chief executives**.
- **From disclosure to explanation: ensuring complete transparency over executive roles and remuneration**: to enable citizens to understand executive remuneration and the nature of executive responsibilities, from 2011–2012 the government should require that all organisations delivering public services disclose in precise numbers the full remuneration of all executives, alongside an explanation of the responsibilities of each role and of how executives' pay reflects individual performance.
- **Enabling citizen analysis of executive pay**: from 2011–2012, the government should require public organisations to submit executive pay data through an online template, and make this data available on data.gov.uk, to allow citizens to access and analyse this data and thus have the information required to hold public service organisations to account.
- **Abandoning arbitrary benchmarks for public service pay**: once this framework of recommendations is in place, the government should refrain from using the pay of the Prime Minister or other politicians as a benchmark for the remuneration of senior public servants, whose pay should reflect their due desert and be proportional to the weight of their roles and their performance.
- **Preventing rewards for failure through earn-back pay for senior public servants**: to allow pay to vary down as well as up with performance, all public service executives should have an element of their basic pay that needs to be earned back each year through meeting pre-agreed objectives with excellent performers who go beyond their objectives eligible for additional pay.
- Extending earn-back pay to high performing middle managers.
- **Sharing the rewards of greater productivity**: to prevent executives monopolising the rewards of productivity increases, and allow all employees who have contributed to share the benefits, government departments should identify ways of offering gainsharing schemes linked to achievement of the efficiency aspects of their business plans. The government should also explore options for gainsharing schemes across public services more widely.
- **Opening up opportunities for future generations of public service leaders**: to increase the supply of candidates for top positions and reinforce public service management as a career, the government should facilitate greater opportunities for managers to move across different public services. By the end of 2011 the government should establish a single online portal for advertisements and applications for public service management roles, and work with major public service employers to establish a passport scheme for middle and senior managers across public services. It should also drive and prioritise ongoing collaboration between public sector graduate recruitment and development programmes.

- **A Fair Pay Code**: to embed fairness principles and ensure fair process in executive remuneration, all public service organisations should adopt the Fair Pay Code proposed by this Review. Government departments should by July 2011 bring forward proposals for the application of this code to all bodies and sectors in which they have an interest.
- **Tracking pay multiples across the economy**: to make tracking pay multiples normal practice across the economy, as part of its commitment to improve corporate reporting, the Government should require listed companies to publish top to median pay multiples in their annual reporting from January 2012.

The DH is likely to accept the recommendations in full and has issued a circular to all foundation trusts inviting them – it cannot require them – to say how they are going to implement them.

Interestingly a number of these recommendations have been echoed in the final report 'Cheques with Balances: why tackling high pay is in the national interest' (November 2011) from The High Pay Commission, which is an independent inquiry into high pay and boardroom pay across the public and private sectors in the UK. The report examines the reasons for the gap between high and low pay in the UK in recent years and why this matters:

> 'Will Hutton's suggestion of a framework for public sector pay, which the private sector might be expected to follow, may provide the beginnings of a more comprehensive approach. But it is absolutely vital that we extend the discussion beyond the public sector, and have a real debate on high pay in the private sector now. Our Commission is gathering evidence so that we can have such a debate. We need a degree of openness and honesty about what we are rewarding when it comes to pay across the spectrum and what is fair pay in a modern corporate environment.'

TEST YOUR KNOWLEDGE 9.2

a What is the proposed Fair Pay Code for senior pay based on?
b How do the recommendations help to improve openness and transparency?
c Why is it vital that the discussion on high pay is extended beyond the public sector?

2 Principles of senior executive remuneration

The UK government have recently announced new measures to curb levels of executive pay and these measures are likely to include:

- making firms' remuneration reports easier to understand, and requiring them to explain executive salaries in relation to the earnings of other employees
- increasing transparency by requiring the publication of all directors' salaries
- giving shareholders a binding vote on executive pay, notice periods and exit packages – at present their say is merely advisory
- encouraging a wider range of people onto company boards, including academics, lawyers, public servants and those who have never served on a board before
- requiring all companies to introduce 'clawback' policies, allowing them to recoup bonuses in cases where they are later shown to be unwarranted.

Principles of remuneration are now included in the corporate governance codes of many countries. In a system of good governance, the remuneration of directors and key senior executives should be sufficient to attract and retain individuals of a suitable calibre. At the same time, the structure of an individual's remuneration package should motivate the individual towards the achievement of performance that is in the best interests of the organisation and its stakeholders, as well as those of the individual.

The *UK Corporate Governance Code* states as a principle that:

'Levels of remuneration should be sufficient to attract, retain and motivate directors of the quality required to run the company successfully, but a company should avoid paying more than is necessary for this purpose. A significant proportion of executive directors' remuneration should be structured so as to link rewards to corporate and individual performance.'

It is widely accepted that senior executives should be able to earn a high level of remuneration in return for the work they do and the responsibilities they carry. If a company does not offer an attractive package, it will not attract individuals of the required calibre. It is also generally accepted that the level of remuneration should be linked in some way to satisfactory performance. If an executive performs well, he should receive more rewards than if he performs only reasonably well. That said, it is widely recognised that the top levels of pay in the public sector are running at between 50% and 55% of the salaries at the top of the private sector. There is then already a very substantial discount being accepted by senior executives who want to work in the public sector and build a career going to the top. There is also the long held belief that people should want to do the job and should not want to do it for the money, so long as the salary pays them a reasonable living.

The central issue for good corporate governance is concerned with the link between pay and performance:

- In the corporate sector the remuneration package should include a performance-related element. If the director successfully achieves predetermined levels of performance, he will be rewarded accordingly. There could be some debate as to how much remuneration should be performance related, but there is a view that a substantial part of a director's total potential remuneration should be linked to performance.
- The purpose of performance-related remuneration is to give a director an incentive to achieve the performance targets. This is why potential performance-related pay should be substantial.
- It is clearly in the interest of good corporate governance that directors should be motivated to perform, but it is equally important that the performance targets set for each individual director are: (1) sufficiently challenging; and (2) related to objectives that are in the interests of the company and its shareholders. Performance targets should therefore be challenging, and large rewards should not be paid for average performance.

Linking remuneration, wholly or in part, to performance is not an easy task, however, as the following shows:

- Unsuitable measures of performance may be selected, so that although the individual executive succeeds in achieving targets that earn high rewards, the company itself and its shareholders do not obtain a comparable benefit.
- Many performance measures are based on the short term, possibly linked to annual results. This may not be in the interests of the company's longer-term development and performance.
- Remuneration systems are normally designed to provide the reward after the performance has been made. This time delay means that if the company has poor results in the current year after having done well in the previous year, an executive may be paid high remuneration (for the previous year) at a time the company is doing badly.

If it is not an easy task for corporate governance, then it becomes even more difficult for health service governance. As this text has already demonstrated there is a great diversity and complexity of stakeholders and their objectives for NHS organisations. Finding suitable measures of performance is a challenge that was highlighted in the *Hutton Review*.

A supporting principle in corporate governance states that the performance-related elements of a remuneration package for a senior executive should be 'stretching' and should also be designed in a way that:

- aligns the interests of the executive with the interests of the shareholders, and
- promotes the long-term success of the company.

The view of the *UK Code* is therefore that the interests of shareholders in the longer term should not be subordinated to short-term considerations.

For health service governance a key principle relates to the public scrutiny and transparency of the remuneration package and the accountability of the executive director.

STOP AND THINK 9.3

In response to the threat of measures by the UK government to levy a higher rate of tax on bonuses for bank executives, UK banks might consider increasing the basic salaries of many of its executives instead. Is this an example of poor government policy, bad corporate governance by the bank, or both?

3 Elements of remuneration for executive directors and other senior executives

3.1 The component elements of executive directors' remuneration

The remuneration package for a senior executive in the corporate sector is likely to consist of a combination of a **fixed pay** element – remuneration received regardless of performance, such as a fixed salary and payments made into a salary related pension scheme – and a **variable pay** element that might consist of **performance related incentives**, which might be tied to short-term performance such as an annual bonus, and longer term incentives such as share option awards.

In addition, executives might enjoy a number of other perks such as free private medical insurance, a company car and the use of a company plane or apartment.

A problem in negotiating a remuneration package with an executive is to decide on the balance between the fixed and the variable elements, and to agree on measures of performance as the basis for deciding on how much the performance-related payments should be.

Short-term incentives are based on annual performance targets. Long-term incentives may be awarded each year, but are linked to performance over a longer period of time, typically three years (or longer). Another problem in deciding a remuneration package is to find a suitable balance between short-term and longer-term incentives.

Not so for the senior executive in the NHS where the remuneration package usually consists of a fixed salary and a final salary related pension. The FTN Remuneration Survey of executive pay confirms this, although some foundation trusts are now adding a car allowance or lease car to their remuneration packages. There is also evidence that some foundation trusts offer a performance related pay scheme in connection with the achievement of trust corporate objectives. These schemes, however, are still in their infancy and small in number.

3.2 Use of remuneration consultants

Companies and NHS organisations often use remuneration consultants, who give advice to the remuneration committee on remuneration packages, including basic salary levels for senior executives. Consultants should not be given responsibility for deciding remuneration; this responsibility should remain with the remuneration committee of the boards.

Consultants may use competitive pay data to recommend a basic package for senior executives. Competitive pay data is simply information about the rewards that are being paid to senior executives in other top companies.

A supporting principle in the *UK Corporate Governance Code* is that the remuneration committee should judge where to position the company relative to other companies, but it should exercise caution in making this judgement 'in view of the risk of an upward ratchet of remuneration levels with no corresponding improvement in performance'. The *UK Code* also states that the remuneration committee should consider pay and employment conditions elsewhere within the group, especially when deciding the annual salary increases for the executive directors. However, remuneration consultants may not offer advice on this matter.

If a UK listed company does use the services of remuneration consultants, it should make available a statement of whether they have any other connection with the company. This statement may help to indicate whether the consultants are independent and provide objective advice.

3.3 Problems with linking rewards to performance

The purpose of incentive schemes is to provide an incentive to an executive director or senior manager to improve the organisation's performance by linking rewards to performance. However, experience has shown that there are a number of severe practical problems in devising a satisfactory scheme:

- There may be disagreement about what the performance targets should be, and at what level they should be set. For example, should short-term incentives be based exclusively on one or more financial targets, or should there be rewards for the achievement of non-financial targets?
- Newly appointed executives might benefit from a 'legacy effect' from their predecessor in the job. The bonuses paid to a new director, for example, might arise because of the effort and work of his predecessor in the job.
- Occasionally, rewards are paid to incentivise directors for doing something that should be a part of their normal responsibilities, such as rewarding a CEO for helping the nominations committee to find a successor to replace him when he retires.

TEST YOUR KNOWLEDGE 9.3

a What are the main component elements of the remuneration package of a senior executive director in the corporate sector? How does this compare to the NHS?
b What does the *UK Corporate Governance Code* state about the general level of senior executive remuneration?
c What are the problems with linking rewards to performance for senior executives?
d What are the advantages and problems with the remuneration committee using the services of remuneration consultants?

4 The design of performance-related remuneration

The *UK Corporate Governance Code* requires that the responsibility for setting the remuneration of executive directors (and possibly other senior executives) should be delegated by the board to a remuneration committee. The remuneration committee is explained in more detail later; however, an Appendix to the *UK Code* sets out provisions for the design of the performance-related elements of a remuneration package that the remuneration committee should apply. Some of these provisions offer a useful insight into how incentive schemes may be structured and approved.

4.1 The *UK Code* and general provisions for the design of remuneration packages

The Appendix to the *UK Code* includes some general provisions about performance-related remuneration:

- Payouts or grants under all incentive schemes should be subject to challenging performance criteria.
- These performance criteria should reflect the company's objectives, including non-financial objectives.
- Remuneration incentives should be compatible with the risk policies and systems of the company and criteria for paying bonuses should be risk-adjusted but does not go into detail about what this means in practice.

The code provisions also state that only the basic salary of the director (a fixed element of remuneration) should be pensionable. A director may be entitled to a pension after retirement, which is based partly on the number of years he has been with the company, and partly on his remuneration in the final year (or final few years) before retirement. Alternatively, a director may receive an annual payment into a personal pension scheme, with the amount of the annual contribution to the pension fund set at a fixed percentage of remuneration during the year. The code states that variable elements of remuneration (bonuses and the value of share grants or options) should be excluded from 'pay' when pension entitlements are decided.

The remuneration committee should also consider the consequences for pension costs of deciding to increase the basic salary of a director, especially for directors close to retirement.

Experience has shown that companies may be committed to very large pension payments to former directors for many years after they have retired, and remuneration committees should try to prevent these costs from becoming even more excessive.

4.2 The *UK Code* and short-term incentives

The Appendix to the *UK Code* states that the remuneration committee should consider whether the directors should be eligible for annual bonuses. If so, performance criteria should be 'relevant, stretching and designed to enhance shareholder value and to promote the long-term success of the company'.

There should be upper limits to annual bonuses, and these limits should be disclosed. There may be a case for an annual bonus to be part-paid in shares, which the director is required to hold for a 'significant period'.

Concern has been expressed that executives may deliberately provide misleading information about the performance of their company to increase their entitlement to bonuses. For example, the CEO and finance director may be tempted to 'window dress' the accounts of the company to boost profits, or to 'hide losses' so that reported profits are higher than they should be. The true situation may become apparent later, but the executives by that time may have received their bonuses. The Appendix to the *UK Code* therefore includes a further provision that consideration should be given by the remuneration committee to the use of provisions in the remuneration agreement for a director 'that permit the company to reclaim variable components in exceptional circumstances of misstatement and misconduct'. This is known as 'claw-back' of bonuses.

An alternative arrangement would be to include in the remuneration agreement with an individual a provision that an annual bonus should be paid over a period of time, say two or even three years. If it is subsequently found that the company's performance was over-stated and the original calculation of the bonus amount was too high, the future bonus payments can be adjusted to their appropriate amount.

4.3 The *UK Code* and longer-term incentives

The Appendix to the *UK Code* states that the remuneration committee should consider whether the directors should be eligible for benefits under long-term incentive schemes:

- Traditional share option schemes should be weighed against other types of long-term incentive scheme.
- Executive share options should not be offered at a discount to the current market price of the shares (except in certain cases permitted by the UK Listing Rules).
- Any proposed new long-term incentive scheme should be approved by the shareholders.
- The total rewards available in any long-term incentive scheme 'should not be excessive'.
- In normal circumstances the benefits under share options schemes and share grant schemes should not be receivable in less than three years.
- Share options should not be exercisable within three years.
- Shares granted to an executive should not 'vest' (be receivable) in less than three years.
- Directors should be encouraged to hold their shares for a further period after they have been granted or after the share options have been exercised (subject to the need to finance any costs of purchase or any associated tax liabilities).

The provisions in the code also suggest that awards of share options and grants of shares should normally be phased over time rather than granted in a single large block. This is to avoid a situation in which the size of the rewards for a director relies excessively on the share price at a particular date.

TEST YOUR KNOWLEDGE 9.4

a What are the general provisions in the *UK Corporate Governance Code* on the design of remuneration packages?
b What are the provisions in the *UK Corporate Governance Code* on short-term and long-term incentive schemes?
c Why, in the interests of good corporate governance, should NEDs be paid a basic annual fee and no incentive?

5 The remuneration committee

It is a well-established principle of 'best practice' in governance that:

- there should be a formal procedure for deciding on remuneration for directors and senior executives, and
- no individual should be involved in setting his own remuneration.

This means that executive directors should not be involved in setting their remuneration packages (although they can negotiate with the individuals who make the decision) and NEDs should not decide their fees.

The remuneration of executive directors was recognised as an important governance issue in the UK in the 1990s with the work of the Greenbury Committee, whose recommendations were subsequently incorporated into the UK governance code in 1998. The Greenbury Committee reached the following conclusions:

- The formulation of remuneration packages for senior executive directors was a fundamental issue for good corporate governance.
- However, the system was open to abuse if executives could decide their own remuneration levels.
- Shareholders are not able to decide directors' remuneration, although they had a right to extensive information about it.
- Remuneration for executive directors should therefore be decided by a remuneration committee of the board consisting entirely of independent NEDs.

These principles have roundly been adopted by health service governance either in the constitution of a foundation trust or the model standing orders prescribed by the DH. It is worth, therefore, considering the provisions of the *UK Code* as they underpin the provisions of health service governance.

Specimen terms of reference for NHS Remuneration Committees can be found on the ICSA website.

5.1 *UK Corporate Governance Code* requirements for a remuneration committee

The *UK Corporate Governance Code* states that:

> 'There should be a formal and transparent procedure for developing policy on executive remuneration and for fixing the remuneration packages of individual directors. No director should be involved in deciding his own remuneration.'

It goes on to make a provision that:

> '[T]he board should establish a remuneration committee . . . [which] should make available its terms of reference, explaining its role and the authority delegated to it by the board.'

The remuneration committee is responsible for both developing remuneration policy and for negotiating the remuneration of individual directors. Although these two matters are related, they are different.

The remuneration committee should consist entirely of independent NEDs. In larger companies, the committee should consist of at least three members, and in smaller companies (i.e. companies below the FTSE 350) at least two members. The company chairman may be a member of the committee, but not its chairman, provided that he was considered to be independent on appointment as company chairman.

The remuneration committee should have delegated responsibility for setting the remuneration for all executive directors and the chairman (including pension rights and any compensation payments or severance payments).

The remuneration committee should also recommend and monitor the level and structure of remuneration for senior management. The definition of 'senior management' is a matter for the board to decide, but it will normally include the first level of management below board level.

However, shareholders should be invited specifically to approve all new long-term incentive schemes (and changes to existing schemes) that are recommended by the remuneration committee and the board.

5.2 Consultation with the chairman or CEO about executive remuneration

The *UK Code* states as a supporting principle that the remuneration committee should consult with the chairman and/or the CEO about their proposals for the remuneration of the other executive directors. This is to ensure that the remuneration committee receives advice about the performance of executive directors from individuals who know about their contributions to the management team and to the work of the board.

- The remuneration committee may ask for advice from other sources, including other senior executives.
- The remuneration committee is responsible for deciding whether to appoint remuneration consultants to advise it.
- If executives or senior managers are involved in giving advice to the remuneration committee, the committee should take care to recognise and avoid any conflicts of interest.
- The remuneration committee should keep the chairman well informed about its decisions on remuneration policy and the remuneration of individual directors, because the chairman should be the point of contact for shareholders who want to ask questions about remuneration or make their opinions known to the company.

5.3 The principal duties of the remuneration committee

A list of duties of the remuneration committee were at one time included as an annex to the UK Combined Code, and they are now indicated in ICSA's guidance note on the terms of reference for a remuneration committee. Typically, the duties of a remuneration committee are as follows:

- The committee should determine and agree with the main board the remuneration policy for the CEO, the board chairman and any other designated executive managers. This policy should provide for executive managers to be given appropriate incentives for enhanced performance.
- To maintain and assure his/her independence, the committee should also decide the remuneration of the company secretary.
- The committee should decide the targets for performance for any performance-related pay schemes operated by the organisation.
- It should decide the policy for and scope of pension arrangements for each executive director.
- It should ensure that the contractual terms for severance payments on termination of office are fair to both the individual and the organisation, that failure is not rewarded and that the director's duty to mitigate losses is fully recognised.
- Within the framework of the agreed remuneration policy, it should determine the remuneration package of each individual executive director, including any bonuses, incentive payments and share options.

- It should be aware of and advise on any major changes in employee benefit structures throughout the organisation or group.
- It should agree the policy for authorising expense claims from the chairman and CEO.
- It should ensure compliance by the organisation with the requirements for disclosure of directors' remuneration in the annual report and accounts.
- It should be responsible for appointing any remuneration consultants to advise the committee.
- In the annual report, it should report the frequency of committee meetings and the attendance by members.
- It should make available to the public its terms of reference, setting out the committee's delegated responsibilities. Where necessary these should be reviewed and updated each year.
- The company secretary (or someone from the company secretary's department) should act as secretary to the remuneration committee, because it is the company secretary's responsibility to ensure that the board and its committees are properly constituted and advised. The company secretary can also play a role as intermediary and co-ordinator between the committee and the main board.

TEST YOUR KNOWLEDGE 9.5

a What are the principal responsibilities of a remuneration committee?
b According to the *UK Code*, what should be the composition of a remuneration committee for a company in the FTSE 350 and who may be its chairman?
c Is it appropriate for a remuneration committee to consult the company chairman or chief executive officer on remuneration packages for individual executive directors?

STOP AND THINK 9.4

What do you think would be the key areas of discussion for the remuneration committee of an NHS organisation if they were going to consider a remuneration package for the chief executive that included bonuses, incentive payments or performance related schemes?

6 The remuneration of non-executive directors (NEDs)

NEDs are not employees. They receive a fee for their services, not a salary. In the UK corporate sector, it is usual for NEDs to receive a fixed annual fee, typically in the region of £20,000 to £60,000 (or possibly more), for attending board meetings, some committee meetings and general meetings of the company. This is substantially less in the health service sector, although, the annual fees in the larger foundation trusts are increasing.

The latest FTN Remuneration Survey of Chairs and NEDs in foundation trusts demonstrates a range of NED remuneration from £6,000 to £17,000. The range for foundation trust chairs is from £35,000 to £62,000. The range in fees demonstrates the range in turnover of trust or number of staff in the trust as these are usually the indicators used to benchmark individual trusts when assessing the level of non-executive fees.

The principle that individuals should not decide their own remuneration applies to NEDs as well as to executive directors. This means that a remuneration committee should not decide the fees of the NEDs. In the corporate sector, deciding the remuneration of the NEDs should be the responsibility of the chairman and the executive directors (or the shareholders if required by the articles of association). Where permitted by the articles the board may delegate this responsibility to a committee, which might include the CEO. A provision in the *UK Corporate Governance Code* is that the level of remuneration for NEDs should reflect the time commitment and responsibilities of the role.

In the NHS the fees of the NED are set either by the Appointments Commission, where levels of remuneration for NEDs can differ between organisations, or in the case of foundation trusts by the council of governor's remuneration committee. Remuneration for NEDs of PCTs and SHAs are around £7,882 a year. The audit committee chair of these organisations receives an additional £5,254 for taking on this additional responsibility. Remuneration for NEDs of NHS trusts is £6,096 a year. This provides the same protection as in the corporate sector so that individuals do not set their own remuneration.

In the corporate sector NEDs may receive other forms of remuneration or reward from the organisation, alongside the basic fee (e.g. payment for additional services) but this could raise questions about their independence. For example, a NED might be paid additionally as a 'consultant' to the company. No matter how genuine and useful these consultancy services are, they put his independence at risk because the size of a consultancy fee is decided by executive management. Management also has the decision about extending or renewing a consultancy agreement.

This kind of arrangement is very unusual in the NHS.

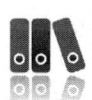

CASE EXAMPLE 9.2

In 2006, Coca-Cola in the US attracted considerable attention for a remuneration initiative for its NEDs. In April, Coca-Cola announced major changes in the remuneration structure for its NEDs. Previously, NEDs had been paid a fixed annual fee of $125,000 ($50,000 in cash, and the rest in Coca-Cola stock) and with extra fees for chairing board committees and attending board meetings and committee meetings. Under the new 'all-or-nothing' arrangement, directors would receive no remuneration unless earnings per share grew by at least 8% compound over three years, and there would be no payments to the NEDs during that time. The aim was to achieve greater alignment of the interests of the NEDs with those of the shareholders.

Critics of the new scheme argued that linking NED pay to company performance could threaten the independence of the directors from executive management, rather than align the interests of NEDs and shareholders. In addition, it was argued that by delaying payment of non-executive remuneration for three years, it would be more difficult for the company to recruit directors from less affluent socio-economic backgrounds (on the assumption that this is a desirable objective).

STOP AND THINK 9.5

Some NEDs, particularly company chairmen, have substantial shareholdings in their company. Would you consider that paying NEDs in shares rather than cash would be likely to compromise their independence?

The *UK Code* makes specific provisions about performance related rewards for NEDs, including the award of share options to NEDs:

- As a general rule the remuneration of NEDs should not include share options or any other performance-related reward.
- In exceptional cases, share options may be granted. However, the approval of the shareholders should be obtained in advance, and if the NED subsequently exercises options to acquire shares in the company, these shares should be held until at least one year after the NED leaves the board.
- Holding share options could affect the determination of whether or not the NED is independent.

7 Compensation for loss of office

7.1 Dismissal of directors and severance payments

Most executive directors have employment contracts with their organisation that provide for an annual review of their remuneration and a minimum period of notice in the event of dismissal. When a company decides to dismiss a director, it is bound by the terms of the employment contract. There are various reasons why an individual might leave the company:

- He might be regarded as having failed to do a good job, and someone else should do the job instead. A high **severance payment** would be seen as 'rewarding failure'.
- There could be a disagreement or falling out between directors, resulting in one or more directors being asked to leave.

The service contract of a director might provide for the payment of compensation for loss of office. Alternatively, a company might be required to give the individual a minimum period of notice, typically one year or six months in the UK. If an individual is asked to leave, he might be paid for the notice period, without having to work out the notice. In addition the individual may be entitled to further bonus payments under the terms of his remuneration package – in spite of being considered a failure in the job.

Shareholder concerns and the wider public concern, in regard to public sector organisations, arise where the compensation for loss of office is paid even though an individual is being dismissed for having performed badly. In the past, severance payments have been high for executives who have been seen to have failed A large compensation payment can seem annoying, because it seems that the individual is being rewarded for failure. Large severance payments reduce company profits and returns to shareholders and in the public sector are viewed as the improper use of public sector monies.

Institutional investor organisations have issued guidelines on the subject, and put pressure on companies to make sure that severance payments ('rewards for failure') are restricted.

In the NHS, the NHS Finance Controllers Office (in the DH) has produced and published detailed guidance on the process for making severance payments (Treasury letter and accompanying document 'Managing Public Money' Annex 4.13). This guidance states that employers should consider why a severance case represents VFM, before a business case for the payment is produced. Guidance has also been issued by NHS employers to assist those handling severance payments to senior managers who are generally covered by the VSM Pay Framework. It also states that it is good practice to apply this guidance to other employees. The NHS Employers Guidance sets out five initial considerations:

1. Is it appropriate to terminate the senior manager's employment? Severance should not be used as an option to avoid management action, disciplinary processes, unwelcome publicity or reputational damage.
2. What is the appropriate method of termination?
   For example, in cases involving performance or misconduct issues, generally the capability or disciplinary procedures are appropriate and should be utilised at the earliest possibility.
3. Have all the circumstances of the case been considered, including the scope for potential litigation and the consequences of this?
4. Is this arrangement in the public interest? Why does the severance payment represent VFM and the best use of public funds?
5. For NHS trusts, social care trusts and PCTs – has the SHA been consulted?

If these steps have been taken and the severance payment is in the best interests of the employer and represents VFM, then the guidance requires a proposal be made to the remuneration committee containing the business case for the severance payment. Written advice from the trust's auditors and legal advisers on the proposed business case and severance payment must be made available to the remuneration committee.

SHAs are required to submit all business cases for severance payments to the NHS Finance Controllers Office in the DH. The NHS Finance Controllers Office then seeks HM Treasury approval for the business case. Foundation trusts must also seek HM Treasury approval, through

Monitor, for all severance payments. Consequently, all severance payments made by NHS employers must be approved by HM Treasury. As part of this approval process, HM Treasury apply their own criteria to assess whether severance payments achieve VFM.

7.2 *UK Corporate Governance Code* and severance payments

The *UK Code* contains two provisions about service contracts and compensation for termination of office:

- When negotiating the terms of appointment of a new director, the remuneration committee should consider what compensation commitments the organisation would have in the event of early termination of office. More specifically, the aim should be to avoid rewarding poor performance. The committee should 'take a robust line' on reducing the amount of compensation to reflect a departing director's obligation to mitigate losses.
- Notice periods in the employment contract of an executive director should be set at one year or less. If it is necessary to offer a longer notice period to a director coming into the organisation from outside, the notice period should subsequently be reduced to one year or less 'after the initial period'.

The reference to taking a robust line on a director's duty to mitigate losses is a suggestion that a director's contract should provide for a payment of compensation in stages, and which would be halted in the event of the director finding employment elsewhere.

Remuneration committees should consider whether the organisation should retain an entitlement to reclaim bonuses if performance achievements are subsequently found to have been materially mis-stated and contracts of employment should not provide for compensation payments to senior executives in the event of a change of control over the company (a takeover).

Remuneration committees should ensure that the benefits of mitigation are obtained when an individual is dismissed. This should include a contractual obligation of the dismissed individual to mitigate the loss incurred through severance by looking for other employment. The contract should provide for the severance payment to be reduced in circumstances where the individual finds alternative employment.

Phased payments are more appropriate than a severance payment as a single lump sum.

Pension arrangements that guarantee pensions, with limited or no abatement in the event of dismissal or early retirement 'are no longer regarded as acceptable' (unless they are available to all employees, which is unlikely).

TEST YOUR KNOWLEDGE 9.6

a What steps must an NHS organisation take with regard to severance payments?
b What are the principles or provisions of the *UK Code* with regard to severance payments for senior executives?

8 Disclosure of directors' remuneration details

The main arguments about directors' remuneration can be summarised as follows. Top executives have to be paid well in order to attract and retain them. A remuneration package for a senior executive should offer incentives for achieving performance targets, and incentive-based payments should be a substantial element in the total package. However, it is very difficult to devise an incentive-based system that properly aligns the interests of top executives with those of the shareholders/stakeholders. Top executives should not be allowed to decide their own remuneration packages. The responsibility for executive remuneration decisions can be given to a remuneration committee of NEDs. This committee should try to find the elusive balance between rewarding their top executives sufficiently, while structuring the reward package to bring the interests of shareholders/stakeholders and executives into alignment. In addition, within the public sector there is a tacit understanding that people should want to do the job and should not be motivated by financial reward.

It is noticeable that within these arguments, the interests of shareholders/stakeholders are mentioned, but there is no suggestion that they should get involved in making remuneration decisions themselves. Shareholder/stakeholder involvement, however, is desirable, and there are two ways in which this might happen: (1) disclosure; and (2) shareholder/stakeholder voting on remuneration.

8.1 Directors' remuneration report

In the UK, quoted companies are required by the Companies Act 2006 to include a directors' remuneration report for each financial year. This report must be approved by the board and signed on its behalf. A copy must be circulated to shareholders in the same way as the annual report and accounts, and it is normal for the remuneration report to be included in the same document.

Similarly the *NHS Foundation Trust Annual Reporting Manual (NHS FT ARM)* and the *NHS Finance Manual* both require a similar report to be made in the organisation's annual report.

Shareholders/stakeholders must vote at the AGM on a resolution (ordinary resolution) to approve the report. This is an advisory vote only. The shareholders cannot, for example, vote against the remuneration package awarded to any individual director. However, a vote against the remuneration report is a way for shareholders/stakeholders to express their strong disapproval of the organisation's remuneration policies and practices.

The auditors, in their audit report (see also Chapter 10), must state whether in their opinion the part of the report to be audited has been prepared properly. For companies, a signed copy of the report must also be filed with the Registrar of Companies, in the same way as the annual accounts, directors' report and auditors' report.

Items to be included in the directors' remuneration report that are not subject to audit are as follows:

- The names of the directors who were members of the remuneration committee, and details about any remuneration consultants that were used (name, nature of services provided).
- A statement of the organisation's policy on directors' remuneration for the next financial years and the years after that (i.e. a forward-looking policy statement).
- Information about the service contract for each director: the date of the contract, its unexpired term and details of any notice periods; any compensation payable for early termination of the contract and any other provisions in the contract affecting the liability of the company in the event of early termination (i.e. severance terms).

Companies must also include:

- A performance graph. This is a line graph showing the total shareholder return (TSR) on the company's shares over a five-year period, and the TSR on a holding of a portfolio of shares over the same period representing a named broad equity market index. The graph can therefore be used to compare shareholder returns on the company's shares with those of a market index. The Act specifies how TSR should be calculated.

The remuneration report must contain the following items, which are subject to audit:

- For each director, the total remuneration for the year, broken down into salary and fees, bonuses, expenses received, compensation for loss of office and other severance payments, and non-cash benefits.
- For each director, details of pension contributions or entitlements. The nature of the disclosures will vary according to whether the pension scheme is a defined benefit scheme or a defined contribution scheme.
- For each director, details of any excess pension benefits received or receivable in the year (i.e. benefits in excess of the director's contractual entitlement).
- Significant payments made during the year to former directors of the company.
- The total amount of any payments made to third parties for the services of any director.
- An explanation and justification of any element of directors' remuneration, other than basic salary, which is pensionable.

Where share options and incentive schemes are utilised, the following must be included:

- For each director, details of interests in share options, both beneficial and non-beneficial. (Beneficial options are options held in the name of the director or a connected person, such as the director's spouse or child under 18.) The information disclosed should include details of options awarded or exercised during the year, options that expired unexercised during the year, and any variations to the terms and conditions relating to the award or exercise of options. For options exercised during the year, the disclosures should show the market price of the shares when the options were exercised. For options not yet expired, the disclosures should give details of the price paid for their award (if any), the exercise price, the date from which the options may be exercised and the date they expire. The market price of the shares at the end of the year, and the highest and lowest market prices reached during the year should also be avoided.
- For each director, details of any long-term incentive schemes (other than share options). These should show the director's interest in each scheme at the start of the year and the end of the year, any changes during the year, and details of when the awards/entitlements can be taken.

The ICSA's Guidance on the Directors' Remuneration Report (2008) commented on the value and significance of the report as follows:

'The requirement to produce a remuneration report as part of the annual report and accounts should not be seen simply in compliance terms. It is an opportunity for the company to demonstrate that remuneration policies and structures have a clear rationale which supports the business strategy and enhances shareholder value. There is significant reputational risk associated with the failure to manage and disclose executive remuneration and the remuneration report is a prominent opportunity to explain the company's position.'

TEST YOUR KNOWLEDGE 9.7

a What are the rules in the UK for the disclosure of details of directors' remuneration by listed companies?
b Why might it be appropriate for shareholders to be allowed to vote on remuneration policy for directors, but not on the remuneration package of individual directors?
c What items are to be included in the directors' remuneration report that are not subject to audit?

9 Further guidance

Additional guidance that is applicable to corporate governance is also useful background in health service governance. In the UK, the associations of institutional investors have developed strong views on directors' remuneration. The ABI and the NAPF have issued guidelines on executive remuneration, and regularly issue **'red top'** notices to their members recommending that they vote against the boards of companies on resolutions relating to pay.

9.1 ABI guidelines on executive remuneration

The ABI has issued principles and guidance for executive remuneration (updated in 2011). These are directed mainly at listed companies, which are encouraged to comply with them. The effect of the ABI guidelines is to notify listed companies about the concerns and expectations of institutional shareholders with regard to pay:

- Boards of directors are appointed by shareholders to run companies and act in their interests. They have a fiduciary duty to act in the best interests of their shareholders when determining remuneration. It is their responsibility to promote the long-term success of the company, taking into account the interests of employees, suppliers, customers, community, the environment and society.

- Executive directors develop and implement strategy for the company. NEDs should constructively challenge and contribute to this process, scrutinise the performance of the executives, and ensure that risk management systems are robust.
- NEDs, particularly those serving on the Remuneration Committee, should oversee executive remuneration.

9.2 Remuneration committees and their responsibilities

The main aspects of ABI guidance on remuneration committees are as follows:

- Shareholders look to the remuneration committee to protect and promote their interests in setting executive remuneration. As directors, committee members are accountable to shareholders for the structure and quantum of remuneration.
- Remuneration committees should set remuneration within the context of overall corporate performance. Structure should be aligned with strategy and agreed **risk appetite**, reward success fairly and avoid paying more than is necessary.
- Remuneration committees should look at executive remuneration in terms of the pay policy of the company as a whole, pay and conditions elsewhere in the Group, and the overall cost to shareholders.

9.3 Base pay, bonuses, pensions and contracts and severance

The ABI's guidelines on remuneration policies and practices go into some detail on specific aspects of remuneration packages. Many of them are consistent with the *UK Corporate Governance Code* guidelines. They include the following:

Base pay and bonuses

Base pay should be set at a level that reflects the role and responsibility of the individual, and should not be more than is necessary:

- The reasons for any proposal by the remuneration committee to increase base pay should be fully disclosed and justified.
- Salary decisions should not be made simply on the basis of benchmarking against median companies. 'The constant chasing of a perceived median has been a major contributor to spiralling levels of pay.'

A significant proportion of remuneration should be performance-related. **Annual bonuses** should incentivise performance. They should be linked to key performance indicators (both financial and non-financial):

- Shareholders discourage the payment of annual bonuses when the company has experienced an 'exceptional negative event', even if some specific performance targets have been met. In these circumstances, shareholders should be consulted on bonus policy and any bonus payments must be carefully explained.
- Following the payment of a bonus, shareholders will expect full details to be included in the remuneration report of the extent to which relevant targets were met.
- Deferring a portion of an annual bonus into shares (paying a bonus in shares instead of cash) 'can create a greater alignment with shareholders'. However, this should not be used as an excuse for increasing the total value of bonuses.

Long-term incentives exist to reward the successful implementation of strategy over a period of time. Shareholders have a strong preference for long-term rewards to be linked to financial measurements of performance and value creation:

- Equity-based long-term incentive schemes (share options or share grant schemes) are the most effective way to align the interests of the individual with the shareholders.
- All new long-term incentive schemes or changes to existing long-term schemes should be subject to prior approval by shareholders.
- Share incentive schemes should not lead to a dilution of shareholdings in excess of the limits acceptable to shareholders.

The total amount of remuneration should be a matter of concern to remuneration committees. 'Levels of pay that do not reflect corporate performance undermine the ability to reward success and represents excess rent extractions . . . Shareholders are likely to object to levels of pay that do not respect the core principles of paying no more than is necessary and a linkage to sustainable long-term value creation.'

9.4 NAPF policy on directors' remuneration

The NAPF supports the ABI guidelines. It has also issued guidelines to its members about situations where poor remuneration practices by a listed company could trigger a vote against the company's remuneration report at the AGM. Practices that could result in a voting sanction include the following:

- Regularly increasing the base pay (fixed pay) of executives by a larger percentage amount than the rate of inflation.
- Guaranteed annual bonuses, discretionary annual bonuses, pensionable annual bonuses or transaction-related bonuses.
- Using inappropriate benchmarks to set base pay.
- The absence of individual limits for annual bonuses or long-term incentive schemes.
- Long-term incentive schemes featuring a performance period of less than three years.
- *Ex gratia* payments or other non-contractual payments.

In a response to a consultation document on senior executive remuneration from the UK Department of Business Innovation and skills, the NAPF commented (2011) that:

- it approved of claw-back of bonuses in the event of incentives being paid on misstated or miscalculated information, but noted that claw-back arrangements were not common in practice
- an alternative approach may be to allow remuneration committees 'downward discretion' to reduce bonuses that appear excessive
- the payments of annual bonuses may be **deferred** and spread over a period of time, and adjusted if the company's performance is found to have been misstated.

As a general principle, institutional shareholders expect to be consulted on executive remuneration, and in the UK the ABI and NAPF are important representatives of their collective opinion. A supporting principle of the *UK Corporate Governance Code*, in relation to remuneration, is that: 'The chairman of the board should ensure that the company maintains contact as required with its principal shareholders about remuneration.'

9.5 EU recommendations on executive remuneration

Some recommendations on senior executive remuneration in EU-listed companies were issued by the European Commission in 2009. The recommendations are not compulsory, but Member States are encouraged to introduce them into their national codes of corporate governance. Many of the recommendations are consistent with current UK practice, but the following suggestions may at some future time find their way into the *UK Code*:

1 Variable pay should be subject to limits and predetermined performance criteria that promote the long-term sustainability of the company. The payment of a major part of the variable components of pay not be paid immediately but should be deferred, and the company should be entitled to reclaim any payments that have been made on the basis of information that has been 'manifestly mis-stated'.
2 When remuneration committees use benchmarking to decide executive remuneration, they should make comparisons not only with peer group companies, but also with the levels of pay of other employees in the company.
3 After executives have acquired shares by exercising share options, they should be required to hold them until the end of their employment with the company.

Further developments in guidelines for the remuneration of directors and senior executives should therefore be expected.

CHAPTER SUMMARY

- Public hostility to excessive remuneration for directors can affect investor confidence in companies and the stock markets. Senior executives should be well rewarded, but not excessively so.
- While the public is very sympathetic to front line delivery staff, it is hostile to the public sector managers responsible and accountable for the effective deployment of resources – and even more hostile to their pay.
- Organisations need effective boards and senior executive management. Remuneration incentives can be used to motivate executives to perform better and to achieve better results, however, remuneration incentives should be designed carefully to align the interests of the organisation and executives as much as possible, in both the short term and the longer term.
- A remuneration package may consist of fixed pay elements (salary, pension contributions) and variable pay elements (annual bonuses, long-term incentives).
- Incentives could be bonus payments linked to short-term performance (e.g. growth in earnings per share) or possibly long-term performance. Unless appropriate incentives are selected, executives could earn a high bonus even when the company performance is disappointing.
- The *Hutton Review* 2011 sets out a proposed new Fair Pay Code for senior public sector pay, to be adopted by all organisations delivering public services, on a 'comply or explain' basis.
- The *UK Corporate Governance Code* includes provisions and guidelines on remuneration.
- A major concern for governance is that remuneration packages do not achieve their intended purpose, which is to attract and retain talented executives, and then to motivate them to achieve performance targets that are in the best interests of the organisation.
- A key health service governance principle relates to the public scrutiny and transparency of the remuneration package and the accountability of the executive director.
- NEDs should be paid a flat fee and in normal circumstances should not be given incentive-linked rewards.
- Individuals should not be allowed to fix their own remuneration. Remuneration for executive directors and other senior executives should be decided by a remuneration committee consisting entirely of independent NEDs, although this committee may consult the chairman and CEO.
- The requirement for a remuneration committee is included in the *UK Corporate Governance Code*.
- These principles have roundly been adopted by health service governance either in the constitution of a foundation trust or the model standing orders prescribed by the DH.
- The *UK Code* also includes provisions relating to severance payments when a director or senior executive leaves the company. The aim should be, as much as possible, to avoid rewarding departing executives for 'failure'.
- Health service governance guidance on severance pay is provided by the DH.
- In the UK, the Companies Act requires listed companies to provide extensive information about directors' remuneration in the annual report and accounts. This report, which should also contain a statement of remuneration policy, should be submitted to the shareholders for approval at the AGM. The shareholders vote is an indicative vote, and has no power to bind the company.
- Similar provisions are contained within the *NHS Finance Manual* and the *NHS FT ARM*.
- In the UK, institutional shareholders have indicated their concerns about the details of directors' remuneration packages, and the ABI and NAPF have issued guidelines on the subject. This is also useful background information for health service governance.

Reporting and the role of audit

■ CONTENTS

1 Reporting and health service governance
2 Directors' duties and responsibilities for financial reporting
3 Relationship between internal and external audit
4 The role and responsibilities of external audit
5 The audit committee
6 Disclosure of governance arrangements
7 The business review

■ INTRODUCTION

This chapter considers the role of audit in ensuring accurate reporting for good health service governance and the range of reporting requirements that are imposed on NHS organisations. In corporate governance the annual report and accounts is seen as the most important communication between a company and its shareholders, but this is not the case for health service governance. While significant, the annual report and accounts is not the sole means of communication for NHS organisations. The wide variety of reporting requirements, which are primarily to the regulators, also provide information to NHS stakeholders.

The chapter outlines the role of audit, inspection and regulation in providing independent assurance to NHS stakeholders. Quality, performance and financial audits, therefore, provide assurance on the stewardship of public money and the corporate governance and performance of NHS organisations. By contrast, inspection (e.g. CQC) provides assurance that services satisfy service users and are achieving levels of performance consistent with national and local performance standards and targets and regulation (e.g. Monitor) provide assurance that regulated bodies are complying with minimum statutory and professional standards and seek to protect the public and/or service recipients from risks associated with any failure to comply with those standards.

The chapter goes on to consider the particular duties and responsibilities of directors relating to financial reporting and outlines the requirements of a going concern statement before examining the relationship between internal and external audit regarding these reporting requirements.

It will then focus specifically on the role and responsibilities of the external auditors, the issue of auditor independence and the responsibilities of the directors for financial reporting. The role of the audit committee will be explored including its composition and responsibilities.

Finally the chapter will explore the *Company Reporting Directive* implications and the requirement to provide a business review within the annual report.

1 Reporting and health service governance

The key areas of reporting for NHS organisations relate to quality, performance and finance. Within each of these areas there are prescribed frameworks and regulations that govern their content and timing.

Trustworthy reporting and auditing is probably the most significant issue for health service governance. Good health service governance should ensure that quality, performance and financial reporting is reliable and honest, and that the opinion of the external auditors is objective and unbiased.

1.1 Quality governance and quality reporting

The significant report relating to quality is the **annual quality account**, which reports on the quality of services provided by an NHS healthcare service. Quality accounts are not marketing documents, but an opportunity for NHS providers to enter into an open and honest dialogue with the public regarding the quality of care in the organisation.

The growing political agenda for assurance on the delivery of quality services and quality outcomes for patients has led to the growth of quality governance as a specialised area of governance. While not strictly health service governance, many NHS company secretaries will find themselves involved in the quality agenda purely because the board is required by its regulators to give regular and specific assurance on the delivery of quality within their organisation.

Quality has been part of government strategy for modernising the NHS for many years. *A First Class Service: quality in the new NHS* published in July 1998 set out the agenda for quality improvement in the NHS. The framework established:

- clear quality standards – through the establishment of NICE to provide clear advice on clinical and cost-effectiveness, and the development of National Service Frameworks (NSFs) to help raise standards of care and reduce unacceptable variations
- effective local delivery of these standards through a system of clinical governance
- strong monitoring mechanisms – including the NHS Performance Assessment Framework, together with a new statutory Commission for Health Improvement (CHI) and a programme of National Patient and User Surveys.

The publication of Lord Darzi's report 'High quality care for all' in 2008, revived and reinforced this strategy. He highlighted four key areas that would demonstrate improving quality of care: patient safety; effectiveness (including clinical outcomes and patient reported outcome measures – PROMs); user experience; and innovation. As a result greater clarity on quality standards was required, metrics had to be developed to measure quality, 'quality accounts' were to be published, the delivery of quality was to be rewarded via Commissioning for Quality Improvement (CQUINs), and standards were to be raised with the creation of the National Quality Board.

Since, ultimately, the board of an NHS organisation is responsible for the quality of care delivered across all services that it provides, this has to be achieved through governance arrangements, which delegate responsibility down to the operating levels in the organisation. In the case of quality, this means that although individuals and clinical teams are at the frontline and responsible for delivering quality care, it is the responsibility of the board to create a culture within the organisation that enables clinicians and clinical teams to work at their best, and to have in place arrangements for measuring and monitoring quality and for escalating issues, including, where needed, to the board. Boards should encourage a culture where services are improved by learning from mistakes, and staff and patients are encouraged to identify areas for improvement, and not afraid to speak out.

The term **quality governance** is used to refer to the values and behaviours and the structures and processes that need to be in place to enable the board to discharge its responsibilities for quality. The board's responsibilities for quality are threefold:

- to ensure that the essential standards of quality and safety (as determined by CQC's registration requirements) are at a minimum being met by every service that the organisation delivers
- to ensure that the organisation is striving for continuous quality improvement and outcomes in every service
- to ensure that every member of staff that has contact with patients, or whose actions directly impact on patient care, is motivated and enabled to deliver effective, safe and person-centred care.

The arrangements for quality governance should complement, and be fully integrated with, the governance arrangements for other aspects of the board's responsibilities, for example, finance governance and research governance.

The National Quality Board sets out the definition of quality governance in terms of its four component parts in its guidance: *Quality Governance in the NHS – A guide for provider boards* (2011), namely:

- strategy
- capabilities and culture
- processes and structures
- measurement.

Quality reports

The details surrounding the form and content of Quality Accounts were designed in partnership between the DH, Monitor, the CQC and NHS East of England. It involved a wide range of people from the NHS, patient organisations and the public, representatives of professional organisations and of the independent and voluntary sector. A consultation ran between September and December 2009 and the responses shaped the framework for the regulations and guidance in 2010.

CASE EXAMPLE 10.1

Quality reports – What are they and what are they for?

- Aim to improve organisational accountability to the public and engage boards in the quality improvement agenda.
- Enable providers to review services, decide and show where they are doing well, but also where improvement is required.
- Enable providers to demonstrate what improvements they plan to make.
- Provide information on the quality of services to patients and the public.
- Demonstrate how providers respond to feedback from patients and the public, as well as other stakeholders.

Source: Department of Health Quality Accounts Toolkit, December 2010

The quality report is published annually by each NHS healthcare provider and is available to the public. Quality accounts aim to enhance accountability to the public and engage the leaders of an organisation in the quality improvement agenda.

All providers of NHS services are required to produce a quality account as set out in the Health Act 2009 and supporting regulations. However, a phased introduction to the requirement has been adopted, community providers were introduced in 2010–2011 while primary care providers will be encouraged to take part at a later stage. The guidance for this is provided in the DH publication 'Quality Accounts Toolkit 2010/2011: Advisory guidance for providers of NHS services producing Quality Accounts for the year 2010/2011' and sets out the following requirements for quality reports:

CASE EXAMPLE 10.2

Requirement for quality reports

Part 1

- **A statement on quality from the chief executive** (or equivalent) of the organisation and a statement from the senior employee outlining that to the best of that person's knowledge the information in the document is accurate (in regulations).

> **Part 2**
>
> - **Priorities for improvement** (in regulations) – the forward looking section of the report is your opportunity to show clearly your plans for quality improvement within your organisation and why you have chosen those priorities for improvement. You should also demonstrate how the organisation is developing quality improvement capacity and capability to deliver these priorities.
> - **Statements relating to quality of NHS services provided** (in regulations) – content common to all providers, which makes the accounts comparable between organisations and provides assurance that the board has reviewed and engaged in cross-cutting initiatives that link strongly to quality improvement. These include:
>   - the number of NHS services provided
>   - income generated by those services
>   - the number of and level of participation in national clinical audits and national confidential enquiries covered by the NHS services that the trust provides.
>   - the level of participation in clinical research
>   - the use of the CQUIN payment framework
>   - data quality
>   - Information Governance Toolkit attainment levels
>   - clinical coding error rate.
>
> **Part 3**
>
> - **Review of quality performance** (for provider determination) – report on the previous year's quality performance offering the reader the opportunity to understand the quality of services in areas specific to your organisation.
> - **An explanation of who you have involved** (for provider determination) and engaged with to determine the content and priorities contained in your **Quality Account** (in line with current equality legislation and the Health Act 2009).
> - **Any statements provided from your commissioning PCT, LINks or OSCs** (in regulations) including an explanation of any changes you made to the final version of your Quality Account after receiving these statements.

Quality reporting and foundation trusts

Monitor, as part of its reporting and regulatory regime, requires NHS foundation trusts to include a report on the quality of care they provide within the annual report. However, they also have to publish a separate quality account each year according to the DH guidance above. The requirements from the DH are more extensive than Monitor's requirements and many foundation trusts insert the DH quality accounts fully into their annual report rather than produce two separate documents.

The Monitor requirements include:

- a review of performance against the priorities the trust set for the previous year, identified in its annual report
- three to five priorities the trust identified for quality improvement in the forthcoming year's annual plans
- sustainability/climate change – providing a commentary, summary of performance and an outline of future priorities and targets
- NHS staff survey – a statement of the trust's approach to staff engagement, results from the survey, with action plans to address areas of concern, and future priorities and targets
- their regulatory ratings from Monitor.

Monitor also requires NHS foundation trusts to include public interest disclosures on the NHS foundation trust's activities and policies in the areas set out below in their annual reports. NHS foundation trusts can decide where these disclosures are to be included and they are often included within the quality reports:

- actions taken by the NHS foundation trust to maintain or develop the provision of information to, and consultation with, employees
- the NHS foundation trust's policies in relation to disabled employees and equal opportunities
- information on health and safety performance and occupational health
- information on policies and procedures with respect to countering fraud and corruption
- a statement describing the better payment practice code, or any other policy adopted on payment of suppliers, and performance achieved, together with disclosure of any interest paid under the Late Payment of Commercial Debts (Interest) Act 1998
- details of any consultations completed in the previous year, consultations in progress at the date of the report, or consultations planned for the coming year;
- consultation with local groups and organisations, including the OSCs of local authorities covering the membership areas
- any other public and patient involvement activities.

The board (or equivalent) is accountable for the quality account and, therefore, it must assure itself and then state publicly within the document that the information presented is accurate.

SAMPLE WORDING 10.1

STATEMENT OF DIRECTORS' RESPONSIBILITIES IN RESPECT OF THE QUALITY ACCOUNT

The directors are required under the Health Act 2009, National Health Service (Quality Accounts) Regulations 2010 and National Health Service (Quality Account) Amendment Regulation 2011 to prepare Quality Accounts for each financial year. The DH has issued guidance on the form and content of annual Quality Accounts (which incorporate the above legal requirements).

In preparing the Quality Account, directors are required to take steps to satisfy themselves that:

- the Quality Accounts presents a balanced picture of the Trust's performance over the period covered;
- the performance information reported in the Quality Account is reliable and accurate;
- there are proper internal controls over the collection and reporting of the measures of performance included in the Quality Account, and these controls are subject to review to confirm that they are working effectively in practice;
- the data underpinning the measures of performance reported in the Quality Account is robust and reliable, conforms to specified data quality standards and prescribed definitions, is subject to appropriate scrutiny and review; and
- the Quality Account has been prepared in accordance with Department of Health guidance.

The directors confirm to the best of their knowledge and belief they have complied with the above requirements in preparing the Quality Account.

By order of the Board

_____ Date   _____ Chairman

_____ Date   _____ Chief Executive

To ensure that the information presented is accurate and fairly interpreted, and that the range of services described and priorities for improvement are representative of the services delivered assurance is required to ensure accuracy. Further assurance is provided by the inclusion of any statement provided by the lead PCT, Local Involvement Network and local overview and scrutiny committee. These stakeholders must have an opportunity to comment on the report ahead of its publication.

Third party assurance has also been introduced with Monitor carrying out a dry run for foundation trusts' 2009–2010 quality accounts. The dry run was successful in developing third-party assurance for foundation trusts. The National Quality Board then asked that a similar dry run be carried out for NHS trusts in 2010–11. The Audit Commission was mandated as DH's appointed auditors to do this work and provide external assurance to management.

In the year ended 31 March 2011, Monitor required all foundation trusts and their auditors to provide:

- a limited assurance report on the content of the quality report, which will be published in foundation trusts' annual reports
- a separate governors' report – prepared by the foundation trust's auditors – covering external assurance on two mandated and one locally selected indicator.

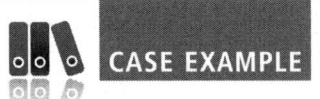

CASE EXAMPLE 10.3

University College London Hospital NHS Foundation Trust

UCLH NHS Foundation Trust has published Quality Accounts for two years now and has developed a format for establishing the quality priorities. First of all a long list of contenders are drawn up. Three of the Trust's Top Ten Objectives are around improving patient safety, experience and clinical outcomes so the long list contains contenders across all these domains. Possible priorities are derived from three sources: the Trust's performance over the past year against its quality and safety indicators; national or regional priorities and finally, from horizon scanning.

For example, last year, the trust drew from its performance scorecard things such as, overall patient satisfaction, falls and medication errors; from national priorities VTE and patient experience and Global trigger Tool from regional priorities. From horizon scanning such things as re-admissions, mortality rate in specific conditions and PROMs were possibilities included in the long list. The list of contenders also had to be in areas that fulfilled most or all of the following criteria:

1 Where the Trust genuinely had a desire or need to drive improvement
2 Known improvement strategies; so that the Trust could hit the ground running in delivering tangible improvement in a defined timeline
3 Have measures either in place or in development
4 Capable of historic or benchmark comparison.

The long list (15) plus the rationale for selection was then discussed and consulted on extensively with groups of internal and external stakeholders to develop a shortlist. In the second year of Quality Accounts a further question had to be asked as part of the discussions; did the Trust want to and was there good reason to carry forward any of the quality priorities from the previous year. The Trust found that the shortlist and final selection became virtually self-selecting following this process in that there was wide consensus on what should be the final priorities.

Once established, the Trust has put delivery strategies in place for all the quality priorities. It has also tracked performance against improvement trajectories at all levels from ward to Board on a monthly basis using the quality scorecard and priority specific improvement charts such as the example below for patient experience.

Extract from DH Quality Accounts Toolkit 2011

Quality Governance Framework

In 2010 Monitor introduced the *Quality Governance Framework* into the assessment process for aspirant foundation trusts and subsequently introduced the framework into the *Compliance Framework* via Board Statement 1 in the Annual Plan. The framework consists of ten questions, which are used to test the robustness of quality governance at applicant trusts through the following evidence:

- boards accurately understand the quality of the care their organisation provides;
- boards are able to assess and mitigate risks to quality
- quality is seen as a responsibility of the entire board, not only the medical and nursing directors
- trusts are committed to continuous quality improvement, and have put in place the tools to address poor performance.

1.2 Performance reporting

The *Operating Framework* (OF) for the NHS in England is published each year and describes the national priorities, system levers and enablers needed for NHS organisations to maintain and improve the quality of services provided, while delivering transformational change and maintaining financial stability. Within the OF are the planning, performance and financial requirements for NHS organisations and the basis on which they will be held to account.

Technical guidance is then issued every year, which describes the indicators in the Integrated Performance Measures and sets out for each measure:

- definitions
- monitoring arrangements
- accountability expectations
- planning requirements, if applicable
- further information.

The Annex to the NHS OF sets out further indicators that will be used nationally to assess the performance of SHA clusters and PCT clusters during the year. The indicators are grouped under three domains:

- quality, covering safety, effectiveness and experience
- resources, covering finance, workforce, capacity and activity
- reform, covering commissioning, provision and patient empowerment.

For foundation trusts, Monitor issues an annual *Compliance Framework*, which sets out the approach Monitor will take to assess the compliance of NHS foundation trusts with their terms of Authorisation ('the Authorisation') and to intervene where necessary. Monitor monitors the performance of foundation trusts against key national performance measures to assess the quality of governance at NHS foundation trusts. These cover acute, mental health and ambulance measures.

Foundation trusts are required to report quarterly to Monitor on their performance and declare a governance risk rating as follows:

- **Red**: likely or actual significant breach of terms of authorisation.
- **Amber-red**: material concerns surrounding terms of authorisation.
- **Amber-green**: limited concerns surrounding terms of authorisation.
- **Green**: no material concerns.

Figure 10.1 (see p. 216) sets out the annual reporting cycle that is required of foundation trusts by Monitor. The cycle requires foundation trusts to report on their performance and finances on a quarterly basis in order that Monitor can assess the trust's delivery of its annual plan.

All of this performance information is publicly available through publications from the regulators and on NHS Choices, which is the UK's biggest health website, providing a comprehensive health information service.

1.3 Financial reporting

NHS organisations are obliged to comply with the determination and directions given by the Secretary of State for Health, in the preparation of their annual report and annual accounts. These directions are set out in the *NHS Finance Manual*, which is published by the DH. In addition the government publishes the *Financial Reporting Manual* (FReM), which is the technical accounting guide to the preparation of financial statements. The manual is prepared following consultation with the Financial Reporting Advisory Board (FRAB) and is issued by the relevant authorities. It complements the guidance in the *NHS Finance Manual*. Foundation Trusts, are required to follow the guidance given by Monitor in the *NHS FT ARM*.

NHS organisations must publish an annual report and (full) audited accounts as one document and present it at a public meeting, whether or not summary financial statements are also produced. Where a NHS body has dissolved, or taken NHS Foundation Trust status, an annual report and audited accounts for its final accounting period must still be published and presented at a public meeting by a successor organisation.

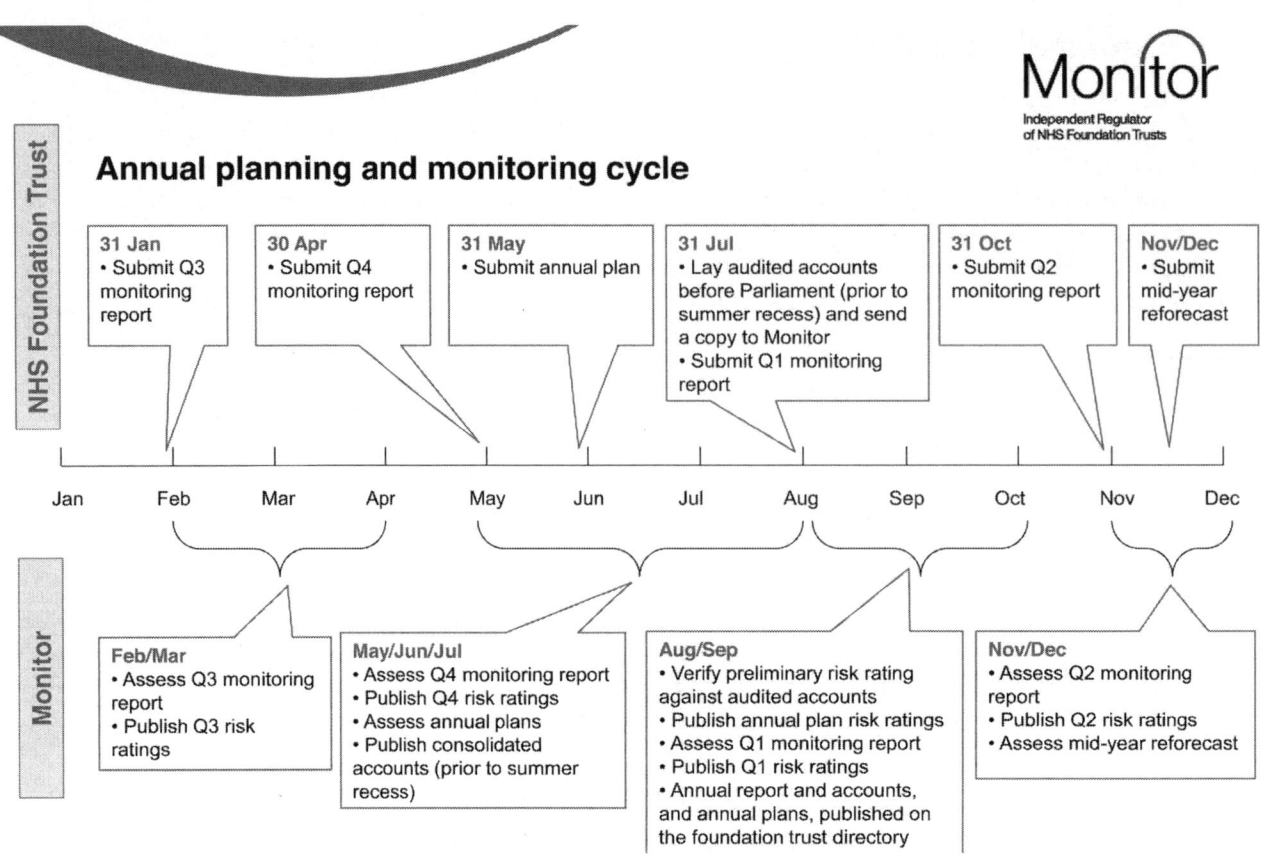

FIGURE 10.1 Monitor annual planning and monitoring cycle
(Source: Monitor, www.monitor-nhsft.gov.uk)

NHS organisations still have the option to prepare and distribute an annual report and summary financial statements, however, this is additional to the annual report and accounts described above which must be available if requested.

For NHS trusts that become NHS foundation trusts part way through the year, part year financial monitoring and accounts forms, must be prepared and submitted to DH in accordance with the timetable in the Manual. Separate accounts and an annual report will be prepared for the NHS Foundation Trust as specified by Monitor. Each set of accounts and annual report must formally be presented at separate public meetings, although these can take place on the same day and at the same venue.

The timetable for the production of the annual accounts is very constrained. For 2010/2011 the deadline for sending unaudited accounts to the external auditors was 21 April 2011 and the deadline for submitting audited accounts to DH was 10 June 2011. The annual accounts of each NHS organisation are summarised as part of the NHS Annual Accounts and laid before Parliament in July of each year.

The annual accounts are made up of:

- the Directors' Statements of Responsibilities (for special health authorities – Accounting Officer's Statement of Responsibilities)
- the auditors' report (which refers to the statement on internal control)
- the statement on internal control,
- four primary statements (Statement of Comprehensive Net Expenditure (or for NHS Trusts, Statement of Comprehensive Income); Statement of Financial Position; Statement of Changes in Taxpayers' Equity; and Statement of Cash Flows), and
- notes to the accounts.

The guidance sets out the minimum content of the annual report. Beyond this however, the entity must take ownership of the annual report and ensure that additional information is included where necessary to reflect the position of the NHS body within the community and give sufficient information to meet the requirements of public accountability.

In assessing the financial performance of foundation trusts Monitor also requires a quarterly financial risk rating to be determined. The risk rating is as follows:

1. highest risk – high probability of significant breach of authorisation in short-term, e.g. <12 months, unless remedial action is taken
2. risk of significant breach in medium-term, e.g. 12 to 18 months, in absence of remedial action
3. regulatory concerns in one or more components. Significant breach unlikely
4. no regulatory concerns
5. lowest risk – no regulatory concerns.

The financial statements report on the financial performance of the organisation over the previous financial year and the financial position of the organisation as at the end of that year. The directors' report and other statements published in the same document provide supporting information, much of it in narrative rather than in numerical form. Stakeholders use the information in the annual report and accounts to assess the stewardship of the directors and the financial health of the organisation.

The annual report and accounts is an important document for health service governance because it is a means by which the directors are made accountable to the stakeholders, and provides a channel of communication from directors to stakeholders. The report and accounts enable the stakeholders to assess how well the organisation has been governed and managed. It should therefore be:

- clear and understandable to a reader with reasonable financial awareness, and
- reliable and 'believable'.

The reliability of the annual report and accounts depends on several factors, including those that follow:

- The honesty of the organisation in preparing them: if allowed to do so by accounting regulations, organisations might indulge in **window dressing** their financial performance or financial position through the use of accounting policies (methods) that hide the true position.
- The care used by directors to satisfy themselves that the financial statements do give a 'true and fair view' and that everything of relevance has been properly reported.
- The opinion of the external auditors, which the stakeholders should be able to rely on as an objective and professional opinion.

If financial statements are produced in a way that is intended deliberately to mislead stakeholders, the persons responsible would be guilty of fraud, which is a crime. Misleading financial statements, however, could only be issued if the:

- audit committee is satisfied with their preparation
- external auditors provide a 'clean' audit report, and
- the board of directors approves the financial statements.

In most organisations, this would require deception by a small group of executives, such as the CEO and finance director.

1.4 Accountability and transparency

The diverse requirements for reporting in health service governance highlight a number of ways in which the organisation's directors are held accountable to stakeholders. The information given can be used to assess the success of the organisation and the effectiveness of its board.

It is therefore essential that the reporting should give a clear presentation of the position and performance of the organisation. In other words, there should be 'transparency' in reporting by organisation, so that the recipients of the reports can see what the organisation has achieved and assess what is likely to happen in the future.

The *UK Corporate Governance Code* states as a main principle that: 'The board should present a balanced and understandable assessment of the company's position and prospects' in its report and accounts and in its interim reports and other public statements. This principle applies to narrative reporting in the annual report as well as to the financial statements.

The *UK Code* also includes a provision that the annual report should contain an explanation of:

- the basis on which the company generates revenue and makes a profit from its operations (its 'business model'), and
- its overall financial strategy.

This information will probably be included in the same part of the annual report as the business review, which is described later. These principles are mirrored in the *NHS Finance Manual*, *FReM* and *NHS FT ARM*.

TEST YOUR KNOWLEDGE 10.1

a What areas of reporting are included in health service governance?
b What guidance is issued in each of these areas?
c Why is openness and transparency important in such reporting?

2 Directors' duties and responsibilities for financial reporting

The organisation's directors are responsible for the preparation and content of the financial statements.

The *UK Corporate Governance Code* states that the directors should explain in the annual report their responsibility for preparing the annual report and financial statements. There should also be a supporting statement by the auditors (in their report) about their reporting responsibilities. The *UK Code* also requires that the directors should include in their annual report an explanation of the:

- basis on which the company generates or preserves value over the longer term (its 'business model'), and
- strategy for delivering the objectives of the company.

2.1 Responsibilities of the directors for financial reporting

There is sometimes confusion and misunderstanding about responsibilities for financial reporting, and a mistaken belief that the external auditors are responsible for the 'true and fair view' in the financial statements. If misleading and incorrect financial statements are produced, it may therefore be supposed that the auditors have been negligent and must be to blame. This view is incorrect. The directors are responsible for the financial statements: they prepare the financial statements and have the primary responsibility for the reliability of the information they provide.

Management and the directors are therefore responsible for identifying and correcting any errors or misrepresentations in the financial statements.

The responsibility of the external auditors is to obtain reasonable assurance, in their professional opinion, that the financial statements are free from material error or mis-statement. They present a professional opinion to the stakeholders, not to the directors of the organisation, and the directors should not rely on the opinion of the external auditors in reaching their own view.

In UK law the directors are also potentially liable for any errors or misleading information in the annual report and accounts. Any person (for example, an investor) suffering a loss because of an error or misstatement in an organisation's report and accounts may sue the organisation, and the organisation may then take legal action against the directors to recover any losses it has occurred from the legal action.

2.2 Going concern statement

A key accounting concept is the 'going concern' concept. This is the view that the organisation will continue to trade for the foreseeable future (at least the next 12 months). The financial statements are therefore prepared on this basis, and assets are valued differently from what there value might be on a break-up basis (in a fire sale, if the organisation went into liquidation).

There are several rules or guidelines that require the directors to make a **going concern statement** in the annual report. This is a statement that in their opinion the organisation is a going concern and will continue to be so for at least the next year.

The *UK Corporate Governance Code* includes a provision that the directors should report in the company's annual and half-yearly financial statements that the company is a going concern, 'with supporting assumptions and qualifications as necessary'. The statement should therefore give reasons why the directors have reached their view, and also indicate any doubts there might be.

Similarly, the UK Listing Rules require the directors to make a statement in the report and accounts that the company is a going concern, together with supporting assumptions and qualifications as necessary.

For other companies, there are requirements in both international and UK accounting standards that the directors should satisfy themselves that it is reasonable for them to conclude that the company is a going concern, so that the financial statements can be prepared in a going concern basis. These requirements are mirrored in the *NHS Finance Manual*, *FReM* and *NHS FT ARM*.

A typical going concern statement within a corporate report might be as follows:

'The directors, on the basis of current financial projections and facilities available, have a reasonable expectation that the organisation and group have adequate resources to continue in operational existence for the foreseeable future. The directors accordingly continue to adopt the going concern basis in the preparation of the group's financial statements.'

In the UK, disclosures about the assumptions or qualifications about going concern status are becoming more extensive. The directors may be personally liable if they make a statement that the organisation is a going concern without giving the matter careful consideration. Liability could arise if the organisation subsequently goes into liquidation within the next 12 months and stakeholders claim that they relied on the going concern statement when making their investment decisions.

Initiative for greater disclosure

There have been concerns about the lack of information about going concern status. At the moment companies are simply required to make a going concern statement, which the auditors review as part of the annual external audit. It does not say anything about how the directors arrived at their judgement about the going concern status of their company, or what the major risks to the business as a going concern might be.

The FRC set up the **Sharman Panel of Enquiry**, to look into going concern statements in the corporate sector. The panel issued a preliminary report in November 2011, which recommended more disclosures that may lead to changes in the reporting requirements. Key recommendations were:

- including the going concern statement in the company's annual report on strategy and principal risks
- disclosing how the directors arrived at their conclusions
- disclosing in the annual report of the audit committee what material risks to the company's going concern status were considered, how they are being addressed and which matters the company has been unable to resolve.

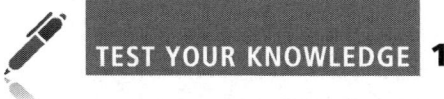
TEST YOUR KNOWLEDGE 10.2

What is a going concern statement?

3 Relationship between internal and external audit

All stakeholders rely on the quality, performance and financial information that is published by the organisation. It is important, therefore, that the information is objective and robust. As a result, the work of both **internal** and **external audit** are vital in making sure that, as far as is reasonably possible, the information is objective and can be relied on. Within NHS organisations the remit of internal and external audit includes the review of quality, performance and financial information. Part of the audit committee's role is to monitor the work of both internal and external auditors and to ensure that the external auditors can place full reliance on the work of internal audit in these three areas of information.

Non-foundation trusts are regulated by the Audit Commission, which is an independent body with statutory responsibilities to regulate the audit of local government and NHS bodies in England, and to promote improvements in the economy, efficiency and effectiveness of public services. The Commission's guidance is contained in the *NHS Code of Audit Practice* (2010). The Commission's responsibilities regarding audit are appointing auditors to local government and NHS bodies, setting the required standards for its appointed auditors and regulating the quality of audits.

Foundation trusts are subject to Monitor's guidance as set out in the *Audit Code for Foundation Trusts* (2010).

3.1 Function and scope of internal audit

Internal audit is defined as 'an independent appraisal activity established within an organisation as a service to it. It is a control that functions by examining and evaluating the adequacy and effectiveness of other controls' (CIMA Official Terminology).

The Chartered Institute of Internal Auditors describes the role as follows:

'The role of internal audit is to provide independent assurance that an organisation's risk management, governance and internal control processes are operating effectively. Internal auditors deal with issues that are fundamentally important to the survival and prosperity of any organisation. Unlike external auditors, they look beyond financial risks and statements to consider wider issues such as the organisation's reputation, growth, its impact on the environment and the way it treats its employees.'

The NHS Accounting Officer Memorandum requires all NHS trusts to have an internal audit function.

An organisation might have an internal audit unit or section, which carries out investigative work. An internal audit function should act independently of executive managers, but normally reports to a senior executive manager such as the finance director.

In the corporate sector, the FRC *Guidance on Audit Committees* suggests that the audit committee should ensure that the internal auditor has direct access to the board chairman and the audit committee, and is also responsible to the audit committee. This means that the internal auditors may be in an unusual position within the organisation. For operational reasons they may have a line reporting responsibility to a senior executive manager such as the finance director. Executive managers may also ask the internal auditors to carry out audits or reviews of the systems or procedures (and internal controls) for which they are responsible. However, the senior internal auditor should have some control over deciding what aspects of the organisation's systems should be investigated or audited, and also has a responsibility for reporting to the audit committee and the chairman of the board.

The work done by any internal audit unit is not prescribed by regulation, but is decided by management or by the board (or audit committee). The possible tasks of internal audit include the following:

- **Reviewing the internal control system**. Traditionally, an internal audit department has carried out independent checks on the financial controls in an organisation, however, this has now extended to include quality and performance controls as well. The checks would be to establish whether suitable quality, performance and financial controls exist and if so, whether they are applied properly and are effective. It is not the function of internal auditors

to manage risks, only to monitor and report them, and to check that risk controls are efficient and cost-effective.
- **Special investigations**. Internal auditors might conduct special investigations into particular aspects of the organisation's operations (systems and procedures), to check the effectiveness of operational controls.
- **Examination of financial and operating information**. Internal auditors might be asked to investigate the timeliness of reporting and the accuracy of the information in reports.
- **VFM audits**. This is an investigation into an operation or activity to establish whether it is economical, efficient and effective.
- **Reviewing compliance by the organisation with particular laws or regulations**. This is an investigation into the effectiveness of compliance controls.
- **Risk assessment**. Internal auditors might be asked to investigate aspects of risk management, and in particular the adequacy of the mechanisms for identifying, assessing and controlling significant risks to the organisation, from both internal and external sources.

A more detailed examination of the role of internal audit is contained in Chapter 12.

3.2 Function and scope of external audit

External audit traditionally has been the process by which the annual accounts of public and private sector bodies are subject to external scrutiny to provide independent assurance that they have been prepared in accordance with relevant legal and professional standards and give a 'true and fair' view of the financial performance and financial position of the audited body. More recently, however, external audit has comprised quality, performance and financial audits. Such audits being delivered through the private firms of auditors that organisations may appoint:

> 'It is one of the basic principles of audit in the public sector, that the scope of the audit should be understood to go beyond giving assurance on the accounts, to include examination of aspects of corporate governance and the use of resources.'
>
> Public Audit Forum, 'The principles of public audit'

External audit in the public sector is characterised by three distinct features:

- auditors are appointed independently from the bodies being audited
- the scope of auditors' work is extended to cover not only the financial statements, but also aspects of corporate governance and arrangements to secure the economic, efficient and effective use of resources
- auditors may report aspects of their work to the public and other key stakeholders.

In addition, external auditors of foundations trusts are also required to satisfy themselves that the quality report has been prepared according to the detailed guidance issued by Monitor.

The statutory responsibilities and powers of appointed auditors for non-foundation trusts are set out in the Audit Commission Act 1998. In discharging these specific statutory responsibilities and powers, auditors are required to carry out their work according to the Audit Commission's *Code of Audit Practice*. This code covers the audits of all local NHS bodies to which the Commission appoints auditors. It does not, however, cover the audits of NHS foundation trusts, which appoint their own auditors under arrangements overseen by Monitor. Nor does it apply to the audits of special health authorities or charitable funds held on trust by NHS bodies.

The auditors of a foundation trust have a primary responsibility to the NHS foundation trust's council of governors. Such auditors may also be responsible to Monitor for the exercise of some functions, and will have responsibilities to the members of the NHS foundation trust, as well as the wider public, in the case of public interest reports.

After completing their annual audit, the auditors are required to prepare a report to the stakeholders of the organisation, which is included in the published report and accounts. The audit report has two main purposes:

- to give an expert and independent opinion on whether the financial statements give a true and fair view of the financial position of the organisation as at the end of the financial year covered by the report, and of its financial performance during the year

- to give an expert and independent opinion on whether the financial statements comply with the relevant laws.

However, in carrying out their audit, external audit must also have regard to aspects of corporate governance and securing economy, efficiency and effectiveness in its use of resources.

Auditors of NHS foundation trusts are required to review the organisation's compliance with the *FT Code of Governance*, and to obtain evidence to support the organisation's compliance statement (in the annual report and accounts) of its compliance with the code. For those trusts that are required to produce quality accounts third party assurance from the external auditors is also required.

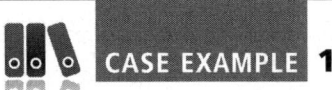

CASE EXAMPLE 10.4

The external assurance engagements undertaken on the 2010/11 Quality Accounts required NHS foundation trust auditors to:

- review the content of the 2010/2011 Quality Report against the content requirements included in the *NHS FT ARM* 2010/2011
- review the content of the 2010/2011 Quality Report for consistency against the other information sources detailed in the guidance
- provide a signed limited assurance report in the Quality Report on whether anything had come to the attention of the auditor that led them to believe that the content of the Quality Report had not been prepared in line with the requirements set out in the *NHS FT ARM* 2010/2011 and was not consistent with the other information sources detailed in the guidance
- undertake substantive sample testing of two mandated performance indicators and one locally selected indicator (to include, but not necessarily be limited to, an evaluation of the key processes and controls for managing and reporting the indicators and sample testing of the data used to calculate the indicator back to supporting documentation)
- provide a report to the NHS foundation trust board of their findings and recommendations for improvements concerning the content of the Quality Report and the mandated indicators
- provide a report to the NHS foundation trust board of their findings and recommendations for improvements concerning the local indicator.

3.3 Reliance on the work of internal audit

The Monitor *Audit Code for NHS Foundation Trusts* (March 2011) states that it is expected that the external auditors will liaise with the internal audit function to obtain a sufficient understanding of internal audit activities to assist in planning the audit and developing an effective audit approach. The auditors may also wish to place reliance upon certain aspects of the work of internal audit in satisfying their statutory responsibilities as set out in the National Health Service Act 2006 and in the Monitor Audit Code. In particular the auditors may wish to consider the work of internal audit when undertaking their procedures in relation to the statement on internal control (which for foundation trusts from 2011/2012 will be known as the annual governance statement (AGS).

The Audit Commission's *Code of Audit Practice* 2010 requires external audit to establish effective coordination arrangements with internal audit. External audit should seek to place maximum reliance on the work of internal audit whenever possible.

This all demonstrates the key relationship between internal and external audit as it is vital for the external auditors to be able to rely on the work undertaken by internal audit, not just on financial controls but on quality and performance controls as well.

4 The role and responsibilities of external audit

4.1 Audit report

The **audit report** is contained in the organisation's annual report and accounts, and is addressed by the auditors to the stakeholders of the organisation. The main purpose of the audit report is to give the users of an organisation's financial statements (and in particular the stakeholders) some reassurance that the information in the statements is believable and that the financial statements present a 'true and fair view' of the organisation's financial position and performance. The opinion of the auditors should be the opinion of independent professional experts, based on an investigation of the organisation's control systems, accounting systems and financial/business transactions.

The audit report itself provides only limited information to stakeholders, even though stakeholders often assume that an unqualified audit report means that the financial statements of the organisation are accurate and reliable.

An unmodified audit report (sometimes called an 'unqualified opinion') is given when the auditor believes that the accounts give a true and fair view of the organisation's financial position and performance. The wording of an unmodified audit report is usually fairly standard, although reports are longer for public companies (where the auditors might also report on some corporate governance statements) and differ between countries.

An unmodified audit report may include an 'emphasis of matter' paragraph. Although the audit report is not modified, and the auditors consider that the financial statements present a true and fair view, there is an item that the auditor wants to bring to the attention of users because it is of some importance for an understanding of the statements.

Auditors may present a **modified audit report**, although this is unusual. If it happens, there is a potentially serious problem with the financial statements and, by implication, the financial condition of the organisation. It also means that the auditors have been unable to agree with the directors of the organisation about what information the financial statements should contain. Because the directors and the auditors cannot agree, the auditors have considered it necessary to give a statement to stakeholders to this effect. There are three types of modified audit opinion:

- a qualified opinion
- an adverse opinion, and
- a disclaimer of opinion.

A qualified audit opinion is sometimes called an 'except for' opinion. It is given when, in the opinion of the auditor, the financial statements would give a true and fair view except for a particular matter, which the auditor explains.

An adverse opinion is given when the auditor considers that there are material mis-statements in the accounts and that these are 'pervasive'. In effect, the auditor is stating that the figures in the accounts are seriously wrong.

A disclaimer of opinion is given in cases where the auditor has been unable to obtain the information that he needs to give an audit opinion. The lack of information means that the auditor is unable to state that the financial statements give a true and fair view, and that there may possibly be serious mis-statements that the auditor has been unable to check.

In the rare circumstances that the auditors give a modified audit report to the stakeholders, a situation has arisen where professional accountants have given an opinion that the stakeholders cannot trust the information that has been given to them by the directors. If the stakeholders cannot trust the directors, the quality of corporate governance could hardly be lower.

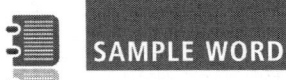

SAMPLE WORDING 10.2

UNMODIFIED AUDIT REPORT
Here is a simplified example of a typical unmodified audit report.

Report on the financial statements
We have audited the accompanying financial statements of XYZ Organisation, which comprise the statement of financial position as at 31 December 20XX, and the statement of comprehensive income, statement of changes in equity, and cash flows for the year then ended, and a summary of significant accounting policies and other explanatory notes.

Management's responsibility for the financial statements
Management is responsible for the preparation and fair presentation of these financial statements in accordance with International Financial Reporting Standards. This responsibility includes: designing, implementing and maintaining internal control relevant to the preparation and fair presentation of financial statements that are free from material misstatement, whether due to fraud or error; selecting and applying appropriate accounting policies; and making accounting estimates that are reasonable in the circumstances.

Auditor's responsibility
Our responsibility is to express an opinion on these financial statements based on our audit. We conducted our audit in accordance with International Standards on Auditing. Those standards require that we comply with ethical requirements and plan and perform the audit to obtain reasonable assurance whether the financial statements are free from material misstatement.

An audit involves performing procedures to obtain audit evidence about the amounts and disclosures in the financial statements. The procedures selected depend on the auditor's judgement, including the assessment of the risks of material misstatement of the financial statements, whether due to fraud or error. In making those risk assessments, the auditor considers internal control relevant to the entity's preparation and fair presentation of the financial statements in order to design audit procedures that are appropriate in the circumstances, but not for the purpose of expressing an opinion on the effectiveness of the entity's internal control. An audit also includes evaluating the appropriateness of accounting policies used and the reasonableness of accounting estimates made by management, as well as evaluating the overall presentation of the financial statements.

We believe that the audit evidence that we have obtained is sufficient and appropriate to provide a basis for our audit opinion.

Opinion
In our opinion, the financial statements give a true and fair view (or present fairly, in all material respects) of the financial position of XYZ Organisation as of December 31 20XX, and of its financial performance and its cash flows for the year then ended in accordance with International Financial Reporting Standards.

Report on other legal and regulatory requirements
[Form and content of this section of the report will vary depending on the nature of the auditor's other reporting responsibilities.]

Signed: (Auditor) _____

Date: _____

4.2 Responsibility for detecting errors and fraud

Stakeholders would probably like to assume that if the auditors provide a favourable audit report, the financial statements must be 'correct', and there has not been any fraud or error that has resulted in:

- incorrect use of accounting policies
- omissions of fact
- misinterpretation of fact.

('Fraud' is intentional; 'error' is unintentional: both lead to incorrect figures in the financial statements, if they have not been discovered.)

This view is based on the belief that if professional accountants have checked the figures, they must be correct – unless the accountants have been negligent and have failed to do their job properly. However, it is a popular misconception that the auditor is responsible for detecting fraud or error in an organisation's financial statements. This is not the case.

The board of directors is responsible for preventing fraud in their organisation, or detecting fraud if it occurs. The organisation's system of internal control, described in Chapter 12, should be designed to limit the risk of fraud and error, and the board is responsible for monitoring the effectiveness of the internal control system. The responsibility of the board (with delegated responsibility of management) for the prevention and detection of fraud and error is a core principle of corporate governance. The directors are fully accountable to the stakeholders and so are fully responsible for the information presented in the annual report and accounts.

It is not the primary responsibility of the external auditors to detect fraud. The auditors will assess the risk or possibility that fraud or error might have caused the financial statements to be materially misleading. The auditors should therefore design audit procedures that will provide reasonable reassurance that material fraud or error has not occurred, and that the financial statements give a true and fair view of the organisation's financial position and performance. The external audit might also act as a deterrent to fraud, because the auditors will carry out checks of control procedures, documents and transactions in the course of their audit work. They might discover fraud during the course of their audit work, in which case it would be their responsibility to report the matter to the directors (unless the fraud is carried out by the directors themselves).

No matter how well an audit is planned and carried out, there will always be some risk that fraud or error has occurred but not been detected. Given the nature of auditing, for which there is only a limited amount of time and resources, and which is carried out through a process of sampling and testing, it would be impossible to ensure that all errors are detected. Accounting systems and internal control procedures are also vulnerable to fraud and error, arising for example from:

- criminal collusion between employees
- decisions by management to override the system of controls.

An area for dispute, however, is whether the auditors ought to be able to identify fraud or a significant error during the course of their audit work, whenever a fraud or error occurs. Although they are not responsible for the financial statements, it can be argued that a failure by the auditors to discover a major fraud or material error might be the result of professional negligence. If they are negligent, they should be held liable to the organisation and its stakeholders.

In the UK, the Companies Act 2006 introduced new rules on auditors' liability for negligence, breach of duty or breach of trust regarding the conduct of the audit. Shareholders of both public and private companies can vote by ordinary resolution to limit the potential liability of the external auditors, by means of a liability limitation agreement (LLA).

The Act states that in considering what is fair and reasonable in the circumstances, the court should have no regard to the possibility or otherwise of recovering compensation from other persons who are jointly or partly responsible for the loss that has been incurred.

Although the Companies Act 2006 provides the possibility of some protection for auditors against liability for negligence or breach of duty with LLAs, it also introduced two new criminal offences for auditors in connection with the auditors' report. It is a criminal offence, punishable by a fine, to:

- knowingly or recklessly cause an audit report to 'include any matter that is misleading, false or deceptive in any material particular', or
- knowingly or recklessly cause an audit report to omit a statement that is required by certain specified sections of the Act.

4.3 Auditors' liability to third parties

The auditors have a legal duty of care to the organisation and its stakeholders. There is some doubt as to whether they might also have a duty of care to other parties. In the UK, the extent of auditor liability to external parties has been tested in two legal cases.

 CASE LAW 10.1

Caparo Industries plc v Dickman (1990)

In the UK legal case *Caparo Industries plc v Dickman and others (1990)*, it was held by the House of Lords that auditors did not owe a duty of care in audit reports to third parties that they did not know at the time. The auditors of a company had negligently audited its accounts, and as a result the company reported a profit of £1.2 million instead of a loss of £400,000. Replying on these accounts, the respondents in the case made a successful takeover bid for the company. They subsequently brought an action against the auditors for breach of duty of care and skill. In ruling in the auditors' favour, the House of Lords held that there was no liability, since the auditors did not owe a duty of care to a member of the public. Their duty was simply to the company and its stakeholders.

As a result of the *Caparo* case, it was considered that the auditors of a company did not hold a duty of care to any third party, until the subject came up for consideration again in the *Royal Bank of Scotland v Bannerman Johnstone Maclay (2002)*. This was a case in the Scottish courts, and so was not binding on English courts, but it drew from leading English court cases and so is considered to have significant legal implications for England and Wales as well as Scotland.

In this case, Bannerman were the auditors of a company that arranged an overdraft facility with the bank. The overdraft facility letter between the bank and the company contained a requirement for the company to send the bank a copy of its audited annual accounts at the end of each year. In 1998, the company went into receivership owing over £13 million to the bank, which claimed that due to fraud, the accounts for the previous year were materially incorrect and the auditors were negligent. The bank also claimed that it had relied on the auditors' unqualified opinion to continue providing the overdraft facility to the company. In its defence, the audit firm claimed that it had no duty of care to the bank. The judge ruled that although there had been no direct contact between the audit firm and the bank, the auditors would have known about the facility letter. The knowledge they would have gained during the course of their audit work was therefore sufficient, in the absence of any disclaimer, to create a duty of care to the bank. In the judge's view, the absence of a disclaimer was a crucial feature of the case.

In response to the outcome of the *Bannerman* case (see Case law 7.1), PricewaterhouseCoopers decided to include a disclaimer of liability to third parties using its audit reports. In January 2003, the Institute of Chartered Accountants in England and Wales recommended the inclusion of a disclaimer in audit reports.

A disclaimer within the audit report might be worded as follows:

'This report, including the opinion, has been prepared for and only for the organisation's members as a body in accordance with the Companies Act 2006 and for no other purpose. We do not, in giving this opinion, accept or assume responsibility for any other purpose or to any other person to whom this report is shown or into whose hands it may come save where expressly agreed by our prior consent in writing.'

> **TEST YOUR KNOWLEDGE 10.3**
>
> a What is the purpose of internal audit?
> b Why is their relationship to external audit important?
> c How has the role of external audit extended in public bodies?
> d Who is responsible for detecting fraud or errors in financial statements?
> e Who is responsible for detecting fraudulent activity within the organisation, by some of its employees or others?
> f What are the responsibilities of the external auditors with regard to the financial statements of an organisation?
> g What types of audit opinion might be given in an audit report? What is the significance of a modified audit opinion?

4.4 Independence of the external auditors

The external auditor should be independent of the client organisation, so that the audit opinion will not be influenced by the relationship between the auditor and the organisation. The auditors are expected to give an unbiased and honest professional opinion to the stakeholders about the financial statements. An unmodified audit report is often seen by investors as a 'clean bill of health' for the organisation. However, doubts are sometimes expressed about the independence of the external auditors.

It could be argued that unless suitable governance measures are in place, a firm of auditors may reach audit opinions and judgements that are heavily influenced by their wish to maintain good relations with the management of a client organisation. If this happens, the auditors are no longer independent and the stakeholders cannot rely on their opinion.

For example, in the corporate sector, an official 2010 report on the collapse of Lehman Brothers in 2008 criticised the external auditors Ernst & Young for allowing the company to account for certain transactions (repo 105 transactions) in a way that misleadingly improved the look of the end-of-quarter balance sheets during 2007 and 2008, in the months before the bank eventually collapsed.

Perhaps the most significant threat to auditor independence is that the audit firm relies on the organisation's management to secure its appointment and re-appointment as the organisation's auditor. Although companies may give their audit committee responsibility for recommending the appointment of the auditors, the opinions of senior management are often decisive in the matter of auditor selection. The auditor is therefore reliant for future audit work from the organisation on the views of the management whose financial statements it is their job to audit. In addition, the audit firm has to rely extensively on management for the information and explanations needed to enable them to carry out their audit work. A UK Ethical Standards Board has commented on this situation that:

> 'Any reasonable and informed third party — for example, a shareholder — is likely to regard this as a significant threat to the auditor's objectivity.'

Professional guidelines are given to auditors by national and international accountancy bodies, notably the International Federation of Accountants (IFAC). The IFAC Code of Ethics for Professional Accountants identifies certain ways in which the integrity, objectivity and independence of the auditors might be put at risk.

An audit firm should not have to rely on a single organisation for a large proportion of its total fee income, because undue dependence on a single audit client could impair objectivity. IFAC does not specify what amounts to 'undue dependence' on a single client. However, in the UK, the rules of the Association of Chartered Certified Accountants (ACCA) state that the fee income from a single audit client should not exceed 15% of the gross annual income of the audit practice.

A risk to objectivity and independence arises when the audit firm or anyone closely associated with it (such as an audit partner) has a mutual business interest with the organisation or any of its officers. Similarly, objectivity could be threatened when there is a close personal relationship between a member of the audit firm and an employee of the organisation.

The audit firm should not have a client organisation in which a partner holds a significant number of stakes.

The IFAC Code does not have any objection in principle to an audit firm providing non-audit services (such as consultancy services) to a client, although the auditor should not perform any management functions in an organisation nor take any management decisions.

The audit profession has identified five categories of potential threats to auditor independence:

- **Self-interest threats**: e.g. if the audit firm earns a large proportion of its revenue from a client organisation, it may be unwilling to annoy that client by challenging the figures and assumptions used by management to prepare the organisation's financial statements.
- **Self-review threat**: this can arise when the audit firm does non-audit work for the organisation, and the annual audit involves checking the work done by the firm's own employees. The auditors may not be as critical of the work, or prepared to challenge it, because this would raise questions about the professional competence of the audit firm.
- **Advocacy threat**: this can arise if the audit form is asked to give its formal support to the organisation by providing public statements on particular issues or supporting the organisation in a legal case. Acting as advocate for an organisation means taking sides, and this implies a loss of independence.
- **Familiarity threat**: a threat to independence occurs when an auditor is familiar with an organisation or one of its directors or senior managers, or becomes familiar with them through a working association over time. Familiarity leads to trust and a willingness to believe what the other person says. The auditor will also be unwilling to think that the other person is capable of making a serious error or committing fraud. A familiarity threat arises through personal association (for example, family connections) and through long association with the organisation and its management.
- **Intimidation threat**: an auditor may feel threatened by the directors or senior management of an organisation. Both real and imagined threats can affect the auditor's independence. Intimidation may result from a domineering and bullying personality on the organisation's board of directors (for example the CEO). An organisation may also threaten to take away the audit or stop giving the firm non-audit work unless the auditor accepts the opinions of management.

Threats to auditor independence must be identified, and measures should be taken to limit the threat to an acceptable level of risk. Two areas of debate about how to ensure auditor independence have been:

- whether auditors should be prevented from carrying out non-audit work for clients, or
- whether the amount of non-audit work they do should be restricted, and whether there should be a regular rotation of either the audit firm or the audit partner and other senior members of the audit team.

4.5 Non-audit work for a client by an audit firm

The codes of conduct of national professional accountancy bodies are similar to the IFAC Code and lack any clear restrictions on the performance of **non-audit work** for an audit client. Suggestions for regulatory measures to ensure auditor independence have included proposals to restrict the amount of non-audit work, or the type of non-audit work, that the firm of auditors is permitted to carry out for a client organisation. Non-audit work might include:

- consultancy on taxation issues, for example helping an organisation to minimise tax liabilities
- investigating targets for a potential takeover bid
- helping an organisation to construct a bid for a major government contract
- providing advice and expert assistance on IT systems
- internal audit services
- valuation and actuarial services
- services relating to litigation
- services relating to recruitment and remuneration.

The main problem with auditors doing non-audit work is that when the firm audits transactions recommended by its consultancy arm, it is unlikely to take an independent view.

The risk to auditor objectivity and independence from carrying out non-audit work became apparent in the wake of the Enron collapse. Arthur Andersen were the auditors of Enron, and in the financial year before the company's collapse in 2001, Andersen earned more fee income from Enron for non-audit work than from audit work. The audit firm was suspected of failing to carry out a proper audit of the company, with two main reasons being suggested:

- It was claimed that the audit firm would have been reluctant to question the accounts of Enron because it would risk losing not just the audit work but also the substantial non-audit fee income.
- In addition, it was suggested that since the information in the company's financial statements reflected the non-audit consultancy advice given by the audit firm, the firm's auditors would be unlikely to challenge the fairness and accuracy of the statements. In other words, Andersen's auditors would not challenge the opinions of Andersen's consultants.

Audit firms have denied that fees from non-audit work will affect their independence, arguing that the individuals who work as consultants for a client organisation (e.g. on IT projects) are not the same individuals who work on the audit. Even so, activist shareholder groups continue to challenge this assertion. In the UK, a well-reported attempt was made several years ago (2002) by some institutional stakeholders to vote against the re-appointment of Deloitte as auditors to Vodafone at the AGM of the company. The 'dissidents' argued their case because the audit firm did too much non-audit work for the company and so could not be considered sufficiently independent.

There are three broad approaches to the regulation of non-audit work by audit firms:

- There should be no restrictions at all on non-audit work by the audit firm.
- There should be a total prohibition on non-audit work for a corporate client by the audit firm.
- There should be a partial prohibition on non-audit work for a corporate client by the audit firm.

A partial restriction could take either of two forms. There could be a prohibition on audit firms from taking on certain types of consultancy work where their independence as auditors could be put at risk, for example tax planning advice work. However, audit firms would be free to carry out other types of non-audit work. The second approach to restricting non-audit work would be to set a limit on the amount of fees an audit firm could earn from non-audit work, expressed perhaps as a proportion of the fees it earns from the audit. For example, a limit might be imposed restricting non-audit fees to, say, 50% of the fees from the audit work.

The difficulty with a partial restriction on non-audit work is that rules have to be devised and agreed as to what permissible and non-permissible non-audit work should be, or what the maximum amount of non-audit fee income should be.

In the UK, the audit profession is governed by ethical principles rather than rules and regulations about non-audit work for audit clients. The Institute of Chartered Accountants in England and Wales (ICAEW) has made the following statements about non-audit work:

'The most effective way to ensure the reality of independence is to provide guidance centred around a framework of principles rather than a detailed set of rules that can be complied with to the letter but circumvented in substance.'

'A blanket prohibition on the provision of non-audit services to audit clients can be inefficient for the client and is neither necessary to ensure independence, nor helpful in contributing to the knowledge necessary to ensure the quality of the audit.'

The need for auditor independence when the audit firm does non-audit work is recognised in the *UK Corporate Governance Code*. The code includes a provision that:

'The annual report should explain to stakeholders how, if the auditor provides non-audit services, auditor objectivity and independence is safeguarded.'

4.6 Rotation of audit firm or audit partner

Another suggestion for protecting auditor independence is that there should be **'rotation'** of auditors. There is an important distinction, however, between the following.

- Rotation of an audit firm, whereby a firm is required to give up the audit for an organisation after a maximum number of years, and the organisation must appoint different auditors.
- Rotation of audit personnel, whereby the audit engagement partner and other key individuals involved in the annual audit should be removed from the audit after a certain number of years, and new individuals assigned to the work.

Rotation of audit firm

Rotation of the audit firm would enhance auditor independence because a firm of auditors would have little to gain by agreeing with the wishes of the client organisation, and carrying out a less than rigorous audit, if it knows that it will soon lose the audit work anyway. The work of outgoing auditors would also be subject to review – and criticism – by the firm of auditors taking their place.

The case for regular rotation of external auditors was strengthened by the accounting fraud at WorldCom in 2002. Its external auditors (Andersen) had been auditors of the firm since 1989, and in the year before fraud was uncovered, the firm was reportedly earning three times as much from WorldCom in consultancy fees as it was earning in audit fees ($12.4 million, compared with $4.4 million).

A disadvantage of **audit firm rotation** is that the incoming firm of auditors might need one or two years to get to know the business of the client organisation, and might be unable to conduct an audit to the same standard as their predecessor.

If the argument in favour of auditor rotation is accepted, however, there is still scope for disagreement about how frequently audit firm rotation should occur. Regular rotation might involve an organisation changing the audit firm every five years or so. An alternative argument is that audit firm rotation should be much more occasional, say every ten or 15 years.

Audit partner rotation

An argument put forward by the major accountancy firms is that the requirement for rotation should apply, not to the firm of auditors, but to the individual partner of a firm in charge of the audit. For example, it might be acceptable for ABC Corporation to retain the services of Ernst & Young indefinitely, provided that the partner in charge of the audit is replaced every, say, five or seven years. Supporters of this argument claim that the independence of the audit is threatened by the personal relationship an audit partner builds up with the client organisation, not the length of association of the audit firm with the organisation.

In the case of large organisations, there is also an argument for a regular rotation of other senior audit managers, as well as the lead partner.

Peter Wyman, former president of the ICAEW, stressed the distinction between audit partner and audit firm rotation. Writing in the *Financial Times* (25 July 2002) he commented that:

> 'Improvements could be made in the area of audit partner and audit firm rotation, although it is vital not to confuse the two. Audit firm rotation achieves the appearance of greater auditor independence but research shows it is likely to produce a reduction in audit quality, particularly in the first two years after the new firm is appointed. Because people rather than organisations are likely to get "cosy" with one another, greater audit independence could be achieved by rotating the audit partner. This approach avoids quality loss, which arises when the entire cumulative knowledge of the audit firm is cast aside when a new firm is appointed.'

A counter-argument, however, is that **audit partner rotation** would not have prevented the problem that arose between Andersen and its clients Enron and WorldCom. Although Andersen as a whole was not over-dependent on Enron, the company was a vital client for the firm's Houston office, which carried out the audit. Similarly, the Andersen office in Jackson, Mississippi was heavily dependent on the work that it did for WorldCom. To prevent loss of audit independence, audit partner rotation would almost certainly have been ineffective, whereas audit firm rotation might have been much more effective.

Currently, regulations in most countries favour audit partner rotation rather than audit firm rotation. In the UK, for example, the ICAEW's ethical standards require the rotation of various members of an audit team, including the rotation of the audit engagement partner at least every five years.

> **TEST YOUR KNOWLEDGE 10.4**
>
> **a** Give examples of non-audit work for an organisation by a firm of auditors.
> **b** What are the five categories of threats to auditor independence?
> **c** What is the difference between audit firm rotation and audit partner rotation?

5 The audit committee

The *UK Corporate Governance Code* requires that a board of directors should establish formal and transparent arrangements for:

- considering how they should apply the corporate reporting and risk management and internal control principles, and
- maintaining an appropriate relationship with the organisation's auditors.

These arrangements should be met by establishing an audit committee, which should be given certain responsibilities by the board.

The formal requirement for every NHS board to establish an audit committee can be found in *Codes of Conduct and Accountability* issued by DH. Foundation trusts are required to have an audit committee by the *FT Code of Governance*.

The role of the audit committee in applying the principles of risk management and **internal audit** is described in Chapters 11 and 12; this chapter concentrates on the role of the audit committee is applying corporate reporting principles and maintaining an appropriate relationship with the external auditors.

5.1 Role and responsibilities of the audit committee

The *NHS Audit Committee Handbook* (HFMA 2011) describes the role of the audit committee as 'critically reviewing the governance and assurance processes on which the board places reliance'.

This is a wider role than the traditional role of financial scrutiny, which is envisaged by the *UK Corporate Governance Code*, and has resulted from the broad range of stakeholder requirements that exist in the NHS. The two key areas that the audit committee should provide assurance to the board on are the Assurance Framework and documents that are to be publicly disclosed (i.e. AGS, registration evidence for the CQC, the annual report and accounts and the quality accounts).

The Assurance Framework provides an organisation with a method for the effective and focused management of the principal risks to meeting its objectives. It also provides a structure for the evidence to support the AGS. It identifies which of the organisation's objectives are at risk because of inadequacies in the operation of controls or where the organisation has insufficient assurance about them. At the same time it provides structured assurances about where risks are being managed effectively and objectives are being delivered. This allows the board to determine where to make efficient use of resources and to address the issues identified to improve the quality and safety of care.

The audit committee should not be responsible for creating the Assurance Framework, instead it is should satisfy itself that this is being carried out appropriately by line management and that the processes and format are valid, relevant and effective. The Committee needs to be satisfied that it contains the high risk areas pertinent to the organisation.

With regard to public disclosure statements the audit committee has an essential role in reviewing these prior to approval by the board. It should be satisfied with the strength of the processes and the quality of data that has been relied upon to produce the statements.

In addition the *UK Corporate Governance Code* lists the role and responsibilities of an audit committee (excluding those concerned with risk management and internal control) as follows.

- To monitor the integrity of the organisation's financial statements and any formal announcements relating to the organisation's financial performance. In doing so, it should review 'significant financial judgements' that these statements and announcements contain.
- To make recommendations to the board in relation to the appointment, re-appointment or removal of the organisation's external auditors, and for putting these recommendations to the stakeholders for approval at a general meeting of the organisation.
- To approve the remuneration and terms of engagement of the external auditors (after they have been negotiated with the auditors by management).
- To review and monitor the independence and objectivity of the external auditors, and also the effectiveness of the audit process, taking into account relevant UK professional and regulatory requirements.
- To develop and implement the organisation's policy on using the external auditors to provide non-audit services. This should take into account any relevant external ethical guidance on the subject. The committee should report to the board, identifying actions or improvements that are needed and recommending the steps to be taken.

The board should decide just what the role of the audit committee should be, and the terms of reference should be tailored to the organisation's particular circumstances. A separate section of the annual report should describe the work of the committee. The audit committee should review its terms of reference and effectiveness annually, and recommend any necessary changes to the board. The board should also review the effectiveness of the audit committee annually.

The core functions of the audit committee are concerned with 'oversight', 'assessment' and 'review' of other functions and systems in the organisation. It is not the committee's duty to carry out those functions; for example, management remains responsible for preparing the financial statements and the auditors remain responsible for preparing the audit plan and carrying out the audit.

However, the high-level oversight function can sometimes lead to more detailed work. For example in a foundation trust recently, where there were concerns over payroll, the audit committee requested a full-scale review of payroll services.

5.2 Composition of the audit committee

The *NHS Audit Committee Handbook* states:

> 'the distinctive characteristic of the audit committee is that it comprises only non-executive directors. This condition of membership provides the basis for the committee to operate . . . independently of any executive management processes and to apply an objective approach in the conduct of its business.'

The chair of the organisation should not be a member of the audit committee and does not normally attend. The CEO and other executive directors only attend when requested. As a matter of good governance practice, the company secretary should act as secretary to the audit committee.

Under the *UK Code* an audit committee should consist of at least three members (or at least two members outside the FTSE 350). All its members should be independent NEDs. The *UK Code* also states that the board should satisfy itself that at least one member of the committee has 'recent and relevant financial experience'. This individual should ideally have a professional qualification from one of the accountancy bodies, and the degree of financial literacy required from the other committee members will vary according to the nature of the company.

The FRC has published *Guidance on Audit Committees* (revised 2010), which suggests that appointments to the committee should be made by the board on the recommendation of the nomination committee, in consultation with the audit committee chairman. Appointments should be made for a period of up to three years, extendable by no more than two additional three-year periods and so long as the director remains independent.

The *UK Corporate Governance Code* states that a separate section of the company's annual report should describe the work of the audit committee. 'This deliberately puts the spotlight on the audit committee and gives it an authority it might otherwise lack.' Similar recommendations are contained in the DH's Model Standing Orders for NHS trusts and in *FT Code of Governance*.

The organisation's management is under an obligation to make sure that the audit committee is kept properly informed and should take the initiative in providing the committee with information, instead of waiting to be asked. The executive directors should also have regard to their common law duty to provide all directors, including the audit committee members, with all the information they need to discharge their duties as directors of the organisation. This guidance is crucial. The audit committee can only do its work properly if it is kept properly informed by the executive management.

5.3 Remuneration, induction and training of committee members

Because audit committees have wide-ranging and time-consuming work to do, organisations must make the necessary resources available. This includes making suitable payments to the members of the audit committee, in view of the responsibilities they have and the time they must commit to the work. The amount of remuneration paid to the audit committee members should take account of the remuneration paid to other members of the board. The committee chairman's responsibilities and time commitments will normally be greater than those of the other committee members, and this should be reflected in their remuneration.

The committee should have the support of the company secretary and should have access to the services of the organisation's secretariat.

Audit committee members must also be given suitable induction and training. Ongoing training should include keeping the committee members up to date on developments in quality, performance and financial reporting and related NHS guidance or legislation. It may, for example, include understanding financial statements, the application of particular accounting standards, the regulatory framework for the organisation's business, the role of internal and external auditing, and risk management. Both induction and training can take various forms, including attendance at formal courses and conferences, internal organisation talks and seminars and briefings by external advisers.

5.4 Audit committee meetings

The audit committee chairman should decide the timing and frequency of committee meetings, in consultation with the company secretary, and there should be as many meetings as the role and responsibilities of the committee require.

The FRC Guidance suggests that there should be no fewer than three committee meetings each year, timed to coincide with key dates in the financial reporting and audit calendar. For example, meetings might be held when the audit plans are available for review and when interim statements, preliminary announcements and the full annual report are near completion. Most audit committee chairmen will probably want to call meetings more frequently. In practice most NHS audit committees meet quarterly, if not bi-monthly, to manage the significant workload carried by the committee. This is reflected in the *NHS Audit Committee Handbook*.

Sufficient time should be allowed between audit committee meetings and meetings of the main board to allow any work arising out of the committee meeting to be carried out and reported to the board as appropriate. This is reflected in the *NHS Audit Committee Handbook*.

Only the audit committee chairman and members are entitled to attend meetings of the committee. It is for the committee to decide whether other individuals should be invited to attend for a particular meeting or a particular agenda item. It is expected that the external and internal audit lead partners and the organisation's finance director will be invited regularly to attend meetings.

At least once a year, the audit committee should meet the external and internal auditors, without management being present, to discuss matters relating to its responsibilities and issues arising from the audit.

5.5 Quality, performance and financial reporting and the audit committee

It is the responsibility of management, not the audit committee, to prepare complete and accurate quality, performance and financial statements. It is the responsibility of the audit committee to review the significant reporting issues and judgements that are made in connection with these statements. Key points:

- The audit committee should consider significant accounting policies used to prepare the financial statements, any changes to them, and any significant estimates or judgements on which the statements have been based.
- Management should inform the committee about the methods they have used to account for significant or unusual transactions, where the accounting treatment is open to different approaches.
- Taking the external auditors' views into consideration, the committee should consider whether the organisation has adopted appropriate accounting policies and made appropriate estimates and judgements.
- The committee should also consider the clarity and completeness of the disclosures in the quality, performance and financial statements.
- If the committee is not satisfied with any aspect of the proposed reporting by the organisation, it should report its views to the board. The committee should also review related information presented with the quality, performance and financial statements, including the business review and the corporate governance statements relating to audit and risk management.

5.6 Appointment and removal of external auditors

Under the *UK Code* the audit committee has the primary responsibility for making a recommendation to the board on the appointment, reappointment or removal of the external auditors. If the audit committee recommends to the board that new external auditors should be selected, the committee should 'oversee' the selection process (FRC Guidance). The committee's recommendation should be based on the following assessments:

- the qualification and expertise of the auditors
- the resources of the auditors
- the independence of the auditors.

In contrast in foundation trusts, while the audit committee may make recommendations as to appointment, re-appointment or removal of the external auditors, it is the board of governors who make the decision. The NHS foundation trust is required to ensure that, as part of the appointment process, their appointed auditors meet the criteria set out by Monitor. The auditors must agree the terms of engagement with the NHS foundation trust in a letter of engagement. If the auditors fail to meet, or have cause to believe that they will not be able to comply with, the criteria set out in the terms of authorisation at any point during their appointment, they must resign as auditors. NHS foundation trusts must provide Monitor with details of their auditors on authorisation and whenever a change to the auditors is made. This information should include the name and address of the organisation. When the auditor's appointment ends, the auditor is required to write to the foundation trust and to Monitor giving notice of resignation and setting out a statement of the circumstances or stating that there are none.

For non-foundation trusts the external auditors are appointed by the Audit Commission.

If the audit committee recommends that new external auditors should be selected, the committee should 'oversee' the selection process (FRC Guidance). The committee's recommendation should be based on the following assessments:

- the qualification and expertise of the auditors
- the resources of the auditors
- the independence of the auditors
- the effectiveness of the audit process.

The assessment should cover all aspects of the audit service provided by the audit firm, and in carrying out the assessment the committee should obtain from the audit firm a report on its own internal quality control procedures.

If the external auditors resign, the audit committee should investigate the issues that led to the resignation, and consider whether any action is needed.

The audit committee should consider the terms of engagement of the external auditors and the remuneration to be paid to the auditors for their audit services. (The committee should consider the terms and remuneration, but is not required to negotiate them itself.) It should satisfy itself that the amount of the fee payable for the audit services is appropriate, and that an effective audit can be carried out for such a fee. The fee should not be too large, but neither should it be too low. A low audit fee creates a risk that the audit might be of an inadequate scope or quality. The audit committee should then make a recommendation to the board of directors (or governors in the case of NHS foundation trusts).

The committee should review and agree the engagement letter issued by the external auditors at the start of each audit, to make sure that it has been updated to reflect any changes in circumstances since the previous year.

The committee should also review the scope of the audit with the auditor. If it is not satisfied that the proposed scope is adequate, the committee should arrange for additional audit work to be undertaken (FRC Guidance).

5.7 Audit committee responsibilities and auditor independence

The *Audit Code for Foundation Trusts* (2011) and *NHS Code of Audit Practice* (2010) gives the audit committee the responsibility for monitoring and ensuring the independence of the external auditors. If the external auditors provide non-audit services to the organisation, the annual report should explain how auditor independence and objectivity are safeguarded.

The audit committee should have procedures for ensuring the independence and objectivity of the external auditors annually. The FRC Guidance recommends:

- The committee should seek reassurance that the auditors and their staff have no family, financial, employment, investment or business relationship with the organisation that could adversely affect their independence or objectivity. The committee should seek from the audit firm, annually, information about the firm's policies and processes for maintaining independence and monitoring compliance with relevant requirements, such as those regarding the rotation of audit partners and staff.
- The committee should agree with the board the organisation's policy on employing former employees of the external auditor. Particular attention should be given to the organisation's policy on former employees of the auditor who were members of the audit team and then moved directly to the organisation. This policy should be drafted, and the audit committee should monitor its application. The committee should monitor the number of former employees of the external auditor who now hold senior positions within the organisation, and consider whether there may be some impairment (or appearance of impairment) in the auditors' judgement and independence with regard to the audit.
- The committee should monitor the audit firm's compliance with ethical guidance in the UK about the rotation of audit partners, and the fees the organisation pays as a proportion of the overall fee income of (1) the firm; (2) the office of the firm responsible for the audit; and (3) the audit partner.
- The audit committee should develop and recommend to the board the organisation's policy relating to the provision of non-audit services by the external auditors. The committee's objective should be to ensure that the provision of such services does not impair the independence or objectivity of the auditors.

5.8 Provision of non-audit services

The audit committee should ensure that the provision of non-audit services by the organisation's audit firm would not impair the objectivity and independence of the auditors. The committee should consider:

- whether the skills and experience of the audit firm make it a suitable supplier of the non-audit services
- whether there are safeguards in place for ensuring that there would be no threat to the objectivity and independence of the auditors arising from the provision of these services
- the nature of the non-audit services and the fees for these services
- the level of fees for individual non-audit services and the fees in aggregate for these services, relative to the size of the audit fee
- the criteria governing the compensation of the individuals who perform the audit.

The audit committee should set and apply a formal policy specifying the types of non-audit work:

- from which the external auditors are excluded
- for which the external auditors can be engaged without referral to the audit committee
- for which a case-by-case decision is necessary. In these cases, it may be appropriate to give a general pre-approval for certain classes of work, subject to a fee limit decided by the audit committee and ratified by the board. If the external auditor subsequently provides any of these services, the engagement of the auditors should then be ratified at the next audit committee meeting.

The policy may also set fee limits generally or for particular classes of non-audit work.

In deciding its policy on the provision of non-audit work by the external auditors, the committee should take into account relevant ethical guidance, but a guiding set of principles should be that the external auditor should not be engaged for non-audit work if the result is that:

- the external auditor would audit work done by its own employees
- the external auditor makes management decisions for the organisation
- a mutuality of interest is created
- the external auditor is put in the role of advocate for the organisation (FRC Guidance).

If the external auditors do provide non-financial services, the annual report should explain to stakeholders how auditor independence and objectivity is safeguarded (*FT Code of Governance*).

TEST YOUR KNOWLEDGE 10.5

a Who should be the members of an audit committee?
b According to the *NHS Audit Committee Handbook* what should be the role of the audit committee?
c What are the provisions of the Monitor Code of Governance with regard to the appointment, re-appointment or removal of the external auditors for foundation trusts?
d What induction or training might be provided for members of an audit committee?
e What does the FRC Guidance say about the frequency of audit committee meetings?
f What measures might an audit committee take to monitor the independence of the external auditors on a regular basis?

5.9 The audit committee and the annual audit cycle

The FRC Guidance goes into some detail on the annual audit cycle, and the relationship between the audit committee and the external auditors during this process.

At the start of each annual audit, the audit committee should ensure that appropriate plans are in place for the audit.

The committee should consider whether the auditors' overall work plan (including the planned levels of materiality and the proposed resources to carry out the audit) seems consistent with the scope of the audit engagement. This assessment should have regard to the seniority, expertise and experience of the audit team.

The audit committee should review, with the external auditors, the findings of their work. As a part of this review, the committee should: (1) discuss with the auditors any major issues that arose during the audit (and whether these have been resolved); (2) review key accounting or audit judgements; and (3) review levels of errors identified during the audit and obtain explanations as to why certain errors might remain unadjusted.

The FRC Guidance states that the audit committee should review the following:

- The audit representation letters from management, before they are signed, and consider whether the information provided is complete and appropriate, based on the knowledge the committee has.
- The management letter from the auditors, and the responsiveness of the organisation's management to the auditors' findings and recommendations.

Representation letters from the organisation's management are a part of the audit evidence collected and considered by the auditors. They contain information from management to the auditors. These deal with matters for which other audit evidence does not exist; therefore, the auditors are relying on what management tell them. Representations are required:

- from the directors, acknowledging their collective responsibility for the financial statements and confirming that they have approved them, and
- with regard to matters where knowledge of the facts is confined to management (e.g. management's intention to sell off a division of the business) or where there is a matter of judgement and opinion (for example, with regard to the trading position of a major customer and debtor, or the likely outcome of litigation in progress).

The audit committee should review these representations from management and assess whether (on the basis of the knowledge of the committee members) the information provided seems complete and appropriate.

At the end of the audit cycle, the audit committee should assess the effectiveness of the audit process. As a part of this assessment, the committee should:

- review whether the auditors have met the agreed audit plan and consider the reasons for any changes
- consider the 'robustness and perceptiveness' of the auditors, in their handling of key accounting and audit judgements, and in their commentary on the appropriateness of the organisation's internal controls
- obtain feedback about the conduct of the auditors from key people within the organisation, such as the finance director and the head of internal audit
- review the auditor's management letter, to assess whether it is based on a good understanding of the business and to establish whether the auditors' recommendations have been acted on (and if not, why not).

5.10 Review of audits and audit committees by the FRC

The FRC is aware of criticisms of company reporting, audits and audit committees and it believes that more should be done to demonstrate that the auditors are achieving the fundamental purpose of an audit, which is to provide shareholders with an objective and professional opinion on the position and performance of the company. In a report 'Effective Company Stewardship: next steps' in September 2011, the FRC indicated that it was considering a number of changes in the future including:

- improvements in narrative reporting
- the requirement that auditors provide an opinion on the entire annual report and accounts of companies, not just the financial statements
- the responsibilities of the audit committee should be extended to cover review of the entire contents of the annual report and accounts
- companies may be required to put their audit out to tender at least every ten years, or explain why they have not done so and the steps taken and the reasons for the decision.

6 Disclosure of governance arrangements

In 2006, the EU adopted a *Company Reporting Directive*, requiring quoted companies to produce a corporate governance statement in their annual reports. The statement must refer to the corporate governance code applied by the company (for example, the *UK Corporate Governance Code*) and explain whether, and to what extent, the company complies with that code. The statement must also include a description of the main features of the company's internal control and risk management systems in relation to the financial reporting process, and provide a description of the composition and operation of the board and its committees.

In the UK, listed companies were already required to report much of the corporate governance information required by the *Company Reporting Directive*, because the UK Listing Rules require companies to include in their annual report a statement of how they have applied the principles of the *UK Corporate Governance Code*. The code includes requirements for disclosures about governance arrangements, such as reports on the composition of board committees and their work.

However, the *Company Reporting Directive* requires that the information should be presented in a separate 'corporate governance statement'. The Directive also requires that the statement should include a description of the main features of the company's internal control and risk management systems relating to the financial reporting process, something not contained in the *UK Code*.

As the *FT Code of Governance* builds on the principles and provisions of the *UK Code*, much of this is true for foundation trusts. It will be interesting to see whether the move towards renaming the Statement on Internal Control as the AGS will also build on the requirements of the *Company Reporting Directive*.

7 The business review

The Companies Act 2006 (section 417) requires companies (with the exception of small companies) to include a business review in their annual report. Companies give a variety of names to this review, including Operating and Financial Review, Business Review or even Directors' Report. This requirement also applies to NHS organisation and is included within the NHS *FReM* and *NHS FT ARM*.

The review should provide a 'balanced and comprehensive analysis' of the development and performance of the business of the organisation during the financial year and the position of the organisation's business as at the end of the year. The review should be consistent with the size and complexity of the business. It must contain:

- a fair review of the business of the organisation, and
- a description of the principal risks and uncertainties that the organisation faces.

A business review is mainly in narrative form, but should also include:

- key financial performance indicators (KPIs), and
- where appropriate, key non-financial performance indicators, including information of environmental and employee matters.

The auditors must state in their audit report whether in their opinion the information given in the directors' report is consistent with the organisation's accounts for the financial year. This includes the information in the business review. Directors could be personally liable for incorrect information in the business review. When a director is found liable for an untrue or misleading statement or an omission, he will be liable to compensate the organisation for any loss it has suffered as a result.

When the requirement for a business review was first introduced into UK law, concerns were expressed about the potential liability of directors for statements they would be required to make in a review, especially statements that are forward-looking and so impossible to make with certainty. To meet general concerns about the potential liability of directors for the contents of reports, the 2006 Act includes so-called **safe harbour provisions** (section 463).

These provisions state that a director can be liable for untrue or misleading statements only if he knew them to be untrue or misleading, or was 'reckless' as to whether they were untrue or misleading. Similarly a director can only be responsible for an omission if he knew the omission to be a 'dishonest' concealment of a material fact.

TEST YOUR KNOWLEDGE 10.6

a In UK law, which companies must publish an annual business review?
b What should business review provide and what must it contain?
c What are safe harbour provisions?

CHAPTER SUMMARY

- The key areas of reporting for NHS organisations relate to quality, performance and finance. Within each of these areas there are prescribed frameworks and regulations that govern their content and timing.
- Quality, performance and financial audits, therefore, provide assurance on the stewardship of public money and the corporate governance and performance of NHS organisations.
- Trustworthy reporting and auditing is probably the most significant issue for health service governance.
- The significant report relating to quality is the annual Quality Account, which reports on the quality of services provided by an NHS healthcare service.
- The OF for the NHS in England is published each year and describes the national priorities, system levers and enablers needed for NHS organisations to maintain and improve the quality of services provided, while delivering transformational change and maintaining financial stability. Within the OF are the planning, performance and financial requirements for NHS organisations and the basis on which they will be held to account.
- NHS organisations are statutorily obliged to comply with the determination and directions given by the Secretary of State for Health, in the preparation of their annual report and annual accounts. These directions are set out in the *NHS Finance Manual*, which is published by DH.
- The diverse requirements for reporting in health service governance highlight a number of ways in which the organisation's directors are held accountable to stakeholders. The information given can be used to assess the success of the organisation and the effectiveness of its board.
- The directors, not the external auditors, are responsible for the financial statements.
- Stakeholders rely on the quality, performance and financial information that is published by an NHS organisation. It is important, therefore, that the information is objective and robust. As a result the work of both internal and external audit are vital in making sure that, as far as reasonably possible, the information is objective and can be relied on.
- Traditionally, an internal audit department has carried out independent checks on the financial controls in an organisation, however, this has now extended to include quality and performance controls as well.
- The scope of the external auditors' work is extended to cover not only the financial statements, but also aspects of governance and arrangements to secure the economic, efficient and effective use of resources.
- The board of directors, who have a responsibility to safeguard the assets of the company, are responsible for the prevention or detection of fraud within the organisation. Fraud may take the form of criminal activity by employees or others (such as theft) or deliberate misrepresentation in published financial statements. Measures to prevent or detect fraud should be a part of the internal control system in the organisation.
- The external auditors do not have a direct responsibility for detecting fraud, but may discover fraud during their annual audit work, which should then be reported to senior management (or the authorities, if senior management appear to be responsible themselves for the fraud). However, if the auditors fail to detect fraud when they should reasonably have been expected to do so, they may be liable for negligence.

- To perform their role, the external auditors must be independent from the company.
- Threats to independence can be classified as self-interest threats, self-review threats, advocacy threats, familiarity threats and intimidation threats. Carrying out non-audit work for an audit client may create self-interest threats (concerns about losing the work and the fees). Familiarity threats can be reduced by audit firm rotation (not common) or audit partner rotation.
- Doubts have been expressed about the independence of auditors from the organisations to which they provide an audit service. The audit firm (through the ethical codes of the profession) and the organisation's board of directors both have a responsibility to protect the independence of the auditors.
- Control over the audit profession is therefore a governance issue.
- An audit committee, properly constituted, could provide a valuable role in improving the relationship between an organisation and its auditors and helping to ensure that the external audit process is satisfactory and that the external auditors remain independent. In Europe, there is now a statutory requirement for quoted companies to have an audit committee.
- An audit committee should consist entirely of independent NEDs. The *FT Code* in accordance with the *UK Code* specifies that at least one member should have recent and relevant financial experience.
- The responsibilities of an NHS audit committee are set out in detail in the *NHS Audit Committee Handbook*.
- In foundation trusts the audit committee makes recommendations as to appointment, re-appointment or removal of the external auditors to the board of governors who make the decision. The external auditors are appointed by the Audit Commission for non-foundation trusts.
- The audit committee should have procedures for ensuring the independence and objectivity of the external auditors annually.
- The objective of the audit committee should be to ensure that the provision of non-audit services by the organisation's audit firm would not impair the objectivity and independence of the auditors.
- A business review, which is largely in narrative form, should include non-financial information as well as financial information, and should be forward-looking as well as commenting on historical performance. In this way it provides more information to stakeholders, and improves both accountability and transparency.

CASE QUESTION 3.1

Review again the case scenario outlined at the beginning of Part Three. The Audit Committee are asked by the Trust Board to consider the implications of the appointment. Having read the contents of Part 3, how would you advise the Chair of Audit Committee? What concerns would you expect to see raised by Internal Audit?

PART **FOUR**

Risk management and internal control

■ LIST OF CHAPTERS

11 Identifying operational and strategic risks
12 Internal control systems

■ OVERVIEW

The fourth part of this study text considers risk and risk management as issues in health service governance. The leaders of NHS organisations are responsible for deciding risk strategies and risk policies, and for ensuring that the internal control system is effective. There are some similarities between a business risk management system and an internal control system, but each has a different purpose and it is important to distinguish between them. The responsibilities of the board of directors for both business risk management and internal control are specified in the *FT Code of Governance* and are implicit in DH guidance for non FTs.

Chapter 11 explains the nature of business risk and the responsibility of the board for deciding how much risk the company should be prepared to accept in order to achieve hoped-for financial returns, and also how much risk the company should be able to tolerate. Exposures to business risk should not exceed the levels determined by the board, and the business risk management system should be effective in ensuring that board strategies and policies are implemented and also reviewed. The chapter describes the elements that may be found in a business risk management system, including the role of a risk committee of the board (or the audit committee) and the measures that may be taken by executive management to implement and monitor risk strategies. The chapter concludes with a brief consideration of how executive remuneration packages might be arranged so that incentive schemes make suitable allowance for risk and risk exposures.

Chapter 12 examines internal control systems. Whereas business risk is an unavoidable aspect of engaging in business activities and is external to an organisation, internal control risks are internal to a company and so within management control. The chapter describes the nature of internal control risks and internal controls that are applied to prevent adverse events from happening, or identifying them and taking corrective measures when they do happen. A board of directors is responsible for ensuring that the system of internal control is effective, and achieves its purpose. The chapter describes the guidance given to UK listed companies on internal control systems (the *Turnbull Guidance*). It then goes on to describe several elements of internal control in more detail: the role of internal audit in internal control (and whether organisations should have an internal audit function); the benefits of disaster recovery planning; and whistleblowing procedures that enable employees to report suspicions of wrongdoing outside normal lines of reporting through the management hierarchy. The chapter concludes with a description of the statutory measures implemented in the US by the SOX to ensure more effective internal control within companies.

■ LEARNING OUTCOMES

Part Four should enable you to:

- apply the principles of risk management
- appraise the significance of risk management for good governance
- advise on the appropriate arrangements for an effective risk management system
- advise on the board's responsibility for internal control to meet good governance guidelines
- appraise the effectiveness of an internal control system
- understand and apply the NHS principles and guidance in relation to internal audit
- develop appropriate policies and procedures to mitigate the impact of operational disaster and devise a whistleblowing procedure.

PART 4 CASE STUDY

Dr Lee Jesson, as medical director, has been involved in developing a series of quality indicators that measure patient outcomes in the outpatients department within the trust. The indicators are produced from the data collected from questionnaires completed within the department. Dr Jesson has worked with a major mobile manufacturer to adapt smartphones to enable them to be used as the questionnaire. All of the responses are collected on the smartphone and the data is then transferred to computer software that collates and analyses the data. The big advantage is that it provides real time feedback on the quality of care being received in the department. The system and the quality improvements in care that are being delivered have been nationally recognised as good practice and Dr Jesson is receiving lots of invitations to demonstrate the system and outline the benefits for patients.

Helen Wrightford, discovers that Dr Jesson and Wilson Ford have been invited to China to visit the manufacturing plant where the smart phones are made. The manufacturer is funding the whole cost of the trip and it includes a trip to see the Great Wall of China. It is also clear that the manufacturer is also funding the hotel and food costs for Dr Jesson whenever he is invited to speak about the system to other NHS organisations.

Identifying operational and strategic risks

■ CONTENTS

1. Risk management and governance
2. The nature of risk
3. Business risks and internal control risks
4. Responsibilities for risk management
5. Risk committees and risk managers
6. Risk management policies, systems and procedures

■ INTRODUCTION

The responsibility of boards for effective risk management came under close scrutiny following the banking crisis in 2007–2009. Many banks were criticised for getting into financial difficulty because of reckless business strategies and failing to recognise the business risks that they were taking.

Within NHS organisations the scrutiny of risk management is also the responsibility of the board, however, there tends to be much closer external scrutiny as well.

Business risks are risks to patient safety and financial security that arise from factors in the business environment, including competition, over which management has no direct control. NHS organisations must take risks in order to deliver healthcare but how much risk should they be prepared to tolerate, and would they be able to withstand 'shocks' in the business environment if an unexpected event or development were to occur? The board has the responsibility for strategic decisions on risk, and an important aspect of health service governance is for the board to recognise its responsibilities and ensure that the risk management system in the organisation is effective.

1 Risk management and governance

1.1 The relevance of business risk for health service governance

The board of directors has a responsibility to govern the organisation in the interests of the stakeholders. A part of this responsibility is to decide the objectives and strategic direction for the organisation, to approve detailed strategic plans put forward by management, and to monitor and review the implementation of those plans. An important objective of a NHS organisation is to make economic, efficient and effective use of public resources in its provision of healthcare, and the organisation's strategies should be directed towards this. However, any business strategy involves taking risks and actual results may be better or worse than expected.

Bad health service governance can result in the collapse of an organisation, and excessive risk-taking is one aspect of poor governance. The board of directors should consider business risk when it makes strategic business decisions. It should choose policies that are expected to deliver the key objectives, but should limit the risks to a level that it considers acceptable. For example, when the board takes major investment decisions itself or decides on corporate strategy, risks as well as expected returns must be properly assessed. The board should also be satisfied that in their decision-making, managers take risk as well as expected outcomes into account.

The Cadbury Report (1992) described risk management as:

'the process by which executive management, under board supervision, identifies the risk arising from business . . . and establishes the priorities for control and particular objectives.'

The significance of risk management for corporate governance was demonstrated forcibly by the global banking crisis in 2007–2009. In the UK, the government initiated **Walker Report** into the failures in the banking industry published in 2009 commented that although there were failures in the regulation of the banking industry, much of the blame for the crisis was attributable to poor governance, and in particular inadequate attention to risk management.

The significance of risk management for health service governance can be demonstrated at Mid Staffordshire NHS Foundation Trust where the trust was found to be in significant breach of two terms of its authorisation in March 2009. This was as a result of significant failings relating to quality of care, governance and leadership within the trust.

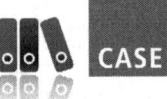

CASE EXAMPLE 11.1

Mid Staffordshire NHS Foundation Trust was authorised by Monitor as an NHS foundation trust in February 2008. In March 2008, the Healthcare Commission started an investigation into mortality rates in emergency care at the trust, publishing a report in March 2009. The investigation identified significant failings relating to quality of care, governance and leadership within the trust. These findings were reinforced by Robert Francis QC's report in February 2010, which looked at the care provided by the trust between 2005 and 2009 and was based on evidence from over 900 patients and families. The report concluded that patients were routinely neglected by a trust that was preoccupied with cost cutting, targets and processes and which had lost sight of its fundamental responsibility to provide safe care.

1.2 Risk appetite and risk tolerance

The board has overall responsibility for risk management and for deciding the organisation's risk appetite.

Risk appetite is the level of risk that an organisation is willing to take in the pursuit of its objectives. Risk appetite can be defined as the combination of the desire to take on risk to obtain a specific return (e.g. financial or quality), **risk capacity** and **risk tolerance**.

The 'desire to take on risk' refers to the amount and type of risk that the board of directors would like the organisation to have exposure to.

Risk capacity is the maximum risk exposures that the organisation can accept without threatening its financial stability.

Risk tolerance is the amount of risk that the organisation is prepared to accept to achieve its financial objectives. Risk tolerance is therefore the amount of risk that an organisation's board of directors allows the organisation to accept.

Risk appetite and risk tolerance are closely related. One is the amount of business risk (and types of business risk) the board would like the organisation to have and the other is the amount of risk that the board is prepared to tolerate. Although the **Walker Report** made recommendations for corporate boards, these should also be considered by the boards of NHS organisations. It recommended that the board should consider risk appetite and risk tolerance, and that much more attention should be given to these issues:

'Board-level engagement in risk oversight should be materially increased, with particular attention to the monitoring of risk and discussion leading to decisions on the entity's risk appetite and tolerance.'

The report went on to state that the board has responsibilities for the determination of risk tolerance and risk appetite through the cycle and in the context of future strategy and, of critical importance, the oversight of risk in real-time in the sense of approving and monitoring appropriate limits on exposures and concentrations. This is largely a forward-looking focus.

Risk appetite should be reviewed regularly by the board, and decisions should be taken about the scale of risk that is desired or acceptable. Risk tolerance could be expressed in numerical terms, such as the maximum loss that the board would be willing to accept on a particular venture if events turn out adversely or in terms of the quality of the service that is provided. Alternatively, risk tolerance could be expressed in terms of a total ban on certain types of business activity or behaviour.

TEST YOUR KNOWLEDGE 11.1

a What is the responsibility of a board of directors for business risk?
b What is risk appetite and risk tolerance?

2 The nature of risk

Risk refers to the possibility that something unexpected or not planned for will happen. In many cases, risk is seen as the possibility that something bad might happen. In everyday life, there is a risk of becoming seriously ill, being involved in a road accident, having a house burgled or flooded, having a motorcar breakdown, and so on. This can be described as **downside risk**, because it is a risk that something will happen that would not normally be expected.

There is **upside risk** too. This is the possibility that actual events might turn out better than expected. In a health service context, an example is the possibility that activity levels will be higher than planned or that working days lost through industrial action will be lower than anticipated.

Another example is investment decisions. Every investment is risky. Actual returns could be lower or higher than expected. In deciding whether to undertake an investment, the risks as well as the potential returns should be considered.

Some risks are easy to recognise, because they are always present and a NHS organisation may have had many years of experience in dealing with them. For example, financial risks include the risk that tariff will be set at a substantially lower level or that the costs of pharmaceutical supplies will increase. Other risks, however, are more difficult to identify and anticipate. The **Walker Report** commented:

> 'While a clear continuing responsibility of the board is to ensure that [recognisable financial] risks are indeed appropriately managed and controlled, different and potentially much more difficult issues arise in the identification and measurement of risks where past experience is an uncertain or potentially misleading guide. When risk materialises, it may do so as a risk previously thought to be understood and managed that turns out to be very different indeed . . .'

TEST YOUR KNOWLEDGE 11.2

a What may be the consequences of failing to consider business risk strategy or establishing an effective **business risk management** system?
b What is business risk and how could it be measured?

3 Business risks and internal control risks

A distinction can be made between business risk and internal control risk (sometimes called governance risk).

Business risks are risks that occur and arise in the external business environment in which an organisation operates. Business risks are usually referred to as **strategic risk**, because the business risks faced by an organisation are determined by the strategies that the organisation pursues.

Internal control risks are risks of losses that arise through ineffective controls within the processes and systems of an organisation's business operations. Internal control risk is risk within an organisation; business risk is risk in the external environment.

This chapter is concerned with the management of business risk. Chapter 12 describes **internal control systems** and the management of internal control risks.

3.1 Categories of business risk

The nature and severity of business risks varies from one organisation to another. Risks also change over time: some become less significant, and new risks emerge.

Business risks are risks that the actual performance of the business could be much worse (or better) than expected, due to unexpected developments in the business environment. For example, when an organisation develops a new service, it will have an expectation of the likely activity level. Actual levels could be higher or lower than expected. With some new services, the risk that activity levels will differ from expectation could be much more severe than with other new services. There are various reasons why activity levels may be less than expected, or may fall unexpectedly. Competitors may take away some of the organisation's market share; an organisation may suffer from bad publicity; there may be new regulations making the provision of a particular service more difficult.

Business risks can be categorised or identified in different ways, but it may help to understand the variety of risks by considering the following sources of risk:

- **Reputation risk**: the risk of loss in customer loyalty or customer support following an event that damages the organisation's reputation.
- **Competition risk**: the risk that business performance will differ from expected performance because of actions taken (or not taken) by other organisations.
- **Business environment risks**: these are risks of significant changes in the business environment from political and regulatory factors, economic factors, social and environmental factors and technology factors (the so-called 'PEST' factors). For example, business performance may be affected by the introduction of new regulations, a change of government, economic decline or growth, environmental issues, unexpected changes in social habits or technological change.
- **Financial risks**: these are risks that financial conditions may change, with adverse changes in tariff or interest rates, higher losses from bad debts or changes in prices from major suppliers.
- **Liquidity risk** is the risk that the organisation will have insufficient cash to settle all its liabilities on time, and so may be forced out of business. The board of directors should monitor this risk regularly and when they prepare their going concern statement for the annual report and accounts.
- **Strategic risks** are the risks of taking decisions on strategy that will result in exposures to excessive business risk and so could lead to losses or even business collapse.

Each industry and each organisation within an industry faces different risks. The questions that management should ask are as follows:

- What risks does this organisation face?
- How can these risks be measured? It may be possible to assess the risk in a business with unpredictable variations in key factors such as sale levels or market prices. High volatility is associated with high business risk.

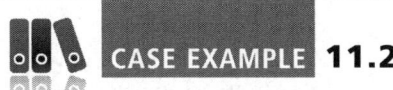

CASE EXAMPLE 11.2

Heart of England NHS Foundation Trust

Heart of England NHS Foundation Trust was the first Foundation Trust to acquire another NHS Trust, Good Hope Hospital, in 2007. The board realised that making an acquisition was a complex process – especially in the NHS – and had to establish clear governance structures to manage the inherent risk in the project. Key areas for consideration were:

- understanding the strategic imperative to acquire
- appraising options
- how to value a trust
- how to negotiate terms
- handling the actual transaction process and interacting with key stakeholders
- planning for post-merger integration
- organisational development post merger to enhance staff morale.

Large-scale mergers and acquisitions have inherent risks and Monitor's role in this area was to ensure that the trust did not jeopardise its quality of services or financial stability. They did this by providing indicative risk ratings of major transactions, leaving the board to put in place strategies and mechanisms to mitigate any material risks.

- For each of these risks, how would the organisation be affected if the worst outcome came about, or if a fairly bad outcome happened?
- What is the likelihood of a bad outcome for that risk item?
- What is the organisation's risk appetite or risk tolerance?
- What should the organisation be doing to manage the risk, either by avoiding it altogether or planning to deal with the problems that will arise in the event of a bad outcome?

TEST YOUR KNOWLEDGE 11.3

a How might business risks be categorised?
b What is the difference between business risk and internal control risk?

4 Responsibilities for risk management

The board is responsible for risk at a 'high level', but responsibilities for the management of risk are delegated to executive management. The board should decide the level of risks that are acceptable at a strategic level, and should ensure that management consider risk in the decisions that they make. The *FT Code* states:

> 'The board of directors' role is to provide effective and proactive leadership of the NHS foundation trust within a framework of processes, procedures and controls which enable risk to be assessed and managed.'

The code also states as a principle that the board should maintain 'a sound system of internal control to safeguard public and private investment, the NHS foundation trust's assets, patient safety and service quality'.

The board should therefore satisfy itself that appropriate systems are in place to identify, evaluate and manage the significant risks faced by the organisation.

The code also requires that, at least annually, the board should also carry out a review of the effectiveness of risk management systems in the organisation. The Code therefore includes requirements for:

- a system of risk management, and
- regular reviews of the system (at least annually) by the board.

(Note: The requirement for NHS organisations to include a business review in their annual directors' report was described in Chapter 10. The review should include a description of the principal risks and uncertainties facing the organisation. However, a requirement to report on significant risks does not necessarily require a formal business risk management system.)

> **TEST YOUR KNOWLEDGE 11.4**
>
> What are the principles and provisions of the Monitor *FT Code* with regard to business risk management?

5 Risk committees and risk managers

5.1 Risk committees

Responsibilities for risk management vary between organisations. An important distinction should be made between the arrangements whereby responsibilities for risk management are fulfilled by:

- the board, and
- executive management.

At board level, responsibility for reviewing the effectiveness of the risk management system may be delegated by the board to the audit committee, which is also likely to have responsibility for reviewing the internal control system. Alternatively, the board may prefer to establish a separate **risk committee** of the board. The advantages of having a separate risk committee are as follows:

- It can focus on risk issues and reviewing the organisation's risk management system, without having to concern itself with other issues (such as the external auditors). It would give advice to the board on matters such as risk appetite and risk strategy.
- The composition of the board is not restricted by requirements of the *FT Code*. A risk committee should ideally consist mainly of NEDs but should also have the finance director as a member. If the audit committee had responsibility for the oversight of risk management, the finance director could not be a committee member (although he could be invited to meetings of the audit committee to give his views).

However, a separate risk committee is probably much more useful for a large public organisation than for a smaller listed organisation.

The Walker Report recommended that there may be another risk committee consisting of senior executives, chaired by the CEO. This committee would be responsible for risk management at an operational level. The responsibilities of this committee and the board risk committee would be very different:

> 'The role of the board risk committee is to advise the board on all high-level risk matters and should not extend into operational matters which are for the executive within the overall risk framework determined by the board. The NEDs on the committee cannot be expected to be able to replicate the industry expertise of the executive team nor will their capacity to contribute be enhanced by information overload. The materials presented to them should be in succinct format, highlighting major issues.'

This provides an interesting consideration for larger NHS organisations where a similar structure may be helpful.

5.2 Risk officers

In common with larger companies some larger NHS organisations may also appoint specialist executive managers with responsibility for risk – a chief risk officer (CRO). The Walker Report recommended that the CRO should:

- report directly to the finance director or CEO but also
- have direct access to the board and should be able to provide advice to the board on all risk issues affecting the organisation.

> 'Alongside an internal reporting line to the chief executive officer or [Chief Financial Officer CFO], the CRO should report to the board risk committee, with explicit, and what is clearly understood to be, direct access to the chairman of the committee in the event of need, for example, if there is a difference of view with the chief executive officer or CFO . . .'

The report emphasises the need to protect the independence of the CRO from the influence of the CEO or finance director, and it also recommends that (like the company secretary) only the board should be able to appoint or dismiss the CRO, and the remuneration of the CRO should be decided by the organisation chairman or the remuneration committee.

Again this provides an interesting consideration for larger NHS organisations where a similar role may be helpful.

TEST YOUR KNOWLEDGE 11.5

a What is the difference between a risk committee of the board and a **risk management committee**?
b What are the responsibilities of the audit committee for business risk and the business risk management system?

6 Risk management policies, systems and procedures

To enable the board of directors to carry out its responsibilities for risk management effectively, there are two essential requirements:

- Board members should have an understanding of risks and risk management.
- There should be a risk management system in place that the board as a whole or the appropriate board committee can review.

6.1 Risk training for board directors

A further consideration for NHS organisations is the requirement of the *UK Corporate Governance Code* that directors should have a personal programme for continuing professional development, and this should include, where necessary, suitable training in risk awareness and risk management systems. This should ensure that they are capable of contributing proactively to board discussions on risk strategy. Training in risk management should be particularly important for members of the board committee (audit committee or risk committee) with responsibility for reviewing the risk management system.

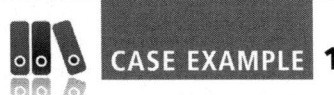

CASE EXAMPLE 11.3

The collapse of Enron has been referred to previously in this text (see, for example, Chapter 1). One of the weaknesses in governance that became apparent after the collapse was the lack of understanding of the risks in the business by the members of the Enron board. Before its collapse, Enron had a good reputation for financial risk management. Because of volatility in prices and supply in the energy industry, Enron used derivative instruments to hedge its long-term exposures to price risk. However, it hedged these risks with special purpose entities (specially created companies) that it owned itself and, as a result, Enron effectively retained the risks itself. These practices were reported to the board, but the board did nothing to stop them or question them, and actually approved resolutions that made some of these dubious 'off balance sheet' hedging transactions possible. After the collapse of the organisation at the end of 2001, it became apparent that the members of the Enron board, although they had been given information about risk management, did not know enough about derivatives and 'off balance sheet' accounting to understand and assess the risks.

6.2 Basic elements in an effective risk management system

There are four basic elements to a risk management system. (These are the same for both business risk management and internal control systems.)

- risk identification
- risk evaluation
- risk management measures
- risk control and review.

These elements are explained here in the context of a business risk management system. They will be described again in Chapter 1 within the context of an internal control system.

Risk identification

An organisation should have a procedure in place for reviewing and identifying the risks it faces. Risks change over time, and risk reviews should therefore be undertaken regularly.

Risk evaluation

The evaluation of risks calls for procedures to assess the potential size of the risk. The expected losses that could occur from adverse events or developments depend on the:

- probability that an adverse outcome will occur
- size of the loss in the event of an adverse outcome.

Where a risk is unlikely to materialise into an adverse outcome, and the loss would in any case be small, no management action might be necessary. Where the risk is higher, measures should be taken to protect the organisation so that the remaining exposure to risk is within the organisation's tolerance level and consistent with its risk appetite.

Risk management measures

The measures taken to deal with each risk are decided by management, which is accountable to the board for the measures they take. In broad terms, business risks can be dealt with by avoiding them or by taking steps to limit the exposure.

Some risks can be avoided but many risks have to be accepted as an inevitable feature of business. For significant risks, an organisation should decide what measures might be necessary to reduce the risk to acceptable proportions. Business risks may be reduced through measures such as stakeholder management and collaborative ventures.

From a health service governance perspective, it should be a responsibility of the board to make sure that risks are reviewed regularly and that management takes suitable measures to deal with them.

Risk control and review

Control systems should be established by executive management to monitor risks. There should be a system for identifying situations that are getting out of control or where significant events have developed or are developing.

6.3 Risk register and other risk management processes

An organisation might use a risk register for:

- recording risks that have been identified
- the evaluation of the risks, and
- the measures that have been taken to deal with them.

The risk register is maintained by executive management, but it can be used by the risk committee of the board (or the audit committee) as a way of reviewing the effectiveness of the risk management system.

Interestingly, the *King III* Code in South Africa is much more explicit about risk management than the *FT Code* and *UK Corporate Governance Code*. Provisions in the *King III Code* relating to risk management (both business risks and internal control risks) include the following:

- The board's risk strategy should be executed by management by means of risk management systems and processes.
- The board should ensure that effective and ongoing **risk assessments** are performed by management.
- Risks should be prioritised and ranked, in order to focus on areas where action is most needed.
- The board should regularly receive and review a register of the organisation's key risks.
- Key risks should be quantified where practicable (for example, in terms of maximum potential loss or expected loss).
- The board should ensure that processes are in place for anticipating unpredictable risks.
- Management should identify and note in the risk register the responses that have been decided upon and taken.
- Management should provide assurances to the board that the risk management plan is integrated into the daily activities of the business.

6.4 Stress testing

Stress testing is widely used by major organisations to assess their ability to withstand extreme 'shocks' or unexpected events in the business environment. This can be done by taking the normal business planning or forecasting model used by the organisation, and altering a key variable, such as the rate of growth (or decline) in economic growth, a very large increase in a major resource such as staff costs, loss of access to a key market for service provision, and so on. The purpose of stress testing is to assess whether the organisation could survive the shock. If there are doubts about this ability, the organisation should consider measures to reduce the risk, perhaps by developing contingency plans, or taking measures to improve their capital or liquidity.

TEST YOUR KNOWLEDGE 11.6

a What are the provisions of the *UK Corporate Governance Code* with regard to training directors in business risk?
b What are the main elements of a business risk management system?
c What is a risk register?
d What is the purpose of stress testing?

CHAPTER SUMMARY

- Business risks are risks to patient safety and financial security that arise from factors in the business environment, including competition, over which management has no direct control.
- The board of directors has a responsibility for making sure that business risks to which the organisation is exposed, or might be exposed in the future, are considered acceptable.
- The board has the responsibility for strategic decisions on risk, and an important aspect of health service governance is for the board to recognise its responsibilities and ensure that the risk management system in the organisation is effective.
- Risk appetite is the amount of exposure to business risk the board wants to take, so that its strategic objectives can be achieved.
- Risk tolerance is the amount of risk that the board is willing to accept. Risk tolerance may be measured quantitatively, so that actual exposures to business risk can be compared with a target or tolerance limit.
- The board should review risk appetite and risk tolerance regularly.
- Business risks are risks that arise from unexpected changes or developments in the business environment that are outside the control of management. These include unexpected initiatives by competitors, unexpected changes in patient demand patterns and changes in the political, regulatory, economic, social, environmental and technological environment. Unexpected changes can be positive as well as negative.
- A measure of high risk is unpredictable variability in key factors such as activity levels or tariff. High volatility is associated with high business risk.
- Business risk should be distinguished from internal control risk. Internal control risk arises from factors within the organisation (or other organisation) that are within the ability of management to control. Business risks are external and cannot be controlled. However, they should be managed.
- Examples of business risk are reputation risk, competition risk, business environment risk, financial risks (such as adverse changes in tariff or interest rates, higher losses from bad debts or changes in prices from major suppliers) and liquidity risk.
- Stress testing may be used to assess the ability of an organisation to withstand unexpected extreme events or developments, so that contingency measures can be planned or risk tolerance levels adjusted.
- The *FT Code* includes a requirement for foundation trusts to have a system of risk management, with regular reviews (at least annually) of the effectiveness of this system.
- There may be a separate risk committee of the board, with special responsibility for monitoring the risk management system.
- Directors must understand business risk and risk management systems. It may be necessary to give them suitable training.
- The basic elements of a risk management system are procedures for identifying risks, evaluation of the risks that have been identified and assessing their significance, taking measures to manage the risks that are consistent with board policy on risk appetite and risk tolerance, control of the system and regular reviews of the effectiveness of the system.

Internal control systems

CONTENTS

1. Elements of an internal control system
2. The UK corporate governance framework for internal control
3. The *Turnbull Guidance* on internal control
4. The Annual Governance Statement (AGS) (previously the SIC)
5. Internal audit
6. Emergency preparedness and business continuity
7. Whistleblowing procedures

INTRODUCTION

An organisation may fail to achieve its objectives because of failures or weaknesses within its systems and operating procedures, or due to human error. These failures and weaknesses could be avoided, or the consequences of failures could be restricted, by means of controls. Internal control risks are the risks of failures in systems and procedures to achieve their intended purpose. Internal controls are measures or arrangements that are intended to prevent failures from happening, limiting their potential effect, or identifying when a failure has occurred so that corrective measures can be taken. This chapter explains the nature of internal control risks and the internal control system, and the responsibilities for internal control within an organisation. Internal control is an aspect of governance, because the board of directors has a responsibility to ensure that the assets of the organisation are not threatened, and the interests of the stakeholders are not damaged, by making sure that an effective system of internal control is in place.

This chapter also explores the processes of recovery and restoration required by NHS organisations to ensure business continuity is embedded in the organisation. The chapter concludes with an outline of the whistleblowing procedures that support the delivery of good governance.

1 Elements of an internal control system

> 'Clear business objectives need to be identified before an effective system of internal control can be established. Without clear objectives, management will be unable to identify and evaluate the risks that threaten the achievement of their objectives and design and operate a system of internal control to manage those risks.'
>
> The Auditing Practices Board

Business risks are risks that arise in the business environment and markets in which an organisation operates. Internal control risks are risks that arise within an organisation because of weaknesses in its systems, procedures, management or personnel. Unless there are controls to deal with them, internal control risks can lead to losses because of operational failures, errors or fraud. The controls for these risks are 'internal controls' and internal controls are applied within an internal control system.

It is the responsibility of the board of directors of an organisation to ensure that the internal control system (and the internal controls within this system) is effective in preventing losses from internal control risks, or identifying losses and taking corrective action when they occur.

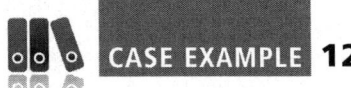

CASE EXAMPLE 12.1

A hospital operated from three separate locations in the same city. At one of these locations, a considerable amount of cash had built up following donations from grateful patients. This was kept in a safe in the manager's office. One day, two uniformed individuals came to the building and said that they had instructions to take the safe to the organisation's head office, which was in a different building. They were allowed to take the safe and the security guard actually helped them to put it into their vehicle, parked outside the front door of the building. The two individuals drove off with the safe, containing over £30,000, and were not seen again.

It should be apparent that the organisation lost £30,000 because of basic mistakes, which point to weaknesses in internal controls:

- Why was there was a lot of money in the safe? Why had most of it not been taken to the bank?
- Why were the two individuals allowed to take the safe without checking their authorisation to take it?
- How did they gain access to the building so easily?

There were weaknesses in the procedures for managing donations, banking cash, building security and authorisation of actions. If suitable internal controls had been in place, the loss of the money would not have occurred.

1.1 Categories of internal control risks

A useful definition of internal control was given by the US Committee of Sponsoring Organizations of the Treadway Commission (COSO). The COSO Framework defines internal control as 'a process, effected by an entity's board of directors, management and other personnel, designed to provide reasonable assurance regarding the achievement of objectives' in the areas of:

- effectiveness and efficiency of operations (through operational controls)
- the reliability of financial reporting (through financial controls)
- compliance with relevant laws and regulations (through compliance controls).

It follows then that internal control risks can be categorised into three broad types:

- **Financial risks**. These are risks of errors or fraud in accounting systems and accounting and finance activities. Errors or fraud could lead to losses for the organisation, or to incorrect financial statements. Weak controls may also mean that financial assets are not properly protected. Examples of financial risks include the risk of failure to record transactions in the book-keeping system, failure to collect money owed by customers, failure to protect cash and mis-reporting (deliberate or unintentional) in the financial statements.
- **Operational risks**. A helpful definition of 'operational risk' is given by the Basel Committee for banking supervision. Although this definition applies to risks in the banking industry, it has a wider application. Operational risk is 'the risk of losses resulting from inadequate or failed internal processes, people and systems, or external events'. Operational risks include the risks of a breakdown in a system due to machine failures or software errors, the risk of losing information from computer files or having confidential information stolen, the risk of a terrorist attack, and losses arising from mistakes or omissions by staff.
- **Compliance risks**. These are risks that important laws or regulations will not be complied with properly. Failure to comply with the law could result in legal action against the organisation and/or fines.

1.2 The purpose of an internal control system and internal controls

An internal control system is the system that an organisation has for identifying internal control risks, applying controls to reduce the risk of losses from these risks and taking corrective action when losses occur:

- There should be controls to ensure that the organisation, its systems and procedures operate in the way that is intended, without disruption or disturbance.
- There should be controls to ensure that assets are safeguarded. For example, there should be controls to ensure that money received is banked and is not stolen, and that operating assets such as items of equipment and computers are not damaged or lost.
- Controls should include measures to reduce the risk of fraud.
- Financial controls should ensure the completeness and accuracy of accounting records, and the timely preparation of financial information.
- Controls should be in place to ensure compliance with key regulations, such as CQC regulations, Monitor regulations or health and safety regulations.

1.3 Financial, operational and compliance controls

In the UK, a committee was set up in 1998 to provide guidance on the board's responsibilities for internal control and risk management. This committee produced the Turnbull Report, since revised and re-named the *Turnbull Guidance*. The Turnbull Report defined an internal control system as 'the policies, processes, tasks, behaviours and other aspects of an organisation' that, taken together:

- help it to operate effectively and efficiently; these operational controls should allow the organisation to respond in an appropriate way to significant risks to achieving the organisation's objectives (this includes the safeguarding of assets from inappropriate use or from loss and fraud and ensuring that liabilities are identified and managed)
- help it to ensure the quality of external and internal financial reporting (financial controls)
- help to ensure compliance with applicable laws and regulations, and also with internal policies for the conduct of business (compliance controls)

In other words, there should be financial, operational and compliance controls for dealing with financial, operational and compliance risks – preventing losses or adverse events from happening, or detecting and correcting the problem when losses or adverse events do occur.

Financial controls

Financial controls are internal accounting controls that are sufficient to provide reasonable assurance that:

- transactions are made only according to the general or specific authorisation of management
- transactions are recorded so that financial statements can be prepared according to accounting standards and generally accepted accounting principles
- transactions are recorded so that assets can be accounted for
- access to assets is only allowed according to the general or specific authorisation of management
- the accounting records for assets are compared with actual assets at reasonable intervals of time
- appropriate action is taken whenever there are found to be differences.

The maintenance of proper accounting records is an important element of internal control. Effective financial controls should ensure:

- the quality of external and internal financial reporting, so that there are no material errors in the accounting records and financial statements
- that no fraud is committed (or that fraud is detected when it occurs)
- that the financial assets of the organisation are not stolen, lost or needlessly damaged, or that these risks are reduced.

A useful method of categorising internal financial controls was used in an old guideline issued by the UK Auditing Practices Board, using the mnemonic SPAMSOAP. In this guideline (no longer in issue) internal financial controls are categorised as follows:

S: **Segregation of duties**. Where possible, duties should be split between two or more people, so that the work done by one person acts as a check on the work done by another. With segregation of duties, it is more difficult for fraud to take place, because several individuals would have to collude in the fraud. It is also more difficult for accidental errors to occur, because when several people are involved in a task, they act as a check on each other.

P: **Physical controls**. Physical controls are measures to ensure the physical safety of assets, such as putting cash in a safe, banking cash receipts immediately, and preventing unauthorised access to computer systems through the use of passwords and internet firewalls.

A: **Authorisation and approval**. All financial transactions should require the authorisation or approval of an appropriate responsible person, and there should be an authorisation limit to how much spending each responsible person can approve.

M: **Management controls**. Management should exercise control over financial systems, for example by preparing a budget and then monitoring actual performance by comparing it with the budget. Management controls can also be exercised by reviewing other financial statements, such as a balance sheet, profit and loss account and cash flow statement.

S: **Supervision**. The day-to-day work of employees should be properly supervised. Good supervision will reduce the likelihood of errors or fraud.

O: **Organisation**. Everyone should be fully aware of his responsibilities, and lines of authority, lines of reporting and levels of responsibility should be clear. Errors and fraud are much more likely where it is uncertain who is responsible for what and who should be reporting to whom.

A: **Arithmetical and accounting controls**. These are procedures in an accounts office to check the accuracy of the records and the numbers. They include the use of control totals and reconciliations.

P: **Personnel**. The quality of internal controls is dependent on the quality of the individuals working in the organisation, and personnel selected to do a job should have the right personal qualities and be properly trained and/or qualified.

This list of different types of control is provided as a guide to the nature of financial controls. Health service governance is concerned with the adequacy of internal controls and the effectiveness of the internal control system; designing and implementing controls is a responsibility of management.

Operational controls

Operational controls are controls that help to reduce operational risks, or identify failures in operational systems when these occur. They are designed to prevent failures in operational procedures, or to detect and correct operational failures if they do occur. Operational failures may be caused by:

- machine breakdowns
- human error
- failures in the performance of systems (possibly due to human error)
- weaknesses in procedures
- poor management.

Operational controls are measures designed to prevent these failures from happening, or identifying and correcting problems that do occur. Regular equipment maintenance, better training of staff, automation of standard procedures, and reporting systems that make managers accountable for their actions are all examples of operational controls.

Compliance controls

Compliance controls are concerned with making sure that an entity complies with all the requirements of relevant legislation and regulations. It can be difficult to understand the nature of internal control risks and internal controls to deal with them. There are many different risks and many controls that are applied.

The following are simple examples:

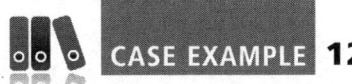 **CASE EXAMPLE 12.2**

A trust had a cumulative deficit of £20 million at 31 March 2008. However, the trust's sights were set firmly on achieving foundation trust status, which meant that the trust's ongoing financial performance had to improve and the cumulative deficit had to be recovered.

Over the past three years the trust has recovered the deficit and is forecasting a £12 million surplus for 2010/2011. The trust has achieved this in a number of ways, notably with significant improvements in its arrangements to manage performance against budgets.

The trust reorganised its management structure, moving from 13 clinical directorates to five clinical divisions, plus a sixth division covering corporate services. Key to this restructuring was the decision to have a clinician as the head of division, who is then accountable to the chief executive. The head of division is paid to manage the division (four sessions per week) as well as undertake clinical activities.

Another key part of the trust's strategy was to minimise its reliance on non-recurrent measures. The financial strategy allows for non-recurrent measures to account for no more than 1% of turnover. If this limit is exceeded, the director of finance works with divisions to replace non-recurrent with recurrent.

The trust has also improved reporting to the board so that key risks are more readily apparent. A new format of finance report to the Trust Board has been introduced, which includes traffic light risk indicators for the high level summary and includes commentary on high level details of the main risks in relation to each division's financial performance.

As a result the trust's budgetary control arrangements have improved considerably over the past three years, which has resulted in the trust being well placed to deliver significant surpluses in the short to medium term and embark on an investment programme to replace all of the trust's facilities that are currently unfit for purpose.

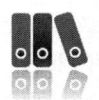 **CASE EXAMPLE 12.3**

Delivering healthcare to satisfy the local population and providing clinically effective treatment requires the extensive use of medicines. External benchmarking suggested that through improved generic prescribing alone, GPs could save at least £350,000 each year. The PCT's Medicines Management team worked closely with GPs in trying to improve prescribing practice both in terms of clinical effectiveness and the assurance of best value. Education, incentive schemes, practice profiling and local drug formularies all helped to improve prescribing habits, but the decision over which drug to prescribe ultimately rested with the GP during their consultation with the patient.

The PCT completed a Business Case for the use of a new software package that tied into the GP's electronic prescribing system. Under the control of the Medicines Management team, a series of protocols were programmed into the system that automatically raised a flag in response to the GP's drug selection. Alternative drug choices were offered, giving the GP an option to accept the recommended alternative(s).

After eight months of full implementation, the PCT reported actual savings in excess of £400,000. In addition to financial savings, the implementation of the software had been a successful means of getting important information to GPs at the moment that they made their prescribing decision. The system provides the PCT with an opportunity to realise financial savings in drug prescribing while at the same time influencing good prescribing practice and supporting clinical effectiveness.

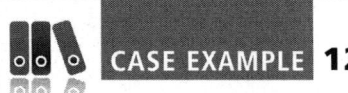

CASE EXAMPLE 12.4

A PCT was seeking to ensure that all levels of staff were provided with knowledge to enable them to display the highest standards of ethical conduct.

The PCT's Corporate Governance Action Plan outlined a range of communications and training methods to be delivered regularly across the year. These included incorporating this area in the essential skills training delivered to staff as part of their KSF training, distributing staff leaflets, including articles in team briefs, incorporating a counter-fraud section into the PCT's website, ensuring posters and leaflets were displayed in all PCT premises and providing standards and fraud training direct to the board.

In addition a series of simple PowerPoint presentations on standards of business conduct, whistleblowing and fraud and corruption were e-mailed to all staff. These presentations ran automatically on opening the e-mail.

As a result of these measures there has been an increased awareness of ethical standards and the methods of reporting concerns. In addition independent contractors have become aware of the PCT's processes for dealing with fraud and have used them to report concerns.

1.4 Elements of an internal control system

Internal controls are an essential part of an internal control system, but an internal control system should also have other elements to be effective and achieve its objectives. An internal control system consists of:

- a 'control environment', and
- control procedures.

The COSO Framework identifies five elements to a system of internal control. (These five elements are also recognised in the Turnbull Report.)

- **A control environment.** A control environment describes the awareness of (and attitude to) internal controls in the organisation, shown by the directors, management and employees generally. It therefore encompasses corporate culture, management style and employee attitudes to control procedures.
- **Risk identification and assessment.** There should be a system or procedures for identifying the risks facing the organisation (and how these are changing) and assessing their significance. Controls or management initiatives should be devised to deal with significant risks.
- **Internal controls.** Controls should be devised and implemented to eliminate, reduce or control risks.
- **Information and communication.** All employees who are responsible for the management of risks should receive information that enables them to fulfil this task.
- **Monitoring.** The effectiveness of risk controls and the internal control system generally should be monitored regularly. Internal audit is one method of monitoring the internal control system. Internal controls are also monitored by executive management and (as part of their annual audit) by the external auditors. The board of directors also has a responsibility to review the effectiveness of the system.

The nature and extent of the internal controls an organisation has in place will depend to a large extent on its size, what controls it can afford and whether the benefits obtained from any particular control measure are sufficient to justify its cost. The internal control system should, however, be sufficiently robust and effective to minimise the risk of serious losses through error or fraud.

In a large organisation, we should expect thousands of different financial operational and compliance controls, each designed to prevent particular financial, operational or compliance failures, or to detect them if they occur.

An important aspect of health service governance is to ensure that the system of internal control (and the internal controls within that system) is adequate and effective in preventing or detecting failures in the system. For example, if the system is ineffective, an organisation may be exposed to a high risk of fraud and also to a high risk that its annual financial statements will not be accurate or reliable.

STOP AND THINK 12.1

The Bribery Act 2010 introduced a corporate offence of failure to prevent bribery by persons working on behalf of a commercial organisation. However, organisations will have a defence against prosecution if they can show that they have adequate procedures in place to prevent bribery. This means that the internal control system needs to take this into consideration.

- What controls would be needed to show a consideration of the risk areas?
- What specific controls might reduce the likelihood of bribery?
- What controls would ensure implementation of anti-bribery policies and practices?

TEST YOUR KNOWLEDGE 12.1

a What are the main elements of a system of internal control?
b Give six examples of financial risk within an organisation.
c What might be the main operational risk or compliance risk concerns for a community services trust?
d For what reason are procedures for the authorisation of expenditures and approval of payments for expenditures an internal control?
e For what reason are procedures for the selection of appropriate applicants to fill job vacancies a part of an internal control system?

2 The UK corporate governance framework for internal control

NHS organisations and health service governance rely upon the provisions in the *UK Corporate Governance Code*, which recognises the connection between good corporate governance and risk management. It is worth therefore setting out these provisions in more detail.

2.1 *UK Corporate Governance Code* requirements

A principle of the *UK Code* is that:

   'The board should maintain sound risk management and internal control systems.'

The board has overall responsibility for the system of internal control, but the responsibility for designing and implementing the system, and for operating it, is delegated to management. (Responsibility for risk management was explained in Chapter 11.) The *UK Code* also includes the following principle and provision:

- **Main principle**. The board is responsible for determining the nature and extent of the significant risks it is willing to take in achieving its strategic objectives.
- **Provision**. The board is required to conduct a review of the effectiveness of the organisation's system of internal controls at least annually, and should report to the stakeholders that they have done so. 'The review should cover all material controls, including financial, operational and compliance controls.' In other words, the board's responsibility for reviewing internal controls (and risk management) extends beyond financial matters to the business operations and regulatory compliance.

Within the NHS this review is known as the Annual Governance Statement (previously known as Statement on Internal Control) and its content is mandated by the DH.

Role of the audit committee

Another principle of the *UK Code* is that the board should establish 'formal and transparent arrangements' for considering how it should apply the corporate governance principles relating to corporate reporting, risk management and internal control and for maintaining a relationship with the external auditors.

- An audit committee should have responsibility for corporate governance matters relating to corporate reporting and the organisation's relationship with its external auditors (as explained in Chapter 10).
- The board may delegate responsibility for the governance aspects of risk management and internal control to either the audit committee or a risk committee of the board. The board may set up a risk committee to deal with risk management matters and give the responsibilities for review of the internal control system to the audit committee. However, delegated responsibilities to board committees may differ between companies.

The *UK Code* states that the responsibilities of the audit committee should include:

- review of the organisation's internal financial controls
- review of the rest of the internal control system (and risk management system), unless this responsibility is given to a separate risk committee of the board
- monitoring and review of the effectiveness of the organisation's internal audit function
- review of the organisation's whistleblowing system.

Internal audit and whistleblowing arrangements are described later in this chapter.

TEST YOUR KNOWLEDGE 12.2

a What are the provisions of the *UK Corporate Governance Code* relating to internal control?
b What are the provisions of the *UK Corporate Governance Code* relating to internal audit?
c What are the responsibilities of an audit committee with respect to internal control and internal audit, as stated in the *UK Code*?

3 The *Turnbull Guidance* on internal control

When principles and provisions relating to internal control and risk management were first introduced into the UK governance code in 1998, a working party, known as the Turnbull Committee, published guidelines to listed companies on how to apply them. These are now known as the **Turnbull Guidance**, and are the responsibility of the FRC. The Guidance applies to the entire system of internal control, including operational and compliance controls as well as financial controls. The introduction to the Guidance makes the following points:

- Internal control should be embedded in the business and its operating systems. Controls should not be applied occasionally and from an external source. They should be applied regularly and automatically, as part of established procedures.
- Controls should remain relevant over time. This means that as circumstances change, controls should be altered or adapted to meet the new requirements.
- The controls that are appropriate to an organisation should take account of its particular circumstances.

This guidance forms the basis of NHS guidance on internal control and internal control systems.

3.1 Maintaining a sound system of internal control

The board of directors is responsible for maintaining a sound system of internal control. The *Turnbull Guidance* states that the board of directors should:

- set appropriate policies on internal control
- seek regular assurance to satisfy itself that the system is operating effectively
- ensure that the system of internal control is effective in managing risks in the way that it has approved.

In deciding its policies for internal control and assessing what constitutes an effective system of internal control, the board should consider:

- the nature and extent of the risks facing the organisation
- the amount of risk and types of risk that it regards as acceptable for the organisation to bear
- the likelihood that the risks will materialise
- the organisation's ability to reduce the impact on the business of the risks that do materialise
- the costs of operating particular controls relative to the benefits to be obtained from managing the risks they control. Controls are not worth having if they cost more than the expected benefits or savings they will provide.

Having identified the responsibilities of the board for maintaining a sound system of internal control, the *Turnbull Guidance* adds the following:

- It is the job of management to implement the board's policies on control. To do this management must have procedures for identifying and evaluating the risks faced by the organisation, and designing, implementing and monitoring a control system to deal with these risks in a way that is consistent with the board's policies.
- In addition all employees have some responsibility for internal control, for example to avoid making mistakes in their work and also to ensure that the control procedures for which they are responsible are properly performed.

3.2 Elements of a sound system of internal control

A sound system of internal control should:

- be embedded in the operations of the organisation and form part of its culture
- be capable of responding quickly to risks to the business as they emerge and develop
- include procedures for reporting immediately to the management responsible and control failings that have been identified and any corrective action that has been undertaken.

The *Turnbull Guidance* emphasises that a sound system of internal control cannot provide certain protection against an organisation suffering losses or breaches of laws or regulations or failing to meet its business objectives. The possibility will always exist of 'poor judgement in decision-making, human error, control processes being deliberately circumvented by employees and others, management overriding controls and the occurrence of unforeseen circumstances'. A sound system of internal control provides reasonable assurance that risks will be suitably controlled, but cannot provide absolute assurance that there will not be any material losses, fraud, errors or breaches of laws and regulations.

3.3 Reviewing the effectiveness of internal control

The *UK Corporate Governance Code* states that the board of directors (or the audit committee) should carry out, at least annually, a review of the effectiveness of the system of internal control (and risk management). In order to review the effectiveness of the system of internal control, there must be procedures for monitoring and review. The *Turnbull Guidance* provides some suggestions. It suggests that 'reviewing the effectiveness of internal control is an essential part of the board's responsibilities'. The board or audit committee needs to form its own view about the effectiveness of the system, based on the information and assurances it receives. The sources of information about internal control are:

- management
- the internal auditors, if the organisation has an internal audit function, and
- the external auditors, who notify management and the audit committee about weaknesses in internal controls that they have discovered in their audit.

The board of directors and the audit committee do not have the time to carry out a detailed review themselves, and they must therefore rely on information provided to them by management and internal auditors. The most regular source of information for the board or audit committee about internal control should be management reports. Additional reporting may be provided, however, by the internal auditors, or by a firm of external accountants or auditors hired to perform a specific internal audit investigation.

In its *Guidance on Audit Committees* (revised 2010), the FRC states that except where the responsibility is retained by the entire board, or delegated to a risk committee:

> 'The audit committee should receive reports from management on the effectiveness of the systems they have established and the conclusions of any testing carried out by internal and external auditors.'

Management reports to the audit committee

Management is accountable to the board (or the audit committee) for monitoring the system of internal control and for providing assurances that it has done so. To be effective, monitoring should be on a regular basis, and management should also provide regular reports to the audit committee (or the board). These regular reports should each deal with a specific aspect of operations and:

- provide an assessment of the significance of the risks and the effectiveness of the system of internal control for dealing with them
- report any significant control weaknesses or failings that have been identified, the impact these have had (or may have) on the organisation and the action that has been taken to deal with the problem.

The board or audit committee may also receive independent reports from the internal auditors. In addition to receiving regular reports from management on internal control, the board (or audit committee) should carry out an annual review of the effectiveness of the internal control system. The annual review should consider the following in particular:

- The changes that have occurred since the previous annual review: in what ways have the significant risks for the organisation changed, and how successful has the organisation been in responding to those changes.
- The scope and quality of monitoring of the control system by management.
- The scope and quality of the investigations by the internal audit function, the weaknesses in the system identified by the internal auditors and the measures taken to implement recommendations of the internal auditors.

4 The Annual Governance Statement (AGS) (previously the SIC)

The SIC was originally developed as part of the DH's NHS Controls Assurance project, and was subsequently introduced across the wider public sector by HM Treasury. This requirement is in line with the *UK Corporate Governance Code*, which states that the board should report to shareholders each year that it has conducted the annual review of the effectiveness of the systems of internal control and risk management. The FSA's Disclosure and Transparency Rules for listed companies also requires companies to report on the main features of their internal control and risk management systems in relation to financial reporting.

All public bodies (including NHS organisations) must provide assurance that they are appropriately managing and controlling the resources for which they are responsible. The SIC was a mandatory disclosure for all central government entities that comply with the *FReM*. It was a primary accountability document. The external auditors do not provide an explicit audit opinion on the content, but it was subject to external audit review to ensure that it had been prepared according to government guidance and that it was consistent with the auditors' knowledge of the entity. The SIC was an important accountability document in communicating these assurances to Parliament and citizens.

NHS foundation trusts are now required to produce an AGS, with enhanced reporting on quality governance, in place of the SIC for reporting periods commencing on or after 1 April 2011. Monitor's *NHS FT ARM* 2011/2012 sets out a model AGS but requires each foundation trust to adapt the model to reflect their own particular circumstance. The AGS also includes reference to quality governance and Monitor's *Quality Governance Framework* may be used for information on good practice in quality governance. The requirement for an AGS rather than the SIC will be rolled out across all NHS organisations during 2012. Further guidance as to its content and format will be issued later in 2012.

The National Audit Office (NAO) issued guidance for public sector audit committees (e.g. NHS audit committees) on the SIC as it is the means by which the accounting officer of each public body declares his or her approach to, and responsibility for, risk management, internal control and corporate governance. It is also the vehicle for highlighting weaknesses that exist in the internal control system within the organisation. It forms part of the Annual Report and Accounts.

The *FReM* set out the expected form and content of the SIC. This was a mix of prescribed text and sections where accounting officers were expected to describe the particular arrangements in their organisations.

The SIC contained disclosures under the following headings:

- scope of responsibility
- the purpose of the system of internal control
- capacity to handle risk
- the risk and control framework
- review of effectiveness.

The audit committee plays a key role in the production of the AGS. It supports the board and accounting officer by reviewing the comprehensiveness of assurances in meeting the board and accounting officer's assurance needs, and reviewing the reliability and integrity of the assurances. The audit committee also advises the board and accounting officer of any control issues that could be considered significant and are therefore appropriate for disclosure in the AGS.

4.1 Elements required to be in place to support the AGS

The annual guidance from the DH continues to set out the key elements that need to be considered when producing the AGS. While NHS organisations will have risk management, control and review processes in place, the detail of these processes vary from one organisation to another depending on circumstances such as size and the complexity of the risks faced. The annual guidance, therefore, offers a summary of characteristics under six high level elements to help with consideration of the completeness of the processes that have been put in place in a particular body.

NHS organisations are required to ensure that they have sufficient evidence to demonstrate that they have implemented processes appropriate to their circumstances under the following seven high level elements:

- scope of responsibility
- the governance framework of the organisation
- risk assessment
- the risk and control framework
- review of the effectiveness of risk management and internal control
- significant issues

4.2 Disclosure of internal control weaknesses

The guidance also requires full disclosure of any significant control issues or weaknesses. This is to deliver assurance that significant internal control issues have been, or are being, addressed and that the AGS is a balanced reflection of the actual control position. Although not required, it may help the disclosure in relation to a significant internal control issue if the description of the weakness and its impact is given to provide context for the actions taken. NHS bodies may exercise discretion in such disclosure to avoid further adverse impacts or exploitation of the weakness.

A single definition of a significant internal control issue is not possible and NHS organisations are required to exercise their judgement in deciding whether or not a particular issue should be regarded as falling into this category. The guidance sets out factors that may be helpful in exercising that judgement, which include:

- the issue seriously prejudiced or prevented achievement of a principal objective
- the issue has had significant one-off financial implications or concerns general financial standing (e.g. deficits)
- the external auditor regards it as having a material impact on the accounts
- the audit committee advises it should be considered significant for this purpose
- the Head of Internal Audit reports on it as significant, for this purpose, in their annual opinion on the whole of risk, control and governance
- the issue, or its impact has attracted significant public interest or has seriously damaged the reputation of the organisation (e.g. an external auditor's public interest report)
- non compliance with CQC core standards
- under achievement against World Class Commissioning assurance
- serious untoward data security incidents
- non-compliance with equality and human rights legislation

4.3 Board Assurance Framework (BAF)

In order to sign off the AGS NHS boards need to be assured that the systems, policies and people they have put in place are operating in a way that is effective, is focused on key risks and is driving the delivery of objectives. There is, however, the potential for a lack of clarity within the board (and beyond) to what is meant by the term 'assurance'. This can extend to uncertainty over the level of assurance required, where that assurance comes from and how the reporting of assurance is managed in a coordinated manner.

Although the process of securing assurance has always been a fundamental principle of good management and accountability, the requirement for all NHS chief executives to sign the AGS, has focused attention on the level of assurance that boards receive. To provide this statement, boards need to be able to demonstrate that they have been properly informed through assurances about the totality of their risks, not just financial, and have arrived at their conclusions based on all the evidence presented to them.

Building the Assurance Framework: a practical guide for NHS Boards by the DH and *Taking it on Trust* by the Audit Commission have contributed further to this discussion. The BAF is a framework that NHS organisations are required to put in place to identify the key risks to the trust's achievement of its strategic objectives and how these risks are being managed. In documented form this would include:

- the trust's strategic objectives
- the key risks to achieving the objectives
- the controls in place to manage the risks
- the assurances that the trust used to provide evidence that the controls were operating effectively
- any gaps in the assurances
- an action plan to address the gaps.

Every NHS organisation must design its own framework, which will relate to the delivery of its own objectives within the context of an understanding of the principle risks that the organisation faces. The BAF should enable the board to:

- establish principal objectives (strategic and directorate)
- identify the principal risks that may threaten the achievement of these objectives – typically in the range of 75–200 depending on the complexity of the organisation
- identify and evaluate the design of key controls intended to manage these principal risks, underpinned by core controls assurance standards
- set out the arrangements for obtaining assurance on the effectiveness of key controls across all areas of principal risk
- evaluate the assurance across all areas of principal risk
- identify positive assurances and areas where there are gaps in controls and/or assurances
- put in place plans to take corrective action where gaps have been identified in relation to principal risks
- maintain dynamic risk management arrangements including, crucially, a well-founded risk register.

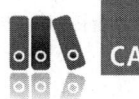

CASE EXAMPLE 12.5

In 2008, the Health Care Commission inspected a service area within a trust and found a number of areas of concern resulting in a series of recommendations for improvement. A year later the trust had failed to make the required level of progress against two of the three recommendations, with some of the recommendations still requiring significant steps in order to be implemented. Two specific problems related to the failure to appoint a consultant and to recruit sufficient staff to ensure the trust operated a service that was safe and effective.

The trust had put in place an action plan to deal with service delivery problems in by the end of 2008. However the board devoted insufficient effort to ensuring that action plan was delivered in a timely manner and there was insufficient evidence of the board driving improvement forward.

In particular the effectiveness of board assurance processes, leadership by the board and clinical leadership within the trust was a cause for concern. The trust remained under enhanced monitoring.

TEST YOUR KNOWLEDGE 12.3

a What are the main recommendations in the Turnbull guidelines?
b How is an AGS different to an SIC?
c What are the main disclosures that must be made in the SIC?

5 Internal audit

The NHS Accounting Officer Memorandum requires all NHS trusts to have an internal audit function.

The formal requirement for every NHS board to establish an audit committee can be found in *Codes of Conduct and Accountability* issued by DH. Foundation trusts are required to have an audit committee by the *FT Code of Governance*. The NHS Internal Audit Standards (Government Internal Audit Audit Standards for foundation trusts) set out the requirements for internal audit and how to assess the service that is delivered.

The *NHS Audit Committee Handbook* states that the audit committee should actively review the plans of both internal and external audit and assess the quality of the services that are provided.

5.1 Function and scope of internal audit

While this has been addressed briefly within Chapter 10 it is worth repeating some of the key issues to set the scene. Internal audit is the 'independent appraisal activity established within an organisation as a service to it. It is a control which functions by examining and evaluating the adequacy and effectiveness of other controls' (CIMA Official Terminology).

The Chartered Institute of Internal Auditors describes the role as being to 'provide independent assurance that an organisation's risk management, governance and internal control processes are operating effectively. Internal auditors deal with issues that are fundamentally important to the survival and prosperity of any organisation.'

The NHS Accounting Officer Memorandum requires all NHS trusts to have an internal audit function.

The work done by any internal audit unit is not prescribed by regulation, but is decided by management or by the board (or audit committee). The possible tasks of internal audit include the following:

- **Reviewing the internal control system.** Traditionally, an internal audit department has carried out independent checks on the financial controls in an organisation; however, this has now extended to include quality and performance controls as well. The checks would be to establish whether suitable quality, performance and financial controls exist and if so, whether they are applied properly and are effective. It is not the function of internal auditors to manage risks, only to monitor and report them, and to check that risk controls are efficient and cost-effective.
- **Special investigations.** Internal auditors might conduct special investigations into particular aspects of the organisation's operations (systems and procedures), to check the effectiveness of operational controls.
- **Examination of financial and operating information.** Internal auditors might be asked to investigate the timeliness of reporting and the accuracy of the information in reports.
- **VFM audits.** This is an investigation into an operation or activity to establish whether it is economical, efficient and effective.
- **Reviewing compliance by the organisation with particular laws or regulations.** This is an investigation into the effectiveness of compliance controls.
- **Risk assessment.** Internal auditors might be asked to investigate aspects of risk management, and in particular the adequacy of the mechanisms for identifying, assessing and controlling significant risks to the organisation, from both internal and external sources.

5.2 Investigation of internal financial controls

Internal auditors are commonly required to check the soundness of internal financial controls. In assessing the effectiveness of individual controls, and of an internal control system generally, the following factors should be considered:

- Whether the controls are manual or automated. Automated controls are by no means error-proof or fraud-proof, but may be more reliable than similar manual controls.
- Whether controls are discretionary or non-discretionary. Non-discretionary controls are checks and procedures that must be carried out. Discretionary controls are those that do not have to be applied, either because they are voluntary or because an individual can choose to disapply them. Risks can infiltrate a system, for example, when senior management chooses to disapply controls and allow unauthorised or unchecked procedures to occur.
- Whether the control can be circumvented easily, because an activity can be carried out in a different way where similar controls do not apply.
- Whether the controls are effective in achieving their purpose. Are they extensive enough or carried out frequently enough? Are the controls applied rigorously? For example, is a supervisor doing his job properly?

Reports by internal auditors can provide reassurance that internal controls are sound and effective, or might recommend changes and improvements where weaknesses are uncovered.

5.3 The objectivity and independence of internal auditors

The manager of a directorate or department should monitor the internal controls within the operation and try to identify and correct weaknesses. They should also report on reviews of the effectiveness of internal control. However, a line manager cannot be properly objective, because they could face 'blame' for control failures in the system or operation for which they are responsible.

In contrast, internal auditors ought to be objective, because they investigate the control systems of other directorates and departments. However, they are also employees within the organisation and report to someone on the organisation structure. If the internal auditors report to the finance director, they will find it difficult to be critical of the finance director. Similarly, if the internal auditors report to the CEO, they will be reluctant to criticise the CEO. In this respect, their independence could be compromised.

In its *Guidance for Audit Committees*, the ICAEW comments that the internal auditors should be separate and independent from line management, but that 'independence' for internal auditors does not have the same meaning as independence for external auditors.

To protect the independence of the internal audit function, the FRC's *Guidance on Audit Committees* suggests that the audit committee should have the responsibility for the appointment of the head of internal audit, and his removal from office.

TEST YOUR KNOWLEDGE 12.4

a What is the purpose of an internal audit function?
b What tasks might be carried out by an internal audit department?
c What should NHS trusts include in their AGS?
d How can the independence of the head of internal audit be protected?

5.4 Review of the effectiveness of the internal audit function

The board or audit committee should review the effectiveness of the internal audit function each year. As part of this review, the *NHS Audit Committee Handbook* suggests that the committee should:

- make sure that the head of internal audit has direct access to the chairman of the board and the audit committee, and is accountable to the audit committee
- review and assess the annual internal audit work plan
- receive reports on the results of work done by the internal auditors
- review and monitor the responses of management to the recommendations made to them by the internal auditors
- meet with the head of internal audit at least once a year without executive management being present.

6 Emergency preparedness and business continuity

Emergency preparedness is a plan of what to do if a disaster that is unconnected with the organisation's business and outside the control of management occurs. Disaster recovery planning goes beyond procedures that should be taken in an emergency, such as a fire or explosion in a building. It is intended to establish what should be done if an extreme disaster threatens the ability of the organisation to maintain its operations. Examples of disasters are natural disasters, such as major fires or flooding or storm damage to key installations or offices, major terrorist attacks and pandemics.

Emergency preparedness plans are vital for NHS organisations as lengthy or widespread overwhelming demand or shutdown of operations could be catastrophic. While the training of appropriate NHS staff regarding such arrangements in the UK is the responsibility of NHS organisations, the DH fund an extensive training programme delivered by the HPA to support the NHS in England in planning and preparing for major incidents. Guidance is given in *The NHS Emergency Planning Guidance 2005*, which sets out general principles to guide all NHS organisations in developing their ability to respond to a major incident or incidents and to manage recovery whether the incident or incidents has effects locally, regionally, or nationally, within the context of the requirements of the Civil Contingencies Act 2004 (the CCA). The guidance contains strategic national guidance for all NHS organisations in England and equivalent guidance is provided by Health Departments in devolved administrations.

The CCA defines an emergency as:

'An event or a situation which threatens serious damage to human welfare in a place in the UK, the environment of a place in the UK, or war or terrorism which threatens serious damage to the security of the UK.'

The definition is concerned with consequences rather than the cause or source.

For the NHS, major incident is the term in general use and is defined as:

'Any occurrence that presents serious threat to the health of the community, disruption to the service or causes (or is likely to cause) such numbers or types of casualties as to require special arrangements to be implemented by hospitals, ambulance trusts or primary care organisations.'

The levels of incident for which NHS organisations are required to develop **emergency preparedness** arrangements are:

- **Major**: individual ambulance trusts and acute trusts are well versed in handling incidents such as multi-vehicle motorway crashes within the long established major incident plans. More patients will be dealt with, probably faster and with fewer resources, than usual but it is possible to maintain the usual levels of service.
- **Mass**: much larger-scale events affecting potentially hundreds rather than tens of people, possibly also involving the closure or evacuation of a major facility (for example, because of fire or contamination) or persistent disruption over many days. These will require a collective response by several or many neighbouring trusts.
- **Catastrophic**: events of potentially catastrophic proportions that severely disrupt health and social care and other functions (for example, mass casualties, power, water, etc.) and that exceed even collective local capability within the NHS.

Although not formally described, there may be events occurring on a national scale, for example fuel strikes, pandemic or multiple events that require the collective capability of the NHS nationally.

In each NHS organisation, the CEO is responsible for ensuring that their organisation has a Major Incident Plan in place that will be built on the principles of **risk assessment**, cooperation with partners, emergency planning, communicating with the public and information sharing. The plan will link into the organisation's arrangements for ensuring business continuity as required by the Civil Contingencies Act 2004.

The CEO will ensure that the board receives regular reports, at least annually, regarding emergency preparedness, including reports on exercises, training and testing undertaken by the organisation, and that adequate resources are made available to allow discharge of these responsibilities. As a minimum requirement, NHS organisations will be required to undertake a live exercise every three years; a table top exercise every year and a test of communications cascades every six months. A review of emergency preparedness plans may therefore be a part of the annual review of the effectiveness of internal control by the board or audit committee.

To support this arrangement the guidance suggests that an executive board director be designated to take responsibility for emergency preparedness on behalf of the organisation. It is further suggested that a NED be nominated to support the executive director lead in this role. In some cases this may be best achieved through the linkage of emergency planning and business continuity to the organisation's Risk Management Committee (or equivalent).

It is considered good practice for NHS organisations to designate an adequately resourced officer, usually referred to as the Emergency Planning Liaison Officer (EPLO), to support the executive in the discharge of their duties for emergency preparedness.

Business continuity management also forms an important part of risk management arrangements and is a further requirement of the Civil Contingencies Act 2004. The aim of

> **STOP AND THINK 12.2**
>
> Why should emergency preparedness planning be a part of the internal control system of an NHS trust?

business continuity management is to ensure that NHS organisations are able to maintain the highest level of service possible whatever might happen to the infrastructure. There is a range of problems that might affect NHS organisations and services at any time, for example, loss of water or power, flooding, or criminal action.

The aim of business continuity planning is to enable planning and reaction in a coordinated manner. While business continuity and major incident planning are usually separate processes within an organisation, a major incident may occur at the same time as a business continuity issue, or be triggered by it.

Business continuity management, including processes for recovery and restoration, should be considered by NHS organisations as part of its everyday business processes requiring a corporate response. Business continuity should be seen as embedded in the culture of the NHS as principles of health and safety, and there must be demonstrable commitment to the process from the boards of NHS organisations. The skills to develop business continuity plans are complementary to those involved in emergency planning and may therefore need to be undertaken by separate officers. It is critical though that both plans are integrated and complementary to each other.

7 Whistleblowing procedures

The *UK Corporate Governance Code* states that the audit committee should 'review arrangements by which staff of the organisation may, in confidence, raise concerns about possible improprieties in matters of financial reporting or other matters'. In other words, the audit committee should be responsible for review of the provisions and procedures for whistleblowing within the organisation. The *UK Code* specifies that the objective of the audit committee should be to ensure that there are satisfactory arrangements in place for:

- the 'proportionate and independent investigation' of allegations by whistleblowers, and
- appropriate follow-up action.

The code is referring to the adequacy of whistleblowing procedures within the organisation.

While a similar provision is not contained within the *NHS Audit Committee Handbook* most NHS whistleblowing policies require either the review of arrangements by the board or the audit committee.

Whistleblowing is also a key aspect in protection against acts of bribery as defined by the Bribery Act 2010.

Reporting acts of bribery

The majority of Trusts should already have an Anti-Fraud and Corruption Policy or equivalent – the reporting of potential acts of bribery should follow the same procedure. It is important that NHS organisations update their whistleblowing policies to cover potential acts of bribery, so employees are aware of what behaviour is unacceptable.

7.1 Whistleblowing and internal control

There is a strong connection between health service governance and whistleblowing. An employee may honestly believe that there is (or has been or could soon be) serious malpractice by someone within the organisation, but feel unable to report his concerns in the normal way. This could be because the individual to whom he normally reports is involved in the suspected malpractice. Serious malpractice or a misdemeanour could be damaging to the organisation.

- It might suffer financial loss if some employees are acting fraudulently.
- It might be incur severe penalties as a consequence of employees breaking the law or regulations.
- There could be damage to the organisation's reputation if the misdemeanour is made public.

The need for whistleblowing arises when normal procedures and internal controls will not reveal the illicit activity, because the individuals responsible for the activity are somehow able to ignore or get round the normal controls.

However, although whistleblowing procedures are an internal control, they are not an embedded control within the organisation's regular procedures, and their effectiveness relies on the willingness of genuine whistleblowers to come forward with their allegations. The incidence of illicit or illegal behaviour should be uncommon; therefore whistleblowing should be an occasional event. Extensive inquiries into the baby heart unit at Bristol Royal Infirmary and into the extraordinary behaviour of the GP Dr Harold Shipman have raised questions about the protection provided to whistleblowers within the health service.

7.2 Whistleblowing: best practice

Cynthia Bower, chief executive of the CQC, said:

> 'Health and social care professionals have a responsibility to raise concerns if they believe that patients or people who use services are being put at risk. The first course of action should be to raise these concerns within your organisation – but if you feel unable to, or if your voice is not being heard, it's important to know that there are other options open to you.'

If an employee has a genuine, honest concern about something happening within the organisation, which he believes to be unsafe or improper, there should be a way for the employee's concerns to be brought to the attention of management and dealt with in a constructive way. Having a system for listening to employees' concerns should be a part of an effective risk management system within the organisation, because diligent employees can act as an early warning system of problems. However, there are several problems with whistleblowing procedures and policies:

- As stated earlier, experience in many organisations appears to show that an individual who reports concerns about illegal or unethical conduct is often victimised by colleagues and management. If the allegations by the whistleblower are rejected, he might not receive the same salary increases as colleagues, or could be overlooked for promotion. The attitude of colleagues and managers might also be hostile, making it difficult for the individual to continue in the job.
- On the other hand, employees may deliberately make false claims about their colleagues or bosses, out of spite or a desire for revenge for some actual or perceived 'wrong'. It would be inappropriate to provide protection for individuals making malicious and intentionally false allegations.

Organisations therefore need to establish a whistleblowing system that:

- encourages employees to report of illegal or unethical behaviour, but
- discourages malicious and unfounded allegations.

An organisation might state its policy on whistleblowing in the following terms:

- An employee is acting correctly if, in good faith, he or she seeks advice about improper behaviour or reports improper behaviour, where it is not possible to resolve the individual's concerns through discussions with colleagues or line management. Whistleblowing is appropriate if the employee does it in good faith and is not being malicious, and there is no other way to resolve the problem.
- The organisation will not tolerate any discrimination by employees or management in the organisation against an individual who has reported in good faith their concerns about illegal or unethical behaviour. This is a policy statement that whistleblowers will be protected if they have made their report in good faith.

- Disciplinary action will be taken against any employee who knowingly makes a false report of illegal or improper behaviour by someone else. Malicious reporting should not be tolerated.

In practice, employees may feel obliged to take their concerns (possibly anonymously) to someone outside the organisation, risking the anger of the employer for breach of proper procedures if he is identified. An employee can be disciplined for making groundless complaints and allegations in bad faith about his employer. On the other hand, there is an 'official' whistleblowing channel that provides a way of reporting concerns to someone outside the employer organisation provided by the government-funded whistleblowing helpline, which changed to a free-phone service in January 2012.

Health staff who raise concerns about poor patient care now receive greater protection following the recent changes in early 2012 to the NHS Constitution. The changes also make it clear that it is the duty of all NHS workers to report bad practice or any mistreatment of patients receiving care from the health service. Changes to the constitution will add:

- an expectation that staff should raise concerns at the earliest opportunity
- a pledge that NHS organisations should support staff by ensuring their concerns are fully investigated and that there is someone independent, outside of their team, to speak to
- clarity around the existing legal right for staff to raise concerns about safety, malpractice or other wrong doing without suffering any detriment.

The consultation report *The NHS Constitution and Whistleblowing* by the DH, which led to these changes outlined that:

'There are two distinct issues in relation to whistleblowing and the legislation relating to it (the Public Interest Disclosure Act 1998 (PIDA)). The first issue is around whether there are sufficient protections under PIDA for those who wish to raise concerns. The second is about creating and encouraging a culture of openness, where individuals who wish to raise concerns, feel confident enough to speak out and employers act upon these concerns as part of good governance.'

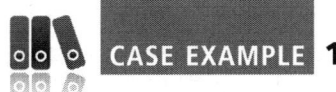

CASE EXAMPLE 12.6

At Queen Elizabeth Hospital Trust, consultant Ramon Neikrash was suspended in 2008 after writing a series of letters to management warning about the impact of cost cutting. An employment tribunal ruled the suspension was unlawful and that Mr Neikrash had been acting as a whistleblower.

7.3 Internal procedures for whistleblowers' allegations

An organisation should have a fair system for dealing internally with accusations from whistleblowers, so that an honest individual does not feel under threat. Employees ought to know what those procedures are. Since whistleblowing is not a regular event, an organisation may simply try to deal with each case on its merits when it arises, without any formal procedures or channels of complaint being established. The employee will therefore not know whom to complain to, and will probably go to the most senior manager available – possibly the CEO.

A problem with dealing with whistleblowing incidents on an ad hoc basis is that the accusations may relate to senior members of staff or the executive directors themselves. An employee who believes the CEO or finance director to be guilty of wrong-doing will have no option other than to resign or take the complaint to an external authority.

It is, therefore, more appropriate to establish a formal internal channel for dealing with whistleblowers, and all NHS organisations will have an established whistleblowing policy. This policy will provide:

- documented internal whistleblowing procedures available to all employees
- the procedures by which an allegation will be investigated
- a named person to whom employees should report their suspicions or concerns

- an independent means of investigation
- a statement that the employer takes malpractice or misconduct seriously, and is committed to a culture of openness in which employees can report legitimate concerns without fear of penalty or punishment
- examples of the type of misconduct for which employees should use the procedure and set out the level of proof that there should be in an allegation. (Although positive proof might not be required, a whistleblower should be able to provide good reasons for his concern.)
- that false or malicious allegations will result in disciplinary action against the individual making them
- that no employee will be victimised for raising a genuine concern. Victimisation for raising a qualified disclosure is a disciplinary offence
- an external whistleblowing route, as well as an internal reporting procedure
- that, as far as possible, whistleblowers will be informed about the outcome of their allegations and the action that has been taken
- that whistleblowers will be promised confidentiality, as far as this is possible.

STOP AND THINK 12.3

As company secretary of an NHS organisation, you have been asked to develop the appropriate internal procedures for dealing with a whistleblower's allegations. What would you advise?

TEST YOUR KNOWLEDGE 12.5

What are the main problems with systems of whistleblowing in the NHS?

7.4 Whistleblowing procedures and the Bribery Act 2010

In the UK, the Bribery Act 2010 introduced a new offence of 'failure of commercial organisations to prevent bribery' by a person associated with them (such as an employee or agent). However an organisation could avoid conviction if it can show that, although bribery may have occurred, it has in place 'adequate processes' to prevent bribery. Having suitable whistleblowing procedures is likely to be a sufficient defence against a criminal charge, provided that the organisation can demonstrate that the procedures work well in practice. It would not be sufficient simply to have a whistleblowing policy in existence, but which no one uses.

CHAPTER SUMMARY

- Internal control risk is the risk of losses arising due to failures or weaknesses in the systems, operating procedures and personnel within an organisation.
- Internal control risks can be categorised into financial risks, operational risks and compliance risks.
- An internal control system should prevent internal control risks, or reduce the potential impact of internal control risks, or should identify failures when they occur and ensure that corrective measures are taken to deal with them. It includes internal controls, which may be categorised as financial controls, operational controls or compliance controls, according to the type of risk they are intended to control.
- An internal control system also includes an appropriate control environment within the organisation, with leadership from the board. There should also be procedures for identifying and assessing internal control risks, designing and implementing suitable internal controls, communication of control information about monitoring of the effectiveness of controls and the control system as a whole.

- The NHS Internal Audit Standards (Government Internal Audit Standards for foundation trusts) set out the requirements for internal audit and how to assess the service that is delivered.
- The board of directors is responsible for ensuring that there is an effective system of internal control and for reviewing the effectiveness of the systems of internal control and risk management.
- The board may delegate the task of carrying out the review of the internal control system and business risk management system to the audit committee (or a risk committee, in the case of the business risk management system).
- The NHS Accounting Officer Memorandum requires all NHS trusts to have an internal audit function.
- The Turnbull Committee issued guidelines on how to establish and maintain a sound system of internal controls. The *Turnbull Guidance* is now the responsibility of the FRC and is periodically reviewed. This guidance forms the basis of NHS guidance on internal control and internal control systems.
- Internal controls should be embedded within operations and procedures, and many are automated. However, some controls are initiated from 'outside' such as internal audit investigations and whistleblowing.
- The review of the effectiveness of the internal control system by the audit committee or the board relies mainly on regular risk reports to the committee (or the board) from management, possibly with occasional additional reports from the internal auditors or external auditors.
- The Statement on Internal Control (SIC) was originally developed as part of the DH's NHS Controls Assurance project. This requirement is in line with the *UK Corporate Governance Code*, which states that the board should report to shareholders each year that it has conducted the annual review of the effectiveness of the systems of internal control and risk management.
- NHS foundation trusts are now required to produce an AGS, with enhanced reporting on quality governance, in place of the statement on internal control for reporting periods commencing on or after 1 April 2011. This will be rolled out to all NHS organisations during 2012.
- In order to sign off the AGS NHS boards need to be assured that the systems, policies and people they have put in place are operating in a way that is effective, is focused on key risks and is driving the delivery of objectives. The BAF is a framework that NHS organisations are required to put in place to identify the key risks to the trust's achievement of its strategic objectives and how these risks are being managed.
- The *NHS Audit Committee Handbook* states that the audit committee should actively review the plans of both internal and external audit and assess the quality of the services that are provided.
- Internal audit can therefore be used to test the effectiveness of internal controls within an organisation's systems and operations, and report to management or the audit committee on their findings and recommendations.
- Internal auditors must be as objective and independent as possible and although the head of internal audit may have a line reporting responsibility to the finance director, they should also have direct access if required to the audit committee.
- The *NHS Audit Committee Handbook* requires the committee to annually review the effectiveness of the internal audit function.
- Emergency preparedness plans are vital for NHS organisations as lengthy or widespread overwhelming demand or shutdown of operations could be catastrophic.
- In each NHS organisation, the CEO is responsible for ensuring that their organisation has a Major Incident Plan in place that will link into the organisation's arrangements for ensuring business continuity as required by the Civil Contingencies Act 2004.
- The *UK Code* requires the board to assess its whistleblowing procedures. While a similar provision is not contained within the *NHS Audit Committee Handbook* most NHS whistleblowing policies require either the review of arrangements by the board or the audit committee.
- Health staff who raise concerns about poor patient care will also receive greater protection in early 2012 when changes to the NHS Constitution will be made. The changes will also make it clear that it is the duty of all NHS workers to report bad practice or any mistreatment of patients receiving care from the health service.

CASE QUESTION 4.1

Review again the case scenario outlined at the beginning of Part 4. Having read the contents of Part Four, how would you advise Helen Wrightford?

APPENDIX 1

The UK Corporate Governance Code

June 2010

THE MAIN PRINCIPLES OF THE CODE

Section A: Leadership

Every company should be headed by an effective board which is collectively responsible for the long-term success of the company.

There should be a clear division of responsibilities at the head of the company between the running of the board and the executive responsibility for the running of the company's business. No one individual should have unfettered powers of decision.

The chairman is responsible for leadership of the board and ensuring its effectiveness on all aspects of its role.

As part of their role as members of a unitary board, non-executive directors should constructively challenge and help develop proposals on strategy.

Section B: Effectiveness

The board and its committees should have the appropriate balance of skills, experience, independence and knowledge of the company to enable them to discharge their respective duties and responsibilities effectively.

There should be a formal, rigorous and transparent procedure for the appointment of new directors to the board.

All directors should be able to allocate sufficient time to the company to discharge their responsibilities effectively.

All directors should receive induction on joining the board and should regularly update and refresh their skills and knowledge.

The board should be supplied in a timely manner with information in a form and of a quality appropriate to enable it to discharge its duties.

The board should undertake a formal and rigorous annual evaluation of its own performance and that of its committees and individual directors.

All directors should be submitted for re-election at regular intervals, subject to continued satisfactory performance.

Section C: Accountability

The board should present a balanced and understandable assessment of the company's position and prospects.

The board is responsible for determining the nature and extent of the significant risks it is willing to take in achieving its strategic objectives. The board should maintain sound risk management and internal control systems.

The board should establish formal and transparent arrangements for considering how they should apply the corporate reporting and risk management and internal control principles and for maintaining an appropriate relationship with the company's auditor.

Section D: Remuneration

Levels of remuneration should be sufficient to attract, retain and motivate directors of the quality required to run the company successfully, but a company should avoid paying more than is necessary for this purpose. A significant proportion of executive directors' remuneration should be structured so as to link rewards to corporate and individual performance.

There should be a formal and transparent procedure for developing policy on executive remuneration and for fixing the remuneration packages of individual directors. No director should be involved in deciding his or her own remuneration.

Section E: Relations with shareholders

There should be a dialogue with shareholders based on the mutual understanding of objectives. The board as a whole has responsibility for ensuring that a satisfactory dialogue with shareholders takes place.

The board should use the AGM to communicate with investors and to encourage their participation.

SECTION A: LEADERSHIP

A.1 The role of the board

Main principle

Every company should be headed by an effective board which is collectively responsible for the long-term success of the company.

Supporting principles

The board's role is to provide entrepreneurial leadership of the company within a framework of prudent and effective controls which enables risk to be assessed and managed. The board should set the company's strategic aims, ensure that the necessary financial and human resources are in place for the company to meet its objectives and review management performance. The board should set the company's values and standards and ensure that its obligations to its shareholders and others are understood and met.

All directors must act in what they consider to be the best interests of the company, consistent with their statutory duties[1].

Code provisions

A.1.1   The board should meet sufficiently regularly to discharge its duties effectively. There should be a formal schedule of matters specifically reserved for its decision. The annual report should include a statement of how the board operates, including a high level statement of which types of decisions are to be taken by the board and which are to be delegated to management.

A.1.2   The annual report should identify the chairman, the deputy chairman (where there is one), the chief executive, the senior independent director and the chairmen and members of the board committees[2]. It should also set out the number of meetings of the board and its committees and individual attendance by directors.

A.1.3   The company should arrange appropriate insurance cover in respect of legal action against its directors.

---

[1] For directors of UK incorporated companies, these duties are set out in the Sections 170 to 177 of the CA 2006.
[2] Provisions A.1.1 and A.1.2 overlap with FSA Rule DTR 7.2.7 R; Provision A.1.2 also overlaps with DTR 7.1.5 R (see Schedule B).

A.2 Division of responsibilities

Main principle
There should be a clear division of responsibilities at the head of the company between the running of the board and the executive responsibility for the running of the company's business. No one individual should have unfettered powers of decision.

Code provision
A.2.1   The roles of chairman and chief executive should not be exercised by the same individual. The division of responsibilities between the chairman and chief executive should be clearly established, set out in writing and agreed by the board.

A.3 The chairman

Main principle
The chairman is responsible for leadership of the board and ensuring its effectiveness on all aspects of its role.

Supporting principle
The chairman is responsible for setting the board's agenda and ensuring that adequate time is available for discussion of all agenda items, in particular strategic issues. The chairman should also promote a culture of openness and debate by facilitating the effective contribution of non-executive directors in particular and ensuring constructive relations between executive and non-executive directors.

The chairman is responsible for ensuring that the directors receive accurate, timely and clear information. The chairman should ensure effective communication with shareholders.

Code provision
A.3.1   The chairman should on appointment meet the independence criteria set out in B.1.1 below. A chief executive should not go on to be chairman of the same company. If, exceptionally, a board decides that a chief executive should become chairman, the board should consult major shareholders in advance and should set out its reasons to shareholders at the time of the appointment and in the next annual report[3].

A.4 Non-executive directors

Main principle
As part of their role as members of a unitary board, non-executive directors should constructively challenge and help develop proposals on strategy.

Supporting principle
Non-executive directors should scrutinise the performance of management in meeting agreed goals and objectives and monitor the reporting of performance. They should satisfy themselves on the integrity of financial information and that financial controls and systems of risk management are robust and defensible. They are responsible for determining appropriate levels of remuneration of executive directors and have a prime role in appointing and, where necessary, removing executive directors, and in succession planning.

Code provisions
A.4.1   The board should appoint one of the independent non-executive directors to be the senior independent director to provide a sounding board for the chairman and to serve as an intermediary for the other directors when necessary. The senior independent director should be available to shareholders if they have concerns which contact through

---

[3] Compliance or otherwise with this provision need only be reported for the year in which the appointment is made.

the normal channels of chairman, chief executive or other executive directors has failed to resolve or for which such contact is inappropriate.

A.4.2 The chairman should hold meetings with the non-executive directors without the executives present. Led by the senior independent director, the non-executive directors should meet without the chairman present at least annually to appraise the chairman's performance and on such other occasions as are deemed appropriate.

A.4.3 Where directors have concerns which cannot be resolved about the running of the company or a proposed action, they should ensure that their concerns are recorded in the board minutes. On resignation, a non-executive director should provide a written statement to the chairman, for circulation to the board, if they have any such concerns.

SECTION B: EFFECTIVENESS

B.1 The composition of the board

Main principle

The board and its committees should have the appropriate balance of skills, experience, independence and knowledge of the company to enable them to discharge their respective duties and responsibilities effectively.

Supporting principles

The board should be of sufficient size that the requirements of the business can be met and that changes to the board's composition and that of its committees can be managed without undue disruption, and should not be so large as to be unwieldy.

The board should include an appropriate combination of executive and non-executive directors (and, in particular, independent non-executive directors) such that no individual or small group of individuals can dominate the board's decision taking.

The value of ensuring that committee membership is refreshed and that undue reliance is not placed on particular individuals should be taken into account in deciding chairmanship and membership of committees.

No one other than the committee chairman and members is entitled to be present at a meeting of the nomination, audit or remuneration committee, but others may attend at the invitation of the committee.

Code provisions

B.1.1 The board should identify in the annual report each non-executive director it considers to be independent[4]. The board should determine whether the director is independent in character and judgement and whether there are relationships or circumstances which are likely to affect, or could appear to affect, the director's judgement. The board should state its reasons if it determines that a director is independent notwithstanding the existence of relationships or circumstances which may appear relevant to its determination, including if the director:

- has been an employee of the company or group within the last five years;
- has, or has had within the last three years, a material business relationship with the company either directly, or as a partner, shareholder, director or senior employee of a body that has such a relationship with the company;
- has received or receives additional remuneration from the company apart from a director's fee, participates in the company's share option or a performance-related pay scheme, or is a member of the company's pension scheme;
- has close family ties with any of the company's advisers, directors or senior employees;
- holds cross-directorships or has significant links with other directors through involvement in other companies or bodies;

---

[4] A.3.1 states that the chairman should, on appointment, meet the independence criteria set out in this provision, but thereafter the test of independence is not appropriate in relation to the chairman.

- represents a significant shareholder; or
- has served on the board for more than nine years from the date of their first election.

B.1.2 Except for smaller companies[5], at least half the board, excluding the chairman, should comprise non-executive directors determined by the board to be independent. A smaller company should have at least two independent non-executive directors.

B.2 Appointments to the board

Main principle
There should be a formal, rigorous and transparent procedure for the appointment of new directors to the board.

Supporting principles
The search for board candidates should be conducted, and appointments made, on merit, against objective criteria and with due regard for the benefits of diversity on the board, including gender.

The board should satisfy itself that plans are in place for orderly succession for appointments to the board and to senior management, so as to maintain an appropriate balance of skills and experience within the company and on the board and to ensure progressive refreshing of the board.

Code provisions
B.2.1 There should be a nomination committee which should lead the process for board appointments and make recommendations to the board. A majority of members of the nomination committee should be independent non-executive directors. The chairman or an independent non-executive director should chair the committee, but the chairman should not chair the nomination committee when it is dealing with the appointment of a successor to the chairmanship. The nomination committee should make available its terms of reference, explaining its role and the authority delegated to it by the board[6].

B.2.2 The nomination committee should evaluate the balance of skills, experience, independence and knowledge on the board and, in the light of this evaluation, prepare a description of the role and capabilities required for a particular appointment.

B.2.3 Non-executive directors should be appointed for specified terms subject to re-election and to statutory provisions relating to the removal of a director. Any term beyond six years for a non-executive director should be subject to particularly rigorous review, and should take into account the need for progressive refreshing of the board.

B.2.4 A separate section of the annual report should describe the work of the nomination committee[7], including the process it has used in relation to board appointments. An explanation should be given if neither an external search consultancy nor open advertising has been used in the appointment of a chairman or a non-executive director.

B.3 Commitment

Main principle
All directors should be able to allocate sufficient time to the company to discharge their responsibilities effectively.

Code provisions
B.3.1 For the appointment of a chairman, the nomination committee should prepare a job specification, including an assessment of the time commitment expected, recognising

---

[5] A smaller company is one that is below the FTSE 350 throughout the year immediately prior to the reporting year.
[6] The requirement to make the information available would be met by including the information on a website that is maintained by or on behalf of the company.
[7] This provision overlaps with FSA Rule DTR 7.2.7 R (see Schedule B).

the need for availability in the event of crises. A chairman's other significant commitments should be disclosed to the board before appointment and included in the annual report. Changes to such commitments should be reported to the board as they arise, and their impact explained in the next annual report.

B.3.2 The terms and conditions of appointment of non-executive directors should be made available for inspection[8]. The letter of appointment should set out the expected time commitment. Non-executive directors should undertake that they will have sufficient time to meet what is expected of them. Their other significant commitments should be disclosed to the board before appointment, with a broad indication of the time involved and the board should be informed of subsequent changes.

B.3.3 The board should not agree to a full time executive director taking on more than one non-executive directorship in a FTSE 100 company nor the chairmanship of such a company.

B.4 Development

Main principle
All directors should receive induction on joining the board and should regularly update and refresh their skills and knowledge.

Supporting principles
The chairman should ensure that the directors continually update their skills and the knowledge and familiarity with the company required to fulfil their role both on the board and on board committees. The company should provide the necessary resources for developing and updating its directors' knowledge and capabilities.

To function effectively, all directors need appropriate knowledge of the company and access to its operations and staff.

Code provisions
B.4.1 The chairman should ensure that new directors receive a full, formal and tailored induction on joining the board. As part of this, directors should avail themselves of opportunities to meet major shareholders.

B.4.2 The chairman should regularly review and agree with each director their training and development needs.

B.5 Information and support

Main principle
The board should be supplied in a timely manner with information in a form and of a quality appropriate to enable it to discharge its duties.

Supporting principles
The chairman is responsible for ensuring that the directors receive accurate, timely and clear information. Management has an obligation to provide such information but directors should seek clarification or amplification where necessary.

Under the direction of the chairman, the company secretary's responsibilities include ensuring good information flows within the board and its committees and between senior management and non-executive directors, as well as facilitating induction and assisting with professional development as required.

The company secretary should be responsible for advising the board through the chairman on all governance matters.

---

[8] The terms and conditions of appointment of non-executive directors should be made available for inspection by any person at the company's registered office during normal business hours and at the AGM (for 15 minutes prior to the meeting and during the meeting).

Code provisions

B.5.1 The board should ensure that directors, especially non-executive directors, have access to independent professional advice at the company's expense where they judge it necessary to discharge their responsibilities as directors. Committees should be provided with sufficient resources to undertake their duties.

B.5.2 All directors should have access to the advice and services of the company secretary, who is responsible to the board for ensuring that board procedures are complied with. Both the appointment and removal of the company secretary should be a matter for the board as a whole.

B.6 Evaluation

Main principle
The board should undertake a formal and rigorous annual evaluation of its own performance and that of its committees and individual directors.

Supporting principles
The chairman should act on the results of the performance evaluation by recognising the strengths and addressing the weaknesses of the board and, where appropriate, proposing new members be appointed to the board or seeking the resignation of directors.

Individual evaluation should aim to show whether each director continues to contribute effectively and to demonstrate commitment to the role (including commitment of time for board and committee meetings and any other duties).

Code provisions

B.6.1 The board should state in the annual report how performance evaluation of the board, its committees and its individual directors has been conducted.

B.6.2 Evaluation of the board of FTSE 350 companies should be externally facilitated at least every three years. A statement should be made available of whether an external facilitator has any other connection with the company[9].

B.6.3 The non-executive directors, led by the senior independent director, should be responsible for performance evaluation of the chairman, taking into account the views of executive directors.

B.7 Re-election

Main principle
All directors should be submitted for re-election at regular intervals, subject to continued satisfactory performance.

Code provisions

B.7.1 All directors of FTSE 350 companies should be subject to annual election by shareholders. All other directors should be subject to election by shareholders at the first annual general meeting after their appointment, and to re-election thereafter at intervals of no more than three years. Non-executive directors who have served longer than nine years should be subject to annual re-election. The names of directors submitted for election or re-election should be accompanied by sufficient biographical details and any other relevant information to enable shareholders to take an informed decision on their election.

B.7.2 The board should set out to shareholders in the papers accompanying a resolution to elect a non-executive director why they believe an individual should be elected. The chairman should confirm to shareholders when proposing re-election that, following formal performance evaluation, the individual's performance continues to be effective and to demonstrate commitment to the role.

---

[9] See footnote 7.

SECTION C: ACCOUNTABILITY

C.1 Financial and business reporting

Main principle

The board should present a balanced and understandable assessment of the company's position and prospects.

Supporting principle

The board's responsibility to present a balanced and understandable assessment extends to interim and other price-sensitive public reports and reports to regulators as well as to information required to be presented by statutory requirements.

Code provisions

C.1.1   The directors should explain in the annual report their responsibility for preparing the annual report and accounts, and there should be a statement by the auditor about their reporting responsibilities[10].

C.1.2   The directors should include in the annual report an explanation of the basis on which the company generates or preserves value over the longer term (the business model) and the strategy for delivering the objectives of the company[11].

C.1.3   The directors should report in annual and half-yearly financial statements that the business is a going concern, with supporting assumptions or qualifications as necessary[12].

C.2 Risk management and internal control[13]

Main principle

The board is responsible for determining the nature and extent of the significant risks it is willing to take in achieving its strategic objectives. The board should maintain sound risk management and internal control systems.

Code provision

C.2.1   The board should, at least annually, conduct a review of the effectiveness of the company's risk management and internal control systems and should report to shareholders that they have done so[14]. The review should cover all material controls, including financial, operational and compliance controls.

---

[10] The requirement may be met by the disclosures about the audit scope and the responsibilities of the auditor included, or referred to, in the auditor's report pursuant to the requirements in paragraph 16 of ISA (UK and Ireland) 700, "The Auditor's Report on Financial Statements". Copies are available at: www.frc.org.uk/apb/publications/pub2102.html.

[11] It would be desirable if the explanation were located in the same part of the annual report as the Business Review required by Section 417 of the CA 2006. Guidance as to the matters that should be considered in an explanation of a business model is provided in paragraphs 30 to 32 of the Accounting Standard Board's Reporting Statement: Operating And Financial Review. Copies are available at: www.frc.org.uk/asb/publications/documents.cfm?cat=7.

[12] 'Going Concern and Liquidity Risk: Guidance for Directors of UK Companies 2009' suggests means of applying this part of the code. Copies are available at: www.frc.org.uk/corporate/goingconcern.cfm.

[13] The Turnbull guidance suggests means of applying this part of the code. Copies are available at www.frc.org.uk/corporate/internalcontrol.cfm.

[14] In addition FSA Rule DTR 7.2.5 R requires companies to describe the main features of the internal control and risk management systems in relation to the financial reporting process.

C.3 Audit committee and auditors[15]

Main principle
The board should establish formal and transparent arrangements for considering how they should apply the corporate reporting and risk management and internal control principles and for maintaining an appropriate relationship with the company's auditor.

Code provisions

C.3.1   The board should establish an audit committee of at least three, or in the case of smaller companies[16] two, independent non-executive directors. In smaller companies the company chairman may be a member of, but not chair, the committee in addition to the independent non-executive directors, provided he or she was considered independent on appointment as chairman. The board should satisfy itself that at least one member of the audit committee has recent and relevant financial experience[17].

C.3.2   The main role and responsibilities of the audit committee should be set out in written terms of reference[18] and should include:

- to monitor the integrity of the financial statements of the company and any formal announcements relating to the company's financial performance, reviewing significant financial reporting judgements contained in them;
- to review the company's internal financial controls and, unless expressly addressed by a separate board risk committee composed of independent directors, or by the board itself, to review the company's internal control and risk management systems;
- to monitor and review the effectiveness of the company's internal audit function;
- to make recommendations to the board, for it to put to the shareholders for their approval in general meeting, in relation to the appointment, re-appointment and removal of the external auditor and to approve the remuneration and terms of engagement of the external auditor;
- to review and monitor the external auditor's independence and objectivity and the effectiveness of the audit process, taking into consideration relevant UK professional and regulatory requirements;
- to develop and implement policy on the engagement of the external auditor to supply non-audit services, taking into account relevant ethical guidance regarding the provision of non-audit services by the external audit firm, and to report to the board, identifying any matters in respect of which it considers that action or improvement is needed and making recommendations as to the steps to be taken.

C.3.3   The terms of reference of the audit committee, including its role and the authority delegated to it by the board, should be made available[19]. A separate section of the annual report should describe the work of the committee in discharging those responsibilities[20].

C.3.4   The audit committee should review arrangements by which staff of the company may, in confidence, raise concerns about possible improprieties in matters of financial reporting or other matters. The audit committee's objective should be to ensure that arrangements are in place for the proportionate and independent investigation of such matters and for appropriate follow-up action.

C.3.5   The audit committee should monitor and review the effectiveness of the internal audit activities. Where there is no internal audit function, the audit committee should consider annually whether there is a need for an internal audit function and make a recommendation to the board, and the reasons for the absence of such a function should be explained in the relevant section of the annual report.

---

[15] The FRC Guidance on Audit Committees suggests means of applying this part of the code. Copies are available at: www.frc.org.uk/corporate/auditcommittees.cfm.
[16] See footnote 6.
[17] This provision overlaps with FSA Rule DTR 7.1.1 R (see Schedule B).
[18] This provision overlaps with FSA Rules DTR 7.1.3 R (see Schedule C).
[19] See footnote 7.
[20] This provision overlaps with FSA Rules DTR 7.1.5 R and 7.2.7 R (see Schedule B).

C.3.6 The audit committee should have primary responsibility for making a recommendation on the appointment, reappointment and removal of the external auditor. If the board does not accept the audit committee's recommendation, it should include in the annual report, and in any papers recommending appointment or re-appointment, a statement from the audit committee explaining the recommendation and should set out reasons why the board has taken a different position.

C.3.7 The annual report should explain to shareholders how, if the auditor provides non-audit services, auditor objectivity and independence is safeguarded.

SECTION D: REMUNERATION

D.1 The level and components of remuneration

Main principle

Levels of remuneration should be sufficient to attract, retain and motivate directors of the quality required to run the company successfully, but a company should avoid paying more than is necessary for this purpose. A significant proportion of executive directors' remuneration should be structured so as to link rewards to corporate and individual performance.

Supporting principle

The performance-related elements of executive directors' remuneration should be stretching and designed to promote the long-term success of the company.

The remuneration committee should judge where to position their company relative to other companies. But they should use such comparisons with caution in view of the risk of an upward ratchet of remuneration levels with no corresponding improvement in performance.

They should also be sensitive to pay and employment conditions elsewhere in the group, especially when determining annual salary increases.

Code provisions

D.1.1 In designing schemes of performance-related remuneration for executive directors, the remuneration committee should follow the provisions in Schedule A to this code.

D.1.2 Where a company releases an executive director to serve as a non-executive director elsewhere, the remuneration report[21] should include a statement as to whether or not the director will retain such earnings and, if so, what the remuneration is.

D.1.3 Levels of remuneration for non-executive directors should reflect the time commitment and responsibilities of the role. Remuneration for non-executive directors should not include share options or other performance-related elements. If, exceptionally, options are granted, shareholder approval should be sought in advance and any shares acquired by exercise of the options should be held until at least one year after the non-executive director leaves the board. Holding of share options could be relevant to the determination of a non-executive director's independence (as set out in provision B.1.1).

D.1.4 The remuneration committee should carefully consider what compensation commitments (including pension contributions and all other elements) their directors' terms of appointment would entail in the event of early termination. The aim should be to avoid rewarding poor performance. They should take a robust line on reducing compensation to reflect departing directors' obligations to mitigate loss.

D.1.5 Notice or contract periods should be set at one year or less. If it is necessary to offer longer notice or contract periods to new directors recruited from outside, such periods should reduce to one year or less after the initial period.

---

[21] As required for UK incorporated companies under the Large and Medium-Sized Companies and Groups (Accounts and Reports) Regulations 2008.

D.2 Procedure

Main principle
There should be a formal and transparent procedure for developing policy on executive remuneration and for fixing the remuneration packages of individual directors. No director should be involved in deciding his or her own remuneration.

Supporting principles
The remuneration committee should consult the chairman and/or chief executive about their proposals relating to the remuneration of other executive directors. The remuneration committee should also be responsible for appointing any consultants in respect of executive director remuneration. Where executive directors or senior management are involved in advising or supporting the remuneration committee, care should be taken to recognise and avoid conflicts of interest.

The chairman of the board should ensure that the company maintains contact as required with its principal shareholders about remuneration.

Code provisions
D.2.1 The board should establish a remuneration committee of at least three, or in the case of smaller companies[22] two, independent non-executive directors. In addition the company chairman may also be a member of, but not chair, the committee if he or she was considered independent on appointment as chairman. The remuneration committee should make available its terms of reference, explaining its role and the authority delegated to it by the board[23]. Where remuneration consultants are appointed, a statement should be made available[24] of whether they have any other connection with the company.

D.2.2 The remuneration committee should have delegated responsibility for setting remuneration for all executive directors and the chairman, including pension rights and any compensation payments. The committee should also recommend and monitor the level and structure of remuneration for senior management. The definition of 'senior management' for this purpose should be determined by the board but should normally include the first layer of management below board level.

D.2.3 The board itself or, where required by the Articles of Association, the shareholders should determine the remuneration of the non-executive directors within the limits set in the Articles of Association. Where permitted by the Articles, the board may however delegate this responsibility to a committee, which might include the chief executive.

D.2.4 Shareholders should be invited specifically to approve all new long-term incentive schemes (as defined in the Listing Rules[25]) and significant changes to existing schemes, save in the circumstances permitted by the Listing Rules.

SECTION E: RELATIONS WITH SHAREHOLDERS

E.1 Dialogue with shareholders

Main principle
There should be a dialogue with shareholders based on the mutual understanding of objectives. The board as a whole has responsibility for ensuring that a satisfactory dialogue with shareholders takes place[26].

---

[22] See footnote 6.
[23] This provision overlaps with FSA Rule DTR 7.2.7 R (see Schedule B).
[24] See footnote 7.
[25] Listing Rules LR 9.4; available at http://fsahandbook.info/FSA/html/handbook/LR/9/4.
[26] Nothing in these principles or provisions should be taken to override the general requirements of law to treat shareholders equally in access to information.

Supporting principles

Whilst recognising that most shareholder contact is with the chief executive and finance director, the chairman should ensure that all directors are made aware of their major shareholders' issues and concerns.

The board should keep in touch with shareholder opinion in whatever ways are most practical and efficient.

Code provisions

E.1.1 The chairman should ensure that the views of shareholders are communicated to the board as a whole. The chairman should discuss governance and strategy with major shareholders. Non-executive directors should be offered the opportunity to attend scheduled meetings with major shareholders and should expect to attend meetings if requested by major shareholders. The senior independent director should attend sufficient meetings with a range of major shareholders to listen to their views in order to help develop a balanced understanding of the issues and concerns of major shareholders.

E.1.2 The board should state in the annual report the steps they have taken to ensure that the members of the board, and, in particular, the non-executive directors, develop an understanding of the views of major shareholders about the company, for example through direct face-to-face contact, analysts' or brokers' briefings and surveys of shareholder opinion.

E.2 Constructive use of the AGM

Main principle

The board should use the AGM to communicate with investors and to encourage their participation.

Code provisions

E.2.1 At any general meeting, the company should propose a separate resolution on each substantially separate issue, and should, in particular, propose a resolution at the AGM relating to the report and accounts. For each resolution, proxy appointment forms should provide shareholders with the option to direct their proxy to vote either for or against the resolution or to withhold their vote. The proxy form and any announcement of the results of a vote should make it clear that a 'vote withheld' is not a vote in law and will not be counted in the calculation of the proportion of the votes for and against the resolution.

E.2.2 The company should ensure that all valid proxy appointments received for general meetings are properly recorded and counted. For each resolution, where a vote has been taken on a show of hands, the company should ensure that the following information is given at the meeting and made available as soon as reasonably practicable on a website which is maintained by or on behalf of the company:

- the number of shares in respect of which proxy appointments have been validly made;
- the number of votes for the resolution;
- the number of votes against the resolution; and
- the number of shares in respect of which the vote was directed to be withheld.

E.2.3 The chairman should arrange for the chairmen of the audit, remuneration and nomination committees to be available to answer questions at the AGM and for all directors to attend.

E.2.4 The company should arrange for the Notice of the AGM and related papers to be sent to shareholders at least 20 working days before the meeting.

SCHEDULE A: THE DESIGN OF PERFORMANCE-RELATED REMUNERATION FOR EXECUTIVE DIRECTORS

The remuneration committee should consider whether the directors should be eligible for annual bonuses. If so, performance conditions should be relevant, stretching and designed to promote the long-term success of the company. Upper limits should be set and disclosed. There may be a case for part payment in shares to be held for a significant period.

The remuneration committee should consider whether the directors should be eligible for benefits under long-term incentive schemes. Traditional share option schemes should be weighed against other kinds of long-term incentive scheme. Executive share options should not be offered at a discount save as permitted by the relevant provisions of the Listing Rules.

In normal circumstances, shares granted or other forms of deferred remuneration should not vest, and options should not be exercisable, in less than three years. Directors should be encouraged to hold their shares for a further period after vesting or exercise, subject to the need to finance any costs of acquisition and associated tax liabilities.

Any new long-term incentive schemes which are proposed should be approved by shareholders and should preferably replace any existing schemes or, at least, form part of a well considered overall plan incorporating existing schemes.

The total potentially available rewards should not be excessive. Payouts or grants under all incentive schemes, including new grants under existing share option schemes, should be subject to challenging performance criteria reflecting the company's objectives, including non-financial performance metrics where appropriate. Remuneration incentives should be compatible with risk policies and systems.

Grants under executive share option and other long-term incentive schemes should normally be phased rather than awarded in one large block.

Consideration should be given to the use of provisions that permit the company to reclaim variable components in exceptional circumstances of misstatement or misconduct.

In general, only basic salary should be pensionable. The remuneration committee should consider the pension consequences and associated costs to the company of basic salary increases and any other changes in pensionable remuneration, especially for directors close to retirement.

SCHEDULE B: DISCLOSURE OF CORPORATE GOVERNANCE ARRANGEMENTS

Corporate governance disclosure requirements are set out in three places:

- FSA Disclosure and Transparency Rules sub-chapters 7.1 and 7.2 (which set out certain mandatory disclosures);
- FSA Listing Rules 9.8.6 R, 9.8.7 R, and 9.8.7A R (which includes the 'comply or explain' requirement); and
- The UK Corporate Governance Code (in addition to providing an explanation where they choose not to comply with a provision, companies must disclose specified information in order to comply with certain provisions).

These requirements are summarised below. The full text of Disclosure and Transparency Rules 7.1 and 7.2 and Listing Rules 9.8.6 R, 9.8.7 R and 9.8.7A R are contained in the relevant chapters of the FSA Handbook, which can be found at http://fsahandbook.info/FSA/html/handbook/.

The Disclosure and Transparency Rules sub-chapters 7.1 and 7.2 apply to issuers whose securities are admitted to trading on a regulated market (this includes all issuers with a Premium or Standard listing). The Listing Rules 9.8.6 R, 9.8.7 R and 9.8.7A R and UK Corporate Governance Code apply to issuers of Premium listed equity shares only.

There is some overlap between the mandatory disclosures required under the Disclosure and Transparency Rules and those expected under the UK Corporate Governance Code. Areas of overlap are summarised in the Appendix to this Schedule. In respect of disclosures relating to the audit committee and the composition and operation of the board and its committees, compliance with the relevant provisions of the Code will result in compliance with the relevant rules.

Disclosure and Transparency Rules

Sub-chapter 7.1 of the Disclosure and Transparency Rules concerns audit committees or bodies carrying out equivalent functions:

- DTR 7.1.1 R to 7.1.3 R set out requirements relating to the composition and functions of the committee or equivalent body:
- DTR 7.1.1 R states than an issuer must have a body which is responsible for performing the functions set out in DTR 7.1.3 R, and that at least one member of that body must be independent and at least one member must have competence in accounting and/or auditing.
- DTR 7.1.2 G states that the requirements for independence and competence in accounting and/or auditing may be satisfied by the same member or by different members of the relevant body.
- DTR 7.1.3 R states that an issuer must ensure that, as a minimum, the relevant body must:
  1) monitor the financial reporting process;
  2) monitor the effectiveness of the issuer's internal control, internal audit where applicable, and risk management systems;
  3) monitor the statutory audit of the annual and consolidated accounts;
  4) review and monitor the independence of the statutory auditor, and in particular the provision of additional services to the issuer.

DTR 7.1.5 R to DTR 7.1.7 G set out what disclosure is required. Specifically:

- DTR 7.1.5 R states that the issuer must make a statement available to the public disclosing which body carries out the functions required by DTR 7.1.3 R and how it is composed.
- DTR 7.1.6 G states that this can be included in the corporate governance statement required under sub-chapter DTR 7.2 (see below).
- DTR 7.1.7 G states that compliance with the relevant provisions of the UK Corporate Governance Code (as set out in the Appendix to this Schedule) will result in compliance with DTR 7.1.1 R to 7.1.5 R.

Sub-chapter 7.2 concerns corporate governance statements. Issuers are required to produce a corporate governance statement that must be either included in the directors' report (DTR 7.2.1 R); or in a separate report published together with the annual report; or on the issuer's website, in which case there must be a cross-reference in the directors' report (DTR 7.2.9 R).

DTR 7.2.2 R requires that the corporate governance statements must contain a reference to the corporate governance code to which the company is subject (for companies with a Premium listing this is the UK Corporate Governance Code). DTR 7.2.3 R requires that, to the extent that it departs from that code, the company must explain which parts of the code it departs from and the reasons for doing so. DTR 7.2.4 G states that compliance with LR 9.8.6 R (6) (the 'comply or explain' rule in relation to the UK Corporate Governance Code) will also satisfy these requirements.

DTR 7.2.5 R to DTR 7.2.10 R set out certain information that must be disclosed in the corporate governance statement:

- DTR 7.2.5 R states that the corporate governance statement must contain a description of the main features of the company's internal control and risk management systems in relation to the financial reporting process. DTR 7.2.10 R states that an issuer which is required to prepare a group directors' report within the meaning of Section 415(2) of the CA 2006 must include in that report a description of the main features of the group's internal control and risk management systems in relation to the process for preparing consolidated accounts.
- DTR 7.2.6 R states that the corporate governance statement must contain the information required by paragraph 13(2)(c), (d), (f), (h) and (i) of Schedule 7 to the Large and Medium-sized Companies and Groups (Accounts and Reports) Regulations 2008 where the issuer is subject to the requirements of that paragraph.

- DTR 7.2.7 R states that the corporate governance statement must contain a description of the composition and operation of the issuer's administrative, management and supervisory bodies and their committees. DTR 7.2.8 G states that compliance with the relevant provisions of the UK Corporate Governance Code (as set out in the Appendix to this Schedule) will satisfy these requirements.

Listing Rules

Listing Rules 9.8.6 R (for UK incorporated companies) and 9.8.7 R (for overseas incorporated companies) state that in the case of a company that has a Premium listing of equity shares, the following items must be included in its annual report and accounts:

- a statement of how the listed company has applied the Main Principles set out in the UK Corporate Governance Code, in a manner that would enable shareholders to evaluate how the principles have been applied;
- a statement as to whether the listed company has:
  - complied throughout the accounting period with all relevant provisions set out in the UK Corporate Governance Code; or
  - not complied throughout the accounting period with all relevant provisions set out in the UK Corporate Governance Code, and if so, setting out:
    i. those provisions, if any, it has not complied with;
    ii. in the case of provisions whose requirements are of a continuing nature, the period within which, if any, it did not comply with some or all of those provisions; and
    iii. the company's reasons for non-compliance.

The UK Corporate Governance Code

In addition to the 'comply or explain' requirement in the Listing Rules, the code includes specific requirements for disclosure which must be provided in order to comply. These are summarised below.

The annual report should include:

- a statement of how the board operates, including a high level statement of which types of decisions are to be taken by the board and which are to be delegated to management (A.1.1);
- the names of the chairman, the deputy chairman (where there is one), the chief executive, the senior independent director and the chairmen and members of the board committees (A.1.2);
- the number of meetings of the board and those committees and individual attendance by directors (A.1.2);
- where a chief executive is appointed chairman, the reasons for their appointment (this only needs to be done in the annual report following the appointment) (A.3.1);
- the names of the non-executive directors whom the board determines to be independent, with reasons where necessary (B.1.1);
- a separate section describing the work of the nomination committee, including the process it has used in relation to board appointments and an explanation if neither external search consultancy nor open advertising has been used in the appointment of a chairman or a non-executive director (B.2.4);
- any changes to the other significant commitments of the chairman during the year (B.3.1);
- a statement of how performance evaluation of the board, its committees and its directors has been conducted (B.6.1);
- an explanation from the directors of their responsibility for preparing the accounts and a statement by the auditors about their reporting responsibilities (C.1.1);
- an explanation from the directors of the basis on which the company generates or preserves value over the longer term (the business model) and the strategy for delivering the objectives of the company (C.1.2);
- a statement from the directors that the business is a going concern, with supporting assumptions or qualifications as necessary (C.1.3);

- a report that the board has conducted a review of the effectiveness of the company's risk management and internal controls systems (C.2.1);
- a separate section describing the work of the audit committee in discharging its responsibilities (C.3.3);
- where there is no internal audit function, the reasons for the absence of such a function (C.3.5);
- where the board does not accept the audit committee's recommendation on the appointment, reappointment or removal of an external auditor, a statement from the audit committee explaining the recommendation and the reasons why the board has taken a different position (C.3.6);
- an explanation of how, if the auditor provides non-audit services, auditor objectivity and independence is safeguarded (C.3.7);
- a description of the work of the remuneration committee as required under the Large and Medium-Sized Companies and Groups (Accounts and Reports) Regulations 2008 including, where an executive director serves as a non-executive director elsewhere, whether or not the director will retain such earnings and, if so, what the remuneration is (D.1.2);
- the steps the board has taken to ensure that members of the board, in particular the non-executive directors, develop an understanding of the views of major shareholders about their company (E.1.2).

The following information should be made available (which may be met by placing the information on a website that is maintained by or on behalf of the company):

- the terms of reference of the nomination, audit and remuneration committees, explaining their role and the authority delegated to them by the board (B.2.1, C.3.3 and D.2.1);
- the terms and conditions of appointment of non-executive directors (B.3.2) (see footnote 9);
- where performance evaluation has been externally facilitated, a statement of whether the facilitator has any other connection with the company (B.6.2); and
- where remuneration consultants are appointed, a statement of whether they have any other connection with the company (D.2.1).

The board should set out to shareholders in the papers accompanying a resolution to elect or re-elect directors:

- sufficient biographical details to enable shareholders to take an informed decision on their election or re-election (B.7.1);
- why they believe an individual should be elected to a non-executive role (B.7.2); and
- on re-election of a non-executive director, confirmation from the chairman that, following formal performance evaluation, the individual's performance continues to be effective and to demonstrate commitment to the role (B.7.2).

The board should set out to shareholders in the papers recommending appointment or reappointment of an external auditor:

- if the board does not accept the audit committee's recommendation, a statement from the audit committee explaining the recommendation and from the board setting out reasons why they have taken a different position (C.3.6).

Additional guidance

The Turnbull Guidance and FRC Guidance on Audit Committees contain further suggestions as to information that might usefully be disclosed in the internal control statement and the report of the audit committee respectively. Both sets of guidance are available on the FRC website at: http://www.frc.org.uk/corporate/ukcgcode.cfm

APPENDIX
OVERLAP BETWEEN THE DISCLOSURE AND TRANSPARENCY RULES AND THE UK CORPORATE GOVERNANCE CODE

DISCLOSURE AND TRANSPARENCY RULES	UK CORPORATE GOVERNANCE CODE
D.T.R 7.1.1 R Sets out minimum requirements on composition of the audit committee or equivalent body.	**Provision C.3.1** Sets out recommended composition of the audit committee.
D.T.R 7.1.3 R Sets out minimum functions of the audit committee or equivalent body.	**Provision C.3.2** Sets out the recommended minimum terms of reference for the audit committee.
D.T.R 7.1.5 R The composition and function of the audit committee or equivalent body must be disclosed in the annual report *DTR 7.1.7 R states that compliance with code provisions A.1.2, C.3.1, C.3.2 and C.3.3 will result in compliance with DTR 7.1.1 R to DTR 7.1.5 R.*	**Provision A.1.2** The annual report should identify members of the board committees. **Provision C.3.3** The annual report should describe the work of the audit committee. Further recommendations on the content of the audit committee report are set out in the FRC Guidance on Audit Committees.
D.T.R 7.2.5 R The corporate governance statement must include a description of the main features of the company's internal control and risk management systems in relation to the financial reporting process. *While this requirement differs from the requirement in the UK Corporate Governance Code, it is envisaged that both could be met by a single internal control statement.*	**Provision C.2.1** The Board must report that a review of the effectiveness of the risk management and internal control systems has been carried out. Further recommendations on the content of the internal control statement are set out in the Turnbull Guidance.
DTR 7.2.7 R The corporate governance statement must include a description of the composition and operation of the administrative, management and supervisory bodies and their committees. *DTR 7.2.8 R states that compliance with code provisions A.1.1, A.1.2, A.4.6, B.2.1 and C.3.3 will result in compliance with DTR 7.2.7 R.*	This requirement overlaps with a number of different provisions of the code: **A.1.1**: the annual report should include a statement of how the board operates. **A.1.2**: the annual report should identify members of the board and board committees. **B.2.4**: the annual report should describe the work of the nomination committee. **C.3.3**: the annual report should describe the work of the audit committee. **D.2.1**: a description of the work of the remuneration committee should be made available. *[Note: in order to comply with DTR 7.2.7 R this information will need to be included in the corporate governance statement].*

APPENDIX 2

NHS Foundation Trust Code of Governance

March 2010

A DIRECTORS

A.1 The board of directors

Main principle

Every NHS foundation trust should be headed by an effective board of directors, since the board is collectively responsible for the exercise of the powers and the performance of the NHS foundation trust.

Supporting principles

- The board of directors' role is to provide effective and proactive leadership of the NHS foundation trust within a framework of processes, procedures and controls which enable risk to be assessed and managed.
- The board of directors is responsible for ensuring compliance by the NHS foundation trust with its terms of authorisation, its constitution, mandatory guidance issued by Monitor, relevant statutory requirements and contractual obligations.
- The board of directors should set the NHS foundation trust's strategic aims at least annually, taking into consideration the views of the board of governors, ensuring that the necessary financial and human resources are in place for the NHS foundation trust to meet its main priorities and objectives and then periodically review progress and management performance.
- The board of directors as a whole is responsible for ensuring the quality and safety of healthcare services, education, training and research delivered by the NHS foundation trust and applying the principles and standards of clinical governance set out by the Department of Health, the Care Quality Commission, and other relevant NHS bodies.
- The board of directors should also ensure that the NHS foundation trust exercises its functions effectively, efficiently and economically.
- The board of directors should set the NHS foundation trust's vision, values and standards of conduct and ensure that its obligations to its members, patients and other stakeholders are understood, clearly communicated and met.
- All directors must take decisions objectively in the interests of the NHS foundation trust.
- All members of the board of directors have joint responsibility for every decision of the board regardless of their individual skills or status. This does not impact upon the particular responsibilities of the chief executive as the accounting officer. The chief executive should refer to the latest guidance from Monitor on the responsibilities and obligations of the accounting officer (NHS Foundation Trust Accounting Officer Memorandum, April 2008).
- The concept of the unitary board refers to the fact that within the board of directors the non-executive directors and the executive directors share the same liability. All directors, executive and non-executive, have responsibility to constructively challenge the decisions of the board and help develop proposals on priorities, risk mitigation, values, standards and strategy.

- As part of their role as members of a unitary board, non-executive directors have a particular duty to ensure appropriate challenge is made. Non-executive directors should scrutinise the performance of the executive management in meeting agreed goals and objectives, receive adequate information and monitor the reporting of performance. They should satisfy themselves as to the integrity of financial, clinical and other information, and that financial and clinical quality controls and systems of risk management and governance are robust and implemented. Non-executive directors are responsible for determining appropriate levels of remuneration of executive directors and have a prime role in appointing, and where necessary removing, executive directors, and in succession planning.

Code provisions

A.1.1 The board of directors should meet sufficiently regularly to discharge its duties effectively. There should be a formal schedule of matters specifically reserved for decision by the board of directors. The schedule of matters reserved for the board of directors should be complemented with a clear statement detailing the roles and responsibilities of the board of governors (as described in B.1.4). There should also be a statement explaining how any disagreements between the board of governors and the board of directors will be resolved. The annual report should include a statement of how the board of directors and the board of governors operate, including a high-level statement of which types of decisions are to be taken by each of the boards and which decisions are to be delegated to the executive management by the board of directors. The developmental nature of the board of governors' role would suggest that any agreements should be kept under review as the role evolves.

A.1.2 The annual report should identify the chairman, the deputy chairman (where there is one), the chief executive, the senior independent director (see A.3.3) and the chairmen and members of the nominations, audit and remuneration committees. A record should be kept of the number of meetings of the board of directors and the attendance of individual directors, and it should be supplied to the board of governors on request.

A.1.3 The chairman should hold meetings with the non-executive directors without the executives present. Led by the senior independent director, the non-executive directors should meet without the chairman at least annually to evaluate the chairman's performance, as part of a process which should be agreed with the board of governors, for appraising the chair and on such other occasions as are deemed appropriate.

A.1.4 The board of directors should make available a statement of the objectives of the NHS foundation trust showing how it intends to balance the interests of patients, the local community and other stakeholders, and use this as the basis for its decision making and forward planning.

A.1.5 The board of directors should ensure that adequate systems and processes are maintained to measure and monitor the NHS foundation trust's effectiveness, efficiency and economy as well as the quality of its healthcare delivery. The board should regularly review the performance of the NHS foundation trust in these areas against regulatory and contractual obligations and approved plans and objectives.

The board of directors should ensure that relevant metrics, measures, milestones and accountabilities are developed and agreed so as to understand and assess progress and delivery of performance. Where appropriate, and in particular in high risk or complex areas, independent advice should be commissioned by the board of directors to provide an adequate and reliable level of assurance.

A.1.6 The board of directors should report on its approach to clinical governance and its plan for the improvement of clinical quality in accordance with guidance set out by the Department of Health, the Care Quality Commission and Monitor.

A.1.7 Where the board or individual directors have concerns which remain unresolved, about the running of the NHS foundation trust or a proposed action, they should ensure that their concerns are recorded in the board minutes.

A.1.8 The chief executive, as the accounting officer, should follow the procedure set out by Monitor (NHS Foundation Trust Accounting Officer Memorandum, April 2008) for advising the board of directors and the board of governors, and for recording and submitting objections to decisions considered or taken by the boards in matters of propriety or regularity, and on issues relating to the wider responsibilities of the accounting officer for economy, efficiency and effectiveness.

A.1.9 The board of directors should establish the values and standards of conduct for the NHS foundation trust and its staff in accordance with NHS values and accepted standards of behaviour in public life, which include the principles of selflessness, integrity, objectivity, accountability, openness, honesty and leadership (The Nolan Principles).

A.1.10 The board of directors should operate a code of conduct that builds on the values of the NHS foundation trust and reflect high standards of probity and responsibility. The board of directors should follow a policy of openness and transparency in its proceedings and decision making unless this conflicts with a need to protect the wider interests of the public or the NHS foundation trust (including commercial-in-confidence matters) and make clear how potential conflicts of interest are dealt with.

A.1.11 The NHS foundation trust should arrange appropriate insurance to cover the risk of legal action against its directors.

A.2 Chairman and chief executive

Main principle

There should be a clear division of responsibilities at the head of the NHS foundation trust between the chairing of the boards of directors and governors and the executive responsibility for the running of the NHS foundation trust's business. No one individual should have unfettered powers of decision.

Supporting principles

- The chairman is responsible for leadership of the board of directors and the board of governors, ensuring their effectiveness on all aspects of their role and setting their agenda.
- The chairman is responsible for ensuring that the two boards work together effectively.
- The chairman is also responsible for ensuring that directors and governors receive accurate, timely and clear information that is appropriate for their respective duties.
- The chairman should ensure effective and open communication with patients, clients, members, staff and other stakeholders.
- The chairman should also facilitate the effective contribution of all executive and non-executive directors and ensure that constructive and productive relations exist between executive and non-executive directors, and between the board of directors and the board of governors.

Code provisions

A.2.1 The division of responsibilities between the chairman and chief executive should be clearly established, set out in writing and agreed by the board of directors.

A.2.2 The chairman should on appointment meet the independence criteria set out in A.3.1 below. A chief executive should not go on to be chairman of the same NHS foundation trust.

A.3 Balance and independence of the board of directors

Main principle

The board of directors should include a balance of executive and non-executive directors (and in particular independent non-executive directors) such that no individual or small group of individuals can dominate the board's decision taking. All directors should be able to exercise one full vote, with the chairman having a second casting vote on occasions where a decision is tied.

Supporting principles

- The board of directors should not be so large as to be unwieldy. The board of directors should be of sufficient size that the balance of skills and experience is appropriate for the requirements of the business and that changes to its composition can be managed without undue disruption.
- To ensure that power and information are not concentrated in one or two individuals, there should be a strong presence on the board of both executive and non-executive directors.
- The value of ensuring that committee membership is refreshed and that undue reliance is not placed on particular individuals should be taken into account in deciding chairmanship and membership of committees.
- Only the committee chairman and relevant members are entitled to be present at a meeting of the nominations, audit or remuneration committees, but others may attend by invitation of the relevant committee.

Code provisions

A.3.1 The board of directors should identify in the annual report each non-executive director it considers to be independent. The board should determine whether the director is independent in character and judgement and whether there are relationships or circumstances which are likely to affect, or could appear to affect, the director's judgement. The board of directors should state its reasons if it determines that a director is independent notwithstanding the existence of relationships or circumstances which may appear relevant to its determination, including if the director:

- has been an employee of the NHS foundation trust within the last five years;
- has, or has had within the last three years, a material business relationship with the NHS foundation trust either directly, or as a partner, shareholder, director or senior employee of a body that has such a relationship with the NHS foundation trust;
- has received or receives additional remuneration from the NHS foundation trust apart from a director's fee, participates in the NHS foundation trust's performance-related pay scheme, or is a member of the NHS foundation trust's pension scheme;
- has close family ties with any of the NHS foundation trust's advisers, directors or senior employees;
- holds cross-directorships or has significant links with other directors through involvement in other companies or bodies;
- has served on the board of the NHS foundation trust for more than six years from the date of their first appointment; or
- is an appointed representative of the NHS foundation trust's university medical or dental school.

A.3.2 At least half the board of directors, excluding the chairman, should comprise non-executive directors determined by the board to be independent.

A.3.3 The board of directors should appoint one of the independent non-executive directors to be the senior independent director, in consultation with the board of governors. The senior independent director should be available to members and governors if they have concerns which contact through the normal channels of chairman, chief executive or finance director has failed to resolve or for which such contact is inappropriate. The senior independent director could be the deputy chairman.

A.3.4 The board of directors should include in its annual report a description of each director's skills, expertise and experience. Alongside this in the annual report, the board should make a clear statement about its own balance, completeness and appropriateness to the requirements of the NHS foundation trust. Both statements should also be available on the NHS foundation trust's website.

A.3.5 No individual should hold, at the same time, positions of director and governor of NHS foundation trusts.

A.3.6 Non-executive directors should receive the necessary information and feel able to raise appropriate challenge of recommendations or decisions of the board, in particular making full use of their skills and experience gained both as a director of the trust and also in other leadership roles. They should expect and apply similar standards of care and quality in their role as a non-executive director of an NHS foundation trust as they would in other similar roles.

B GOVERNORS

Schedule 7 to the 2006 Act sets out the various powers of, and obligations upon, governors of NHS foundation trusts. The code does not provide prescriptive guidance on the extent and interpretation of these powers and obligations. However, Monitor has described in this section of the code those areas of the governor's role that are relevant and which NHS foundation trusts might find helpful. In addition, in October 2009, Monitor published a separate document which examines how governors can deliver their duties: *Your Statutory Duties: A Reference Guide for NHS Foundation Trust Governors*.

B.1 The board of governors

Main principle

Every NHS foundation trust will have a board of governors which is responsible for representing the interests of NHS foundation trust members and partner organisations in the local health economy in the governance of the NHS foundation trust. Governors must act in the best interests of the NHS foundation trust and should adhere to its values and code of conduct. The board of governors should hold the board of directors to account for the performance of the trust, including ensuring the board of directors acts so that the foundation trust does not breach the terms of its authorisation. It remains the responsibility of the board of directors to design and then implement agreed priorities, objectives and the overall strategy of the NHS foundation trust.

Governors are responsible for regularly feeding back information about the trust, its vision and its performance to the constituencies and the stakeholder organisations that either elected or appointed them.

Supporting principles

- Governors should discuss and agree with the board of directors how they will undertake these and any other additional roles, giving due consideration to the circumstances of the NHS foundation trust and the needs of the local community and emerging best practice.
- Governors should work closely with the board of directors and must be presented with, for consideration, the annual report and accounts and the annual plan at a general meeting. The governors can expect to be consulted on the development of forward plans for the trust and any significant changes to the delivery of the trust's business plan.

Code provisions

B.1.1 The board of governors should meet sufficiently regularly to discharge its duties. Typically the board of governors would be expected to meet as a full board at least four times per year. Governors should where practicable make every effort to attend the meetings of the board of governors. The NHS foundation trust should take appropriate steps to facilitate attendance.

B.1.2 The board of governors should not be so large as to be unwieldy. The board of governors should be of sufficient size for the requirements of its duties. The roles, structure, composition, and procedures of the board of governors should be reviewed regularly as described in provision D.2.2.

B.1.3 The annual report should identify the members of the board of governors, including a description of the constituency or organisation that they represent, whether they were elected or appointed, and the duration of their appointments. The annual report should also identify the nominated lead governor. A record should be kept of the number of meetings of the board and the attendance of individual governors and it should be made available to members on request.

B.1.4 The roles and responsibilities of the board of governors should be set out in a written document. This statement should include a clear explanation of the responsibilities of the board of governors towards members and other stakeholders and how governors will seek their views and inform them.

B.1.5 The board of governors should receive and consider other appropriate information required to enable it to discharge its duties, for example, clinical and operational data.

B.1.6 The chairman is responsible for leadership of both boards (see A.2) but the governors also have a responsibility to make the arrangements work and should take the lead in inviting the chief executive to their meetings and inviting attendance by other executives and non-executives as appropriate. In these meetings other members of the board of governors may raise questions of the chairman or his/her deputy or any other director present at the meeting about the affairs of the NHS foundation trust.

B.1.7 The board of governors should establish a policy for engagement with the board of directors for those circumstances when they have concerns about the performance of the board of directors, compliance with the terms of authorisation or other matters related to the general wellbeing of the NHS foundation trust. The board of governors should consider the advantages of there being a senior independent director on the board of directors (see A.3.3).

B.1.8 The board of governors should ensure its interaction and relationship with the board of directors is appropriate and effective, in particular, by agreeing the availability and timely communication of relevant information, discussion and the setting in advance of meeting agendas and use, where possible, of clear, unambiguous language.

B.1.9 Governors should acknowledge the overall responsibility of the board of directors for running the NHS foundation trust and should not use the powers of the board of governors to veto the decisions of the board of directors or otherwise obstruct the implementation of agreed actions and strategies. Through the nominated lead governor, the board of governors should communicate directly with Monitor if the NHS foundation trust is at risk of significantly breaching the terms of its authorisation and if these concerns cannot be satisfactorily resolved.

B.1.10 The board of governors should only exercise its power to remove the chairman or any non-executive directors after exhausting all other means of engagement with the board of directors.

C APPOINTMENT, RESIGNATION AND TERMS OF OFFICE

C.1 Appointment to the board of directors

Main principle

The 2006 Act sets out how appointments to the board of directors are made. There should be a formal, rigorous and transparent procedure for the appointment of directors.

Supporting principles

- Appointments to the board of directors should be made on merit and based on objective criteria.
- Care should be taken to ensure that new appointees have relevant skills and experience to complement other members of the board and enough time to devote to the job. This is particularly important in the case of chairmanships.
- The board of directors should also satisfy itself that plans are in place for orderly succession of appointments to the board so as to maintain an appropriate balance of skills and experience within the NHS foundation trust and on the board.

Code provisions

C.1.1 The nominations committee or committees, with external advice as appropriate, are responsible for the identification and nomination of executive and non-executive directors. The nominations committee should give full consideration to succession planning, taking into account the future challenges, risks and opportunities facing the NHS foundation trust and the skills and expertise required within the board of directors to meet them.

C.1.2 There may be one or two nominations committees. If there are two committees, one will be responsible for considering nominations for executive directors and the other for non-executive directors (including the chairman). The nominations committee(s) should regularly review the structure, size and composition of the board of directors and make recommendations for changes where appropriate. In particular, the nominations committee(s) should evaluate the balance of skills, knowledge and experience on the board of directors and, in the light of this evaluation, prepare a description of the role and capabilities required for appointment of both executive and non-executive directors, including the chairman.

C.1.3 The chairman or an independent non-executive director should chair the nominations committee(s).

C.1.4 The governors are responsible at a general meeting for the appointment, re-appointment and removal of the chairman and the other non-executive directors. They should agree with the nominations committee a clear process for the nomination of a new chair and non-executive directors. Once suitable candidates have been identified the nominations committee should make recommendations to the board of governors.

C.1.5 Where an NHS foundation trust has two nominations committees, the nominations committee responsible for the appointment of non-executive directors should consist of a majority of governors. If only one nominations committee exists, when nominations for non-executives, including the appointment of a chairman or a deputy chairman, are being discussed, there should be a majority of governors on the committee and also a majority governor representation on the interview panel.

C.1.6 When considering the appointment of non-executive directors, the board of governors should take into account the views of the board of directors on the qualifications, skills and experience required for each position.

C.1.7 For the appointment of a chairman, the nominations committee should prepare a job specification defining the role and capabilities required including an assessment of the time commitment expected, recognising the need for availability in the event of emergencies. A chairman's other significant commitments should be disclosed to the board of governors before appointment and included in the annual report. Changes to such commitments should be reported to the board of governors as they arise, and included in the next annual report. No individual, simultaneously while being a chairman of an NHS foundation trust, should be the substantive chairman of another NHS foundation trust.

C.1.8 The terms and conditions of appointment of non-executive directors should be made available for inspection. The letter of appointment should set out the expected time commitment. Non-executive directors should undertake that they will have sufficient time to meet what is expected of them. Their other significant commitments should be disclosed to the board of governors before appointment, with a broad indication of the time involved and the board of governors should be informed of subsequent changes.

C.1.9 The annual report should describe the process followed by the board of governors in relation to appointments of the chairman and non-executive directors.

C.1.10 It is a requirement of the 2006 Act that the chairman, the other non-executive directors and – except in the case of the appointment of a chief executive – the chief executive, are responsible for deciding the appointment of executive directors. The nominations committee with responsibility for executive director nominations should identify suitable candidates to fill executive director vacancies as they arise and make recommendations to the chairman, the other non-executives directors and, except in the case of the appointment of a chief executive, the chief executive.

C.1.11 It is for the non-executive directors to appoint and remove the chief executive. The appointment of a chief executive requires the approval of the board of governors.

C.1.12 An independent external adviser should not be a member of or have a vote on the nominations committee(s).

C.1.13 The board of directors should not agree to a full-time executive director taking on more than one non-executive directorship of an NHS foundation trust or another organisation of comparable size and complexity, nor the chairmanship of such an organisation.

C.1.14 A separate section of the annual report should describe the work of the nominations committee(s), including the process it has used in relation to board appointments.

C.2 Re-appointment of directors and re-election of governors

Main principle

All non-executive directors and elected governors should be submitted for re-appointment or re-election at regular intervals. The performance of executive directors of the board should be subject to regular appraisal and review. The board of directors should ensure planned and progressive refreshing of the board.

Code provisions

C.2.1 Approval by the board of governors of the appointment of a chief executive should be a subject of the first general meeting after the appointment by a committee of the chairman and non-executive directors. All other executive directors should be appointed by a committee of the chief executive, the chairman and non-executive directors.

C.2.2 Non-executive directors, including the chairman, should be appointed by the board of governors for specified terms subject to re-appointment thereafter at intervals of no more than three years and to the 2006 Act provisions relating to the removal of a director. The chairman should confirm to the governors that, following formal performance evaluation, the performance of the individual proposed for re-appointment continues to be effective and to demonstrate commitment to the role. Any term beyond six years (e.g. two three-year terms) for a non-executive director should be subject to particularly rigorous review, and should take into account the need for progressive refreshing of the board. Non-executive directors may in exceptional circumstances serve longer than six years (e.g. two three-year terms following authorisation of the NHS foundation trust), but subject to annual re-appointment. Serving more than six years could be relevant to the determination of a non-executive director's independence (as set out in provision A.3.1).

C.2.3 Elected governors must be subject to re-election by the members of their constituency at regular intervals not exceeding three years. The names of governors submitted for election or re-election should be accompanied by sufficient biographical details and any other relevant information to enable members to take an informed decision on their election. This should include prior performance information such as attendance records at governor meetings and other relevant events organised by the NHS foundation trust for governors.

C.3 Resignation of directors

Main principle

The board of directors is responsible for ensuring ongoing compliance by the NHS foundation trust with its terms of authorisation, its constitution, mandatory guidance issued by Monitor, relevant statutory requirements and contractual obligations. In so doing, it should ensure it retains the necessary skills within its board of directors, and puts in place appropriate succession planning.

Code provision

C.3.1 The board of directors should not agree to an executive member of the board leaving the employment of an NHS foundation trust, except in accordance with the terms of their contract of employment, including but not limited to service of their full notice period and/ or material reductions in their time commitment to the role, without the board first having completed and approved a full risk assessment.

D INFORMATION, DEVELOPMENT AND EVALUATION

D.1 Information and professional development

Main principle

The board of directors and the board of governors should be supplied in a timely manner with relevant information in a form and of a quality appropriate to enable them to discharge their respective duties.

All directors and governors should receive appropriate induction on joining their respective boards and should regularly update and refresh their skills and knowledge.

Supporting principles

- The chairman is responsible for ensuring that the directors and governors receive accurate, timely and clear information. Management has an obligation to provide such information but directors and governors should seek clarification or amplification where necessary.
- The chairman should ensure that the directors and governors continually update their skills, knowledge and familiarity with the NHS foundation trust and its obligations, to fulfil their role both on their respective boards and on board committees. The NHS foundation trust should provide the necessary resources for developing and updating its directors' and governors' knowledge and capabilities.
- The responsibilities of the chairman include ensuring good information flows in the boards and their committees, between directors and governors, and between senior management and non-executive directors, as well as facilitating appropriate induction and assisting with professional development as required.

Code provisions

D.1.1 The chairman should ensure that new directors and governors receive a full, formal and appropriate induction on joining their respective boards.

D.1.2 The board should ensure that directors, especially non-executive directors, have access to independent professional advice, at the NHS foundation trust's expense, where they judge it necessary to discharge their responsibilities as directors. Directors should also have access, at the NHS foundation trust's expense, to training courses and/or materials that are consistent with their individual and collective development programme as described in provision D.2. Decisions to appoint an external adviser should be the collective decision of the majority of non-executive directors. The availability of independent external sources of advice should be made clear at the time of appointment. Committees should be provided with sufficient resources to undertake their duties. The board of directors should also ensure that the board of governors is provided with sufficient resources to undertake its duties, with such arrangements agreed in advance.

D.1.3 The board of directors and the board of governors should be provided with high quality information appropriate to the respective functions of the boards and relevant to the decisions they have to make. The board of directors and the board of governors should agree their respective information needs with the executive directors. The information for the boards should be concise, objective, accurate and timely, and it should be accompanied by clear explanations of complex issues. The board of directors should have complete access to any information about the NHS foundation trust that it deems necessary to discharge its duties, including access to senior management and other employees.

D.1.4 The board of directors, and in particular non-executive directors, may reasonably wish to challenge assurances received from the executive management. They need not seek to appoint a relevant adviser for each and every subject area that comes before the board of directors, although they should wherever possible ensure that they have sufficient information and understanding to take decisions on an informed basis. When complex or high risk issues arise the first course of action should normally be to encourage further and deeper analysis to be carried out, in a timely manner, within the NHS foundation trust. On occasion, non-executives may reasonably decide that external assurance is appropriate.

D.1.5 Governors should canvass the opinion of their members, and for appointed governors the body they represent, on the NHS foundation trust's forward plan, including its objectives, priorities and strategy, and their views should be communicated to the board of directors.

D.1.6 The board of directors should consider and take account of the views of the board of governors on the NHS foundation trust's forward plan. Where appropriate, the board of directors should communicate to the board of governors where their views have been incorporated in the NHS foundation trust's plans, and, if not, the reasons for this.

D.2 Performance evaluation

Main principles

The board of directors should undertake a formal and rigorous annual evaluation of its own performance and that of its committees and individual directors. The board of directors should state in the annual report how performance evaluation of the board, its committees and its individual directors including the chairman, has been conducted, bearing in mind the desirability for independent assessment, and the reason why the NHS foundation trust adopted a particular method of performance evaluation. The outcomes of the evaluation of the executive directors should be reported to the board of directors. The chief executive should take the lead on the evaluation of the executive directors. The board of governors, which is responsible for the appointment and re-appointment of non-executive directors, should take the lead on agreeing a process for the evaluation of the chairman and the non-executives, with the chairman and the non-executives. The outcomes of the evaluation of the chairman and the non-executive directors should be agreed by the governors. The governors should bear in mind the desirability of using the senior independent director to lead the non-executive directors in an evaluation of the chairman.

The board of governors should assess its own collective performance and its impact in the NHS foundation trust.

Supporting principles

- Individual evaluation of directors should aim to show whether each director continues to contribute effectively, to demonstrate commitment and has the relevant skills for the role (including commitment of time for board and committee meetings and any other duties) going forwards. The chairman should act on the results of the performance evaluation by recognising the strengths and addressing the weaknesses of the board, identifying individual and collective development needs and, where appropriate, proposing new members be appointed to the board or seeking the resignation of directors.
- The focus of the chairman's appraisal will be his/her performance as leader of the board of directors. The appraisal should carefully consider that performance against pre-defined objectives that support the design and delivery of the NHS foundation trust's priorities and strategy described in its forward plan.

Code provisions

D.2.1 The chairman, with the assistance of the secretary of the boards if applicable, should use the performance evaluations as the basis for determining individual and collective professional development programmes for directors relevant to their duties as board members.

D.2.2 Led by the chairman, the board of governors should periodically assess their collective performance and they should regularly communicate to members details on how they have discharged their responsibilities, including their impact and effectiveness on:

- contributing to the development of forward plans of the NHS foundation trust; and
- communicating with their member constituencies and transmitting their views to the board of directors.

The board of governors should use this process to review its roles, structure, composition and procedures, taking into account emerging best practice. Further information can be found in Monitor's publication: Your Statutory Duties: A Reference Guide for NHS Foundation Trust Governors.

D.2.3 There should be a clear policy and a fair process for the removal from the board of any governor who consistently and unjustifiably fails to attend the meetings of the board of governors or has an actual or potential conflict of interest which prevents the proper exercise of their duties. In addition removal from the board of governors may be appropriate where behaviours or actions by a governor or group of governors may be incompatible with the values and behaviours of the NHS foundation trust. Where there is any disagreement as to whether the proposal for removal is justified, an independent assessor agreeable to both parties should be requested to consider the evidence and conclude whether the proposed removal is reasonable or otherwise.

E DIRECTOR REMUNERATION

E.1 The level and make-up of remuneration

Main principle

Levels of remuneration should be sufficient to attract, retain and motivate directors of the quality and with the skills and experience required to lead the NHS foundation trust successfully, but an NHS foundation trust should avoid paying more than is necessary for this purpose.

Supporting principles

- The remuneration committee should decide if a proportion of executive directors' remuneration should be structured so as to link reward to corporate and individual performance. The remuneration committee should judge where to position its NHS foundation trust relative to other NHS foundation trusts and comparable organisations. Such comparisons, however, should be used with caution to avoid any risk of an increase in remuneration levels with no corresponding improvement in performance.
- The remuneration committee should also be sensitive to pay and employment conditions elsewhere in the NHS foundation trust, especially when determining annual salary increases.

Code provisions

Remuneration policy

E.1.1 Any performance-related elements of the remuneration of executive directors should be designed to align their interests with those of patients, service users and taxpayers and to give these directors keen incentives to perform at the highest levels. In designing schemes of performance-related remuneration, the remuneration committee should follow the following provisions:

(i) The remuneration committee should consider whether the directors should be eligible for annual bonuses. If so, performance conditions should be relevant, stretching and designed to match the long term interests of the public and patients.
(ii) Payouts or grants under all incentive schemes should be subject to challenging performance criteria reflecting the objectives of the NHS foundation trust. Consideration should be given to criteria which reflect the performance of the NHS foundation trust relative to a group of comparator trusts in some key indicators, and the taking of independent and expert advice where appropriate.
(iii) Performance criteria and any upper limits for annual bonuses and incentive schemes should be set and disclosed.
(iv) The remuneration committee should consider the pension consequences and associated costs to the NHS foundation trust of basic salary increases and any other changes in pensionable remuneration, especially for directors close to retirement. In general, only basic salary should be pensionable.

E.1.2 Levels of remuneration for the chairman and other non-executive directors should reflect the time commitment and responsibilities of their roles.

E.1.3 Where an NHS foundation trust releases an executive director, for example to serve as a non-executive director elsewhere, the remuneration disclosures of the annual report should include a statement on whether or not the director will retain such earnings.

Service contracts and compensation

E.1.4 The remuneration committee should carefully consider what compensation commitments (including pension contributions and all other elements) their directors' terms of appointment would give rise to in the event of early termination. The aim should be to avoid rewarding poor performance. In an early termination, compensation should be reduced to reflect a departing director's obligation to mitigate loss.

E.2 Procedure

Main principle

There should be a formal and transparent procedure for developing policy on executive remuneration and for fixing the remuneration packages of individual directors. No director should be involved in deciding his or her own remuneration.

Supporting principles

- The remuneration committee should consult the chairman and/or chief executive about its proposals relating to the remuneration of other executive directors.
- The remuneration committee should also be responsible for appointing any independent consultants in respect of executive director remuneration.
- Where executive directors or senior management are involved in advising or supporting the remuneration committee, care should be taken to recognise and avoid conflicts of interest.

Code provisions

E.2.1 The board of directors must establish a remuneration committee composed of non-executive directors which should include at least three independent non-executive directors. The remuneration committee should make available its terms of reference, explaining its role and the authority delegated to it by the board of directors. Where remuneration consultants are appointed, a statement should be made available of whether they have any other connection with the NHS foundation trust.

E.2.2 The remuneration committee should have delegated responsibility for setting remuneration for all executive directors, including pension rights and any compensation payments. The committee should also recommend and monitor the level and structure of remuneration for senior management. The definition of senior management for this purpose should be determined by the board but should normally include the first layer of management below board level.

E.2.3 The board of governors is responsible for setting the remuneration of non-executive directors and the chairman. The board of governors should consult external professional advisers to market-test the remuneration levels of the chairman and other non-executives at least once every three years and when they intend to make a material change to the remuneration of a non-executive.

F ACCOUNTABILITY AND AUDIT

F.1 Financial, quality and operational reporting

Main principle

The board of directors should present a balanced and understandable assessment of the NHS foundation trust's position and prospects.

Supporting principle

The responsibility of the board of directors to present a balanced and understandable assessment extends to all public statements and reports to regulators and inspectors, as well as information required to be presented by statutory requirements.

Code provisions

F.1.1 The directors should explain in the annual report their responsibility for preparing the accounts and there should be a statement by the external auditors about their reporting responsibilities.

F.1.2 The directors should report that the NHS foundation trust is a going concern, with supporting assumptions or qualifications as necessary.

F.1.3 (a) The board of directors must notify Monitor and the board of governors without delay, and should consider whether it is in the public interest to bring to the public attention, any major new developments in the NHS foundation trust's sphere of activity which are not public knowledge which may lead, by virtue of their effect on its assets and liabilities or financial position or on the general course of its business, to a substantial change to the financial wellbeing, healthcare delivery performance or reputation and standing of the NHS foundation trust.

(b) The board of directors must notify Monitor and the board of governors without delay and should consider whether it is in the public interest to bring to public attention all relevant information which is not public knowledge concerning a material change:

- in the NHS foundation trust's financial condition;
- in the performance of its business; and/or
- in the NHS foundation trust's expectations as to its performance which, if made public, would be likely to lead to a substantial change to the financial wellbeing, healthcare delivery performance or reputation and standing of the NHS foundation trust.

F.1.4 At least annually, the board of directors should set out clearly its financial, quality and operating objectives for the NHS foundation trust and disclose sufficient information, both quantitative and qualitative, of the NHS foundation trust's business and operations, including clinical outcome data, to allow members and governors to evaluate its performance. Further requirements are included in the NHS Foundation Trust Annual Reporting Manual (previously the NHS Foundation Trust Financial Reporting Manual).

F.2 Internal control

Main principle

The board of directors should maintain a sound system of internal control to safeguard public and private investment, the NHS foundation trust's assets, patient safety and service quality.

Code provision

F.2.1 The board should conduct, at least annually, a review of the effectiveness of the NHS foundation trust's system of internal control and should report to members that they have done so. The review should cover all material controls, including financial, clinical, operational and compliance controls and risk management systems.

F.3 Audit committee and auditors

Main principle

The board should establish formal and transparent arrangements for considering how it should apply the financial reporting and internal control principles and for maintaining an appropriate relationship with the NHS foundation trust's auditors.

Monitor's publications, *Audit Code for NHS Foundation Trusts, Your Statutory Duties: A Reference Guide for NHS Foundation Trust Governors*, and *Guide for Governors: Audit Code for NHS Foundation Trusts* provide further guidance.

Code provisions

F.3.1 The board must establish an audit committee composed of non-executive directors which should include at least three independent non-executive directors. The board should satisfy itself that at least one member of the audit committee has recent and relevant financial experience.

F.3.2 The main role and responsibilities of the audit committee should be set out in written terms of reference and should include details of how it will:

- monitor the integrity of the financial statements of the NHS foundation trust, and any formal announcements relating to the trust's financial performance, reviewing significant financial reporting judgements contained in them;
- review the NHS foundation trust's internal financial controls and, unless expressly addressed by a separate board risk committee composed of independent directors, or by the board itself, review the trust's internal control and risk management systems;
- monitor and review the effectiveness of the NHS foundation trust's internal audit function;
- review and monitor the external auditor's independence and objectivity and the effectiveness of the audit process, taking into consideration relevant UK professional and regulatory requirements;
- develop and implement policy on the engagement of the external auditor to supply non-audit services, taking into account relevant ethical guidance regarding the provision of non-audit services by the external audit firm; and
- report to the board of governors, identifying any matters in respect of which it considers that action or improvement is needed and making recommendations as to the steps to be taken.

F.3.3 The terms of reference of the audit committee, including its role and the authority delegated to it by the board of directors and by the board of governors, should be made publicly available. A separate section of the annual report should describe the work of the committee in discharging those responsibilities.

F.3.4 The board of governors should take the lead in agreeing with the audit committee the criteria for appointing, reappointing and removing external auditors.

F.3.5 The audit committee should make a report to the board of governors in relation to the performance of the external auditor, including detail such as the quality and value of the work, and the timeliness of reporting and fees, to enable the board of governors to consider whether or not to reappoint them. The audit committee should also make recommendations to the board of governors in relation to the appointment, re-appointment and removal of the external auditor and approve the remuneration and terms of engagement of the external auditor.

If the board of governors does not accept the audit committee's recommendation, the board of directors should include in the annual report a statement from the audit committee explaining the recommendation and should set out reasons why the board of governors has taken a different position.

F.3.6 The NHS foundation trust should appoint an external auditor for a period of time which allows the auditor to develop a strong understanding of the finances, operations and forward plans of the NHS foundation trust. The current best practice is for a three to five year period of appointment.

F.3.7 When the board of governors ends an external auditor's appointment in disputed circumstances, the chairman should write to Monitor informing it of the reasons behind the decision.

F.3.8 The annual report should explain to members how, if the external auditor provides non-audit services, auditor objectivity and independence is safeguarded.

F.3.9 The audit committee should review arrangements by which staff of the NHS foundation trust may raise, in confidence, concerns about possible improprieties in matters of financial reporting and control, clinical quality, patient safety or other matters. The audit committee's objective should be to ensure that arrangements are in place for the proportionate and independent investigation of such matters and for appropriate follow-up action.

G RELATIONSHIPS WITH STAKEHOLDERS

G.1 Dialogue with members, patients and the local community

Main principle

The board of directors should appropriately consult and involve members, patients and the local community. Notwithstanding the complementary role of the governors in this consultation, the board of directors as a whole has responsibility for ensuring that regular and open dialogue with its stakeholders takes place.

Supporting principles

- The board of directors should keep in touch with the opinion of members, patients and the local community in whatever ways are most practical and efficient. There should be a members' meeting at least annually.
- The chairman (and the senior independent director and other directors as appropriate) should maintain regular contact with governors to understand their issues and concerns.

Code provisions

G.1.1 The board of directors should make available a public document that sets out its policy on the involvement of members, patients and the local community at large, including a description of the kind of issues it will consult on.

G.1.2 The board of directors should clarify in writing how the public interests of patients and the local community will be represented, including its approach for addressing the overlap and interface between governors and any local consultative forums already in place (e.g. Local Involvement Networks, the Overview and Scrutiny Committee, the local League of Friends, and staff groups).

G.1.3 The chairman should ensure that the views of governors and members are communicated to the board as a whole. The chairman should discuss the affairs of the NHS foundation trust with governors. Non-executive directors should be offered the opportunity to attend meetings with governors and should expect to attend them if requested by governors. The senior independent director should attend sufficient meetings with governors to listen to their views in order to help develop a balanced understanding of the issues and concerns of governors.

G.1.4 The board of directors should ensure that the NHS foundation trust provides effective mechanisms for communication between governors and members from its constituencies. Contact procedures for members who wish to communicate with governors and/or directors should be made clearly available to members on the NHS foundation trust's website and in the annual report.

G.1.5 The board of directors should state in the annual report the steps they have taken to ensure that the members of the board, and in particular the non-executive directors, develop an understanding of the views of governors and members about the NHS foundation trust, for example through attendance at meetings of the board of governors, direct face-to-face contact, surveys of member opinion and consultations.

G.1.6 The board of directors should monitor how representative the NHS foundation trust's membership is and the level and effectiveness of member engagement. This information should be used to review the trust's membership strategy, taking into account any emerging best practice from the sector.

G.2 Co-operation with third parties with roles in relation to NHS foundation trusts

Main principle

The board of directors is responsible for ensuring that the NHS foundation trust co-operates with other NHS bodies, local authorities and other relevant organisations with an interest in the local health economy.

Supporting principle

The board of directors should enter a dialogue at an appropriate level with a range of third party stakeholders and other interested organisations with roles in relation to NHS foundation trusts based on the mutual understanding of objectives.

Code provisions

G.2.1 The board of directors should maintain a schedule of the specific third party bodies in relation to which the NHS foundation trust has a duty to co-operate (refer to Monitor's Compliance Framework for a generic non-exhaustive list of third party bodies). The board of directors should be clear of the form and scope of the co-operation required with each of these third party bodies in order to discharge their statutory duties.

G.2.2 The board of directors should ensure that effective mechanisms are in place to cooperate with relevant third party bodies and that collaborative and productive relationships are maintained with relevant stakeholders at appropriate levels of seniority in each. Periodically, the board of directors should review the effectiveness of these processes and relationships and, where necessary, take proactive steps to improve them.

APPENDIX 3

The Healthy NHS Board

Principles for good governance

**National Leadership Council,
February 2010**

1 INTRODUCTION

This chapter explains the purpose of this Principles guidance and provides a visual summary to help readers navigate through the document. It also describes the online resources that accompany it.

Purpose of this guidance

1 This document sets out the guiding principles that will allow NHS board members to understand the:

- Collective role of the board.
- Governance role within the wider health system.
- Activities and approaches that are most likely to improve board effectiveness.
- Contribution expected of them as individual board members.

2 It is hoped that NHS board members will find this guidance valuable and will focus effort in ways that the evidence suggests should be most productive.

3 This guidance is intended for boards of all NHS organisations. Some interpretation will be required for organisations operating at a national or regional level.

4 This guidance will also be of interest to those aspiring to be NHS board members, to governors of Foundation Trusts and to those who support and work with NHS boards.

How to use the document

5 This document describes the enduring principles of high quality governance, which transcend immediate policy imperatives and the more pressing features of the current health care environment.

6 Alongside this statement of principles, a regularly updated digital compendium sets the principles in the context of the current policy and organisational landscape. It describes recent developments and offers up to date case studies with examples to help board members put the principles into practice. The compendium is accessible at http://www.nhsleadership.org.uk/boarddevelopment.

7 The material in the compendium is complemented by a range of practical resources to support board effectiveness. These resources are available for download. Regular contributions of new tools, approaches, case studies and good practice from the service will be actively sought to ensure that this collection of resources remains current and relevant. This is represented in Figure 1. If you find a resource that merits inclusion please send a copy or a link to board development@nhsleadership.org.uk.

8 This document can be used by board members as an introduction to the subject of governance in the NHS. Since it is designed to be enduring, it can be kept as a reference – a first place to turn – in the future. The compendium should be consulted when more detail is needed on specific issues, or to understand details of underlying guidance and references.

9 The development of this guide and its accompanying resources was underpinned by a comprehensive review of governance literature and an extensive process of engagement with the NHS. In all, some 1,000 NHS staff and board members took part in this consultation, and the shape and content of the guide reflect their contributions. In addition, the literature review, entitled 'The Healthy NHS Board: a review of guidance and research evidence', considered over 140 sources; it is available for download at http://www.nhsleadership.org.uk/boarddevelopment.

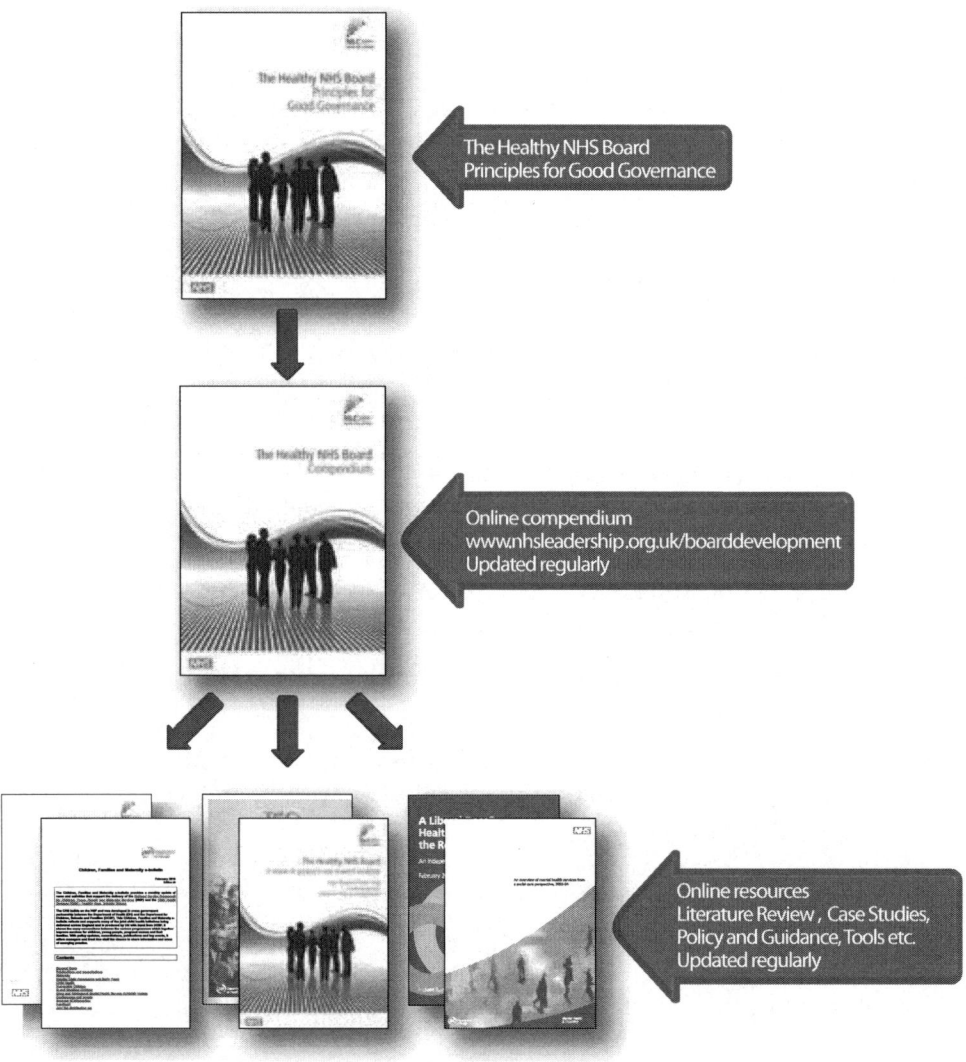

FIGURE 1 Structure of this guidance

2 PURPOSE AND ROLE OF NHS BOARDS

The purpose and role of NHS boards is set out in this chapter, helping board members to navigate through the wide range of guidance available.

10   The purpose of NHS boards is to govern effectively and in doing so to build public and stakeholder confidence that their health and healthcare is in safe hands. This fundamental accountability to the public and stakeholders is delivered by building confidence:

- In the quality and safety of health services.
- That resources are invested in a way that delivers optimal health outcomes.
- In the accessibility and responsiveness of health services.
- That the public can appropriately shape health services to meet their needs.

11   There are a range of models of governance in use in both the public and private sectors, a number of which are summarised in Appendix 1.

12   This guide aims to provide board members with an overarching and durable framework that will allow them to make sense, and effective use, of the wide range of available advice and guidance both in the United Kingdom and internationally. It draws on established good practice in governance and a wide-ranging review of more recent literature, from all sectors.

13   The role of NHS boards is described below and is illustrated in Figure 2.

> 14   Effective NHS boards demonstrate leadership by undertaking three key roles:
>
> - Formulating strategy for the organisation.
> - Ensuring accountability by holding the organisation to account for the delivery of the strategy and through seeking assurance that systems of control are robust and reliable.
> - Shaping a positive culture for the board and the organisation.

Underpinning these three roles are three building blocks that allow boards to exercise their role. Effective boards:

- Are informed by the external context within which they must operate.
- Are informed by, and shape, the intelligence which provides trend and comparative information on how the organisation is performing together with an understanding of local people's needs, market and stakeholder analyses.
- Give priority to engagement with key stakeholders and opinion formers within and beyond the organisation; the emphasis here is on building a healthy dialogue with, and being accountable to, patients, the public, and staff, including clinicians.

15   The three roles of the board and the three building blocks all interconnect and influence one another. This is shown in Figure 2.

16   The roles and building blocks shown in Figure 2 are examined in more detail in the next sections.

> *"The board's role is to articulate the ambition for the organisation and to manage the risk that that ambition contains."*
>
> SHA chair

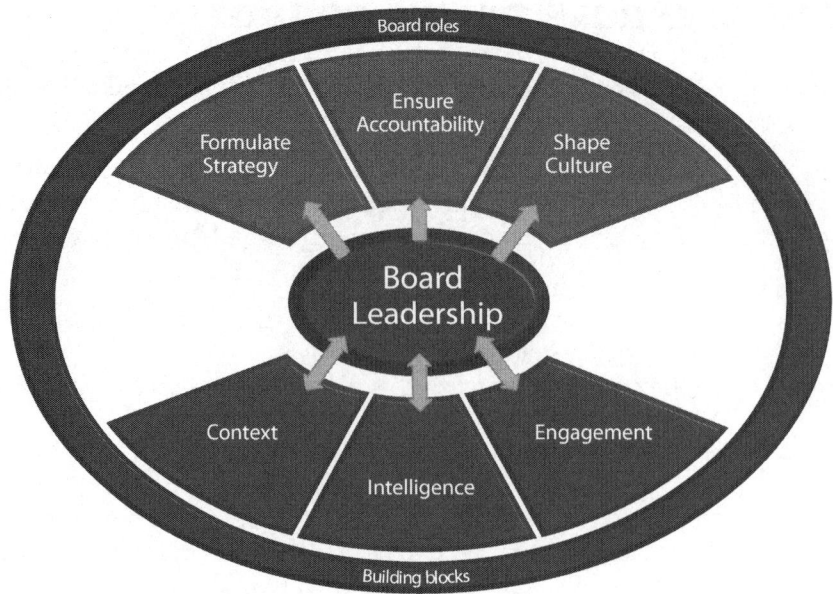

FIGURE 2 Roles and building blocks of NHS boards

Roles of the board

Formulate strategy

17 The first of the three roles of the board is formulating strategy. There are three main elements to consider:

- The process of developing strategy.
- The hallmarks of an effective strategy.
- The approach to strategic decision-making.

> *"Some of the processes that build towards strategic options or hypotheses will not directly engage the whole board – what matters is that there is an open and engaged process by which the board tests the emerging hypotheses."*
>
> PCT chair

> *"In our organization there are two key tests that we apply to all the decisions that we make – Would you spend your own money this way and would you wish to use this service? In this way we ensure that we have the taxpayer on one shoulder and the patient on the other."*
>
> PCT chief executive

18 In general, an effective strategic process:

- Ensures that the strategy is demonstrably shaped and owned by the board.
- Provides for the active involvement of and influence by clinicians and staff.
- Ensures that there have been open, transparent, accountable consultation and involvement processes with patients, the community, members, governors (in the case of Foundation Trusts) and key institutional stakeholders.
- Is underpinned by regular strategic discourse in the board, throughout the year. Strategy needs to be dynamic in responding to changes in the external environment.

19 Some of the hallmarks of an effective strategy include:

- A compelling vision for the future underpinned with clear strategic objectives that are reflected in an explicit statement of desired outcomes and key performance indicators.
- An organisational vision that puts quality and patient safety at its heart
- A clear statement of the organisation's purpose.

- An approach that takes appropriate account of the external context in which the organisation is operating.
- A perspective which balances the priority given to national and local performance indicators and targets.
- Evidence that the strategy has been shaped by the 'intelligence' made available to the board.
- A longer term view (with at least a 3 to 5 year planning horizon)
- A long term financial model and risk analysis.
- A long term workforce model that sets out the organisational arrangements required to deliver the strategy and identifies the workforce implications of strategic choices.
- Demonstrable links to the needs of users, patients and communities.
- An integrated approach to prevention and health promotion.
- Inclusion at its heart so that services that are commissioned or delivered produce accessible, fair and b equitable services and outcomes for all sections of the population served.
- Commitment to treating patients, service users and staff with equity
- Explicit attention paid to the ability to implement the strategy successfully.

20 Strategic decision-making is an integral part of the board's role in formulating strategy. Good practice here includes:

- Strategic decisions which are aligned to overall strategic direction, and are expressly identified as such.
- A formal statement that specifies the types of strategic decisions, including levels of investment and those representing significant service changes that are expressly reserved for the board, and those that are delegated to committees or the executive.
- Early involvement of board members in debating and shaping strategic decisions and appropriate consultation with internal and external stakeholders.
- For significant strategic decisions: consideration by the board of options and analyses of those options.
- Criteria and rationale for decision making that are transparent, objective and evidence based.

Ensure accountability

21 The second core role of NHS boards is ensuring accountability. This has two main aspects:

- Holding the organisation to account for the delivery of the strategy.
- Seeking assurance that the systems of control are robust and reliable.

Holding the organisation to account for its performance in the delivery of strategy

22 This aspect is at the heart of the board's role in pursuing high performance for its organisation. It is important that boards are not too readily assured or reassured. Where issues arise they need to be addressed – swiftly, decisively and knowledgeably – by the whole corporate board. A robust but fair approach is important, particularly where there are problems of underperformance. Effective boards recognize that 'the buck stops with the board'.

23 The Audit Commission reviewed how boards of NHS Trusts and Foundation Trusts get their assurance and developed a checklist against which boards can assess the reliability of their systems of control.[1] A key observation in this review is 'there has been no lack of guidance ... the challenge for boards is therefore not finding out what to do, but instead translating the theory into an approach that works in their trust and then following through with appropriate rigour'.

24 The fundamentals for the board in holding the organisation to account for performance include:

- Drawing on board 'intelligence' – the board monitors the performance of the organisation in an effective way and satisfies itself that appropriate action is taken to remedy problems as they arise.
- Looking beyond written intelligence to develop an understanding of the daily reality for patients and staff, to make data more meaningful.

- Seeking assurance where remedial action has been required to address performance concerns.
- Offering appreciation and encouragement where performance is excellent.
- Taking account of independent scrutiny of performance, including from governors (for Foundation Trusts), regulators and overview and scrutiny committees.
- Rigorous but constructive challenge from all board members, executive and non-executive as corporate board members.

"It is important not to mistake reassurance for assurance."

NHS chair

"Good corporate governance overall depends critically on the abilities and experience of individuals and the effectiveness of their collaboration in the enterprise. Despite the need for hard rules in some areas, this will not be assured by overly-specific prescription that generates box-ticking conformity."

David Walker Review[2]

"Processes without intelligent and rigorous scrutiny are not enough. Governance arrangements that are persuasive on paper must work in practice. The aim of board assurance is to give confidence that the trust is providing (or commissioning) high quality care, in a safe environment for patients by staff who have received appropriate training; that it is complying with legal and regulatory requirements and that it is meeting its strategic objectives."

Taking it on Trust

Seeking assurance that the systems of control are robust and reliable

25 This second aspect of accountability has seven elements:

- Quality assurance and clinical governance
- Financial Stewardship
- Risk Management
- Legality
- Decision-making
- Probity
- Corporate Trustee.

Quality assurance and clinical governance

26 The board has a key role in safeguarding quality, and therefore needs to give appropriate scrutiny to the three key facets of quality – effectiveness, patient safety and patient experience. Effective scrutiny relies primarily on the provision of clear, comprehensible summary information to the board, set out for everyone to see, for example, in the form of quality accounts.

> A recent US study reported that boards of 'high performing' healthcare organisations are significantly more likely to receive and use a quality dashboard.[3]

27 The board has a statutory duty of quality.[4] In support of this, good practice suggests that:

- All board members need to understand their ultimate accountability for quality.
- There is a clear organisational structure that clarifies responsibility for delivering quality performance from the board to the point of care and back to the board.
- Quality is a core part of main board meetings both as a standing agenda item and as an integrated element of all major discussions and decisions.
- Quality performance is discussed in more detail regularly by a quality committee with a stable, regularly attending membership.
- The board becomes a driving force for continuous quality improvement across the full range of services.

28 Boards are also required to endorse and sign off declarations of assurance to regulators in relation to quality, and comply with the registration requirements of the quality regulator.

29 But ensuring accountability in relation to quality is facilitated by more than regular scrutiny of information on quality – however exemplary. Research suggests that governance of quality can be improved if board members periodically step outside of the boardroom to gain first-hand knowledge of the staff and patient experience. It is also important to ensure that clinical leaders are properly empowered to lead on issues relating to clinical quality. Boards benefit from regular opportunities both to take advice from clinical leaders and to reflect on innovative practice in relation to quality improvement.

Financial stewardship

30 The exercise of effective financial stewardship requires that the board assures itself that the organisation is operating effectively, efficiently, economically and with probity in the use of resources. The board has a statutory duty to balance the books[5]. It is also required to ensure that financial reporting and internal control principles are applied, and appropriate relationships with the Trust's internal and external auditors are maintained.

Risk management

31 The role of the board in risk management is twofold:

- First, within the board itself an informed consideration of risk should underpin organisational strategy, decision-making and the allocation of resources.
- Second, the board is responsible for ensuring that the organisation has appropriate risk management processes in place to deliver the annual plan/commissioning plan and comply with the registration requirements of the quality regulator. This includes systematically assessing and managing its risks. These include financial, corporate and clinical risks. For Foundation Trusts, this also includes risks to compliance with the terms of authorisation.

32 Risk management by the board is underpinned by four interlocking systems of control:

- The Board Assurance Framework: This is a document that sets out strategic objectives, identifies risks in relation to each strategic objective along with controls in place and assurances available on their operation. The most effective boards use this as a dynamic tool to drive the board agenda. Formats vary but the framework generally includes:
    - Objective
    - Principal risk
    - Key controls
    - Sources of assurance
    - Gaps in control/assurance
    - Action plans for addressing gaps.
    - Organisational Risk Management: Strategic risks are reflected in the Board Assurance Framework. A more detailed operational risk register will be in use within the organisation.

The board needs to be assured that an effective risk management approach is in operation within the organisation. This involves both the design of appropriate processes and ensuring that they are properly embedded into the operations and culture of the organisation.

- Audit: External and internal auditors play an important role in board assurance on internal controls. There needs to be a clear line of sight from the Board Assurance Framework to the programme of internal audit. While clinical audit is primarily a management tool, the advice in 'Taking it on Trust' suggests that 'it would be reasonable to expect it to appear (in the Board Assurance Framework) as a significant source of assurance'.
- The statement on internal control: This is signed by the chief executive as Accountable Officer and comprehensively sets out the overall organisational approach to internal control. It should be scrutinised by the board to ensure that the assertions within it are supported by a robust body of evidence.

33 The approach to risk management needs to be systematic and rigorous. However, it is crucial that boards do not allow too much effort to be expended on processes. What matters substantively is recognition of, and reaction to, real risks – not unthinking pursuance of bureaucratic processes.

> An international consultation[6] in the wake of the financial crisis that began in 2007 suggests widespread failure of risk management was due to disconnection of the risk management system from strategy and other management systems.

Legality

34 The board seeks assurance that the organization is operating within the law and in accordance with its statutory duties.

Decision making

35 The board seeks assurance that processes for operational decision making are robust and are in accordance with agreed schemes of delegation.

Probity

36 The board adheres to the seven principles of public life. This includes implementing a transparent and explicit approach to the declaration and handling of conflicts of interest. Good practice here includes the maintenance and publication of a register of interest for all board members. Board meeting agendas include an opportunity to declare any conflict at the beginning.

Seven Principles of Public Life
Selflessness
Integrity
Objectivity
Accountability
Openness
Honesty
Leadership

37 Another key area in relation to probity relates to the effective oversight of top level remuneration. Boards are expected to adhere to HM Treasury guidance and to document and explain all decisions made.

38 Corporate trustee

- Finally, if the organisation holds NHS charitable funds as sole corporate trustee the board members of that body are jointly responsible for the management and control of those charitable funds, and are accountable to the Charity Commission.
- Some NHS organisations have a separate trustee body which manages the charitable funds linked to the work of the NHS body. Where this applies the board does not have responsibility for the charitable funds.

Committees of the board that support accountability

39 In order to enable accountability, boards are statutorily required to establish committees[7] responsible for audit and remuneration. In addition the boards of NHS organisations have a statutory duty of quality. Over time NHS organisations have configured board committees in a variety of ways to discharge these functions. For ease of reference, these are described as three core committees. Good practice in respect of the configuration of the membership of board committees can be found in the compendium. The three core committees are:

1. **Audit Committee**: This committee's focus is to seek assurance that financial reporting and internal control principles are applied, and to maintain an appropriate relationship with the organisation's auditors, both internal and external. The Audit Committee offers advice to the board about the reliability and robustness of the processes of internal control. This includes

the power to review any other committees' work, including in relation to quality, and to provide assurance to the board with regard to internal controls. The Audit
Committee may also have responsibility for the oversight of risk management. Ultimately however the responsibility for effective stewardship of the organisation belongs to the board as a whole.

2. **Remuneration Committee**: The duties of this committee are to make recommendations to the board on the remuneration and terms of service for the chief executive and other executive directors; and to monitor and evaluate the performance of the executive directors and to oversee contractual arrangements, including proper calculation and scrutiny of termination payments. The Remuneration Committee should take into account relevant nationally determined parameters on pay, pensions and compensation payments. No director should be involved in deciding his/her own remuneration. The committee may additionally have a role in succession planning for executive level roles.

3. **Quality Committee**: There is a trend for boards to delegate responsibility for seeking assurance that there are effective arrangements for monitoring and continually improving the quality of healthcare provided to or commissioned on behalf of patients. Evidence suggests that Quality Committees are becoming more common and that they can enhance board oversight of quality performance by ensuring input from people with quality expertise, such as clinical, nursing, management and non-healthcare domains. This provides a real opportunity to probe and scrutinise performance in relation to quality. However, the ultimate accountability for quality rests with the board.

> "Committees (are established) 'only to help the board do its job'."
>
> John Carver

> "One PCT had established 17 committees of the board. No board requires 17 committees to do its job!"
>
> SHA chair

40 All board committees normally have a nonexecutive chair. Audit Committee members are all non-executive directors with executives in attendance as appropriate. At least one member of the Audit Committee must have a financial background. Checks and balances need to be maintained in committee membership. So, for example, the board chair cannot be a member of the Audit Committee, nor can the Audit Committee chair be the senior independent director. Best practice suggests that the vice chair of the organization should not chair the Audit Committee in order to avoid potential conflicts of interest.

41 Effective boards minimise the number of standing board committees. However, boards may establish other committees. Examples include investment committees, risk committees[8] and Charitable Funds Committees.

Shape culture

42 The third core role of the board is shaping a positive culture for the board and the organisation. This recognises that good governance flows from a shared ethos or culture, as well as from systems and structures. The board also takes the lead in establishing and promoting values and standards of conduct for the organisation and its staff.

43 Over recent years there has been an increasing drive to change the culture of the NHS to be more patient-centred and user-centred. Boards play a key role in creating a diverse, plural, and responsive culture that can deliver services that meet the needs of individual patients and communities.

Shaping organisational culture

44 Effective boards shape a culture for the organisation which is ambitious, self-directed, nimble, responsive, and encourages innovation. A commitment to openness and transparency means that boards are more likely to give priority to the organisation's relationship and reputation with patients, the public and partners as the primary means by which it meets policy and/or regulatory requirements. As such it puts patients and communities at the centre.

45 Boards need to recognise the importance of ensuring that the culture of their organization reflects the NHS values, as defined in the NHS Constitution. These are:

Respect and dignity
Commitment to quality of care
Compassion
Improving lives
Working together for patients
Everyone counts

46 If shaping the culture of the organisation is a vital role for boards, then embedding the culture, so that it becomes a lived reality is equally important and arguably the most challenging part of the role.

47 Embedding a new culture in an organisationrequires sustained effort and consistency of approach, often over a number of years. International research provides some helpful points on how boards can play a role in achieving desired culture change in a health context.

> CULTURE AND QUALITY: Research with hospital boards in Canada[9] suggests that the prominence of quality and safety as organisational values increase when they are set by the board. This is reflected in an increased focus on quality on the ground, in the form of team priorities, improvement initiatives and resources.
>
> CULTURE AND SAFETY: Board influence on organisational 'safety culture' is well-recognised in guidance10. Research in the US, Canada and the UK indicates that boards can contribute to this through visible engagement with the quality agenda, for example by participating in 'walk rounds' where board members discuss safety issues with frontline staff; by hearing patient stories at the board; by distributing 'safety briefings' across the organisation, covering key issues and performance data; and by establishing quality training and education programmes for all staff.
>
> CULTURE and INNOVATION: Research in the UK, in the NHS and in industry[7], has demonstrated that boards have a responsibility to embed innovation in the organisation's culture. Innovation friendly organisations have decentralised but clearly defined structures, which encourage frontline and managerial staff to innovate by allowing them freedom to make their own decision and take risks (but not at the expense of safety). Their boards avoid a top-down, rule driven approach, but do monitor, evaluate and learn. These boards actively support innovation and innovators.

Board's role in exemplifying and modelling culture

48 So far the focus in this section has been on the board's role in shaping the values and culture for the organisation.

49 An outward looking board leadership culture that actively embraces change, fosters innovation and maintains an unswerving commitment to quality and patient safety offers the best prospect of navigating effectively through a demanding and rapidly changing environment.

50 The board needs to be seen as champions of these values in the way the board itself operates and behaves. There are a number of facets to this. Effective boards and their members:

- Exemplify the seven principles of public life
- Reflect a drive to challenge discrimination, promote equity of access and quality of services and respect and protect human rights
- Ensure that their approach to strategy, accountability and engagement are consistent with the values they seek to promote for the organisation.

> "Objectives appear to have focused insufficiently on service quality and patient safety: national targets, including financial balance, and a drive to gain Foundation Trust status, took priority. This analysis was evidenced by analysis of board minutes, the board placing financial performance ahead of addressing staff shortages, and further supported by the views of nursing and medical staff."
>
> Quality regulator investigation into major quality failures in a Foundation Trust

> "The board was 'insulated from the reality of poor care."
>
> From a regulator report on a failing NHS Trust

An approach to shaping culture

51 Boards may wish to consider adopting a culture shaping process that is gaining prominence among third sector boards in North America. It involves an active but focused process of dialogue and engagement with staff and service users. This approach has a great deal to offer NHS boards as they seek to shape organisational culture and, in turn, use their learning from staff and user experience to set strategy and ensure accountability. It is described in Appendix 1.

52 As boards undertake their strategy development role, this approach could involve an interactive process of direct engagement with key stakeholders, clinicians, staff, members and patients, at key stages in the strategy development process. This ensures that the board as a whole is listening, learning and shaping, rather than just receiving draft strategies for approval. This approach is more likely to achieve a viable and responsive direction, build commitment and buy in, enrich board discussion and challenge board group think.

53 Similarly, when ensuring accountability, a more interactive style of governance could move beyond paper reporting. Examples of such an approach could include patient safety walk rounds, hearing patient stories at the board andnstaff focus groups.

54 While the importance of board visibility in the organisation has long been recognised, a more interactive process allows board members, staff and users to shape organisational values and culture through direct engagement. It also ensures that board members take back to the boardroom an enriched understanding of the lived reality for staff, users and partners.

Building blocks

Context

55 The first building block requires that boards have a comprehensive understanding of the external national and regional context in which they operate.

56 While many of the fundamental principles of good governance are common across a range of different types of organisations (both private and public sector), the complexity of the statutory, accountability and organizational context in which NHS boards operate is a key difference that must be fully understood by all board members. Boards operate in a demanding environment. Some of the challenges are illustrated here in figure 3. In addressing these challenges it is important that Boards listen to the voices of citizens and patients.

> "It has taken quite some time to learn enough about the context within which the NHS operates to be able to contribute effectively as a board member."
>
> FoundationTrust Non-Executive Director

57 The areas that boards will need to consider when developing an understanding of context are set out below:

58 Policy: It is important for boards to have a good understanding of the current and emerging policy direction, and the strategies for the NHS and its key partners.

59 Economy: Boards need to be aware of information on the economic environment for public services, and the wider economy. This assists boards in understanding the implications for future funding as well as the potential impact of economic changes on the health of the public and the demand for health services.

60 Legislation: NHS bodies are subject to a wide range of legislation, from central government and from the European Union. This includes statutes, regulations and a variety of directives and Secretary of State directions.

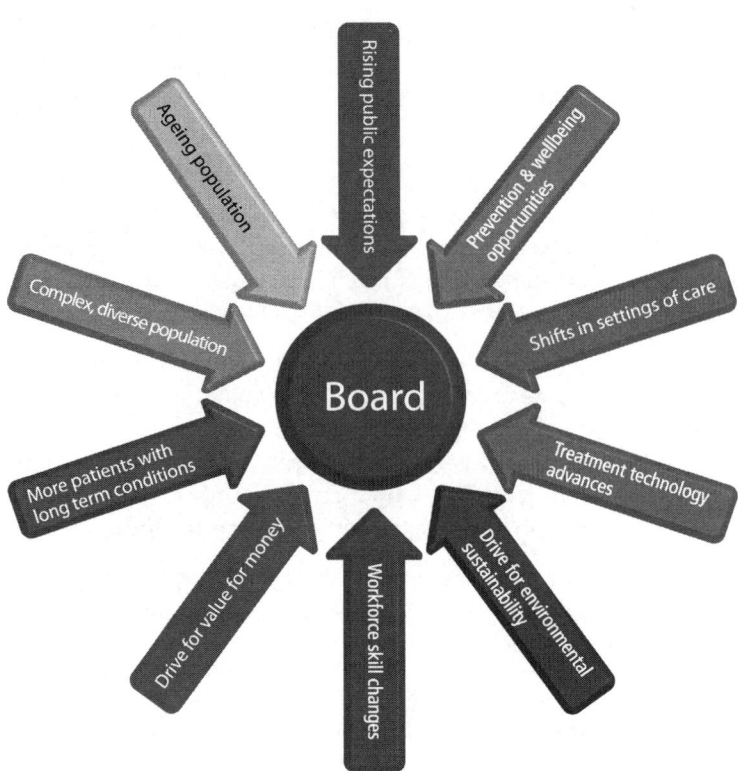

FIGURE 3 Challenges on NHS boards

61 Institutional landscape: An understanding of the structures and institutions of the NHS and those with whom the NHS does business is essential for boards to undertake their role effectively. This includes central and local government and other public and voluntary services which contribute to health and well being.

62 Regulation: NHS bodies are subject to oversight from several regulators. Developing a good understanding of the most significant regulators and their requirements and expectations of NHS bodies will greatly assist boards as they steer the organisation.

63 Public Expectations: Expectations of all public services are rising; arguably this is most pronounced in relation to the NHS. Even the most stretching national targets and standards have struggled to keep pace with mounting public expectations. The most effective NHS boards energetically develop their own understanding of trends in public and patient expectation and ensure that this actively informs their strategic choices.

64 An understanding of the wider determinants of health status: It is important for boards to develop an understanding of the wide range of factors that impact on health status. These include poor housing, neighbourhood deprivation, limited employment and educational opportunities, as well as the effects of affluence. This understanding helps inform the board's strategic response and shapes its whole system and partnership working.

Intelligence

65 Intelligence is the second key building block. It includes performance information, which can be both quantitative (such as performance metrics) and qualitative (such as staff, patient and stakeholder perspectives). It also includes information on the external local environment.

66 Boards need to be provided with information that is timely, reliable and comprehensive. The Intelligent Board series[11,12,13,14,15] continues to offer excellent guidance to boards, and some of the key elements of this advice are summarized below. More details can be found in the compendium. However, guidance can never be a substitute for discussion in the board aimed at evaluating the usefulness of current intelligence and shaping future intelligence requirements.

67 Intelligence that boards need to consider falls under two headings:

- Performance Information.
- Intelligence on the external local environment.

Performance information

68 This describes how the organisation is performing both strategically and operationally. The key requirement here is that the intelligence:

- Allows the board to arrive at judgments about organisational performance in the delivery of strategy.
- Allows the board to scrutinise operational performance 'in the round' – bringing together its appraisal of organizational performance in relation to operational activity, quality, finance and the workforce.

> *"The challenge for our board has been to maintain a driving focus on our own, locally determined strategic objectives as the framework for holding the organisation to account. The reporting demands placed on the organisation, by regulators and central government, are onerous and it is easy to succumb to the temptation to confuse the performance information requirements of these external stakeholders with those of the board."*
>
> PCT Non-Executive Director

> *"It is important to be able to state performance criteria in a simple, crisp way, we want to measure against the following characteristics 'prompt, safe, effective, efficient, considerate'."*
>
> NHS chair

69 Intelligence about **strategic performance** needs to:

- Be structured around an explicit set of strategic goals.
- Show trends in performance in terms of quality; the experience and satisfaction of patients; business development; and finance.
- Provide forecasts and anticipate future performance issues
- Encourage an external focus.
- Enable comparison with the performance of similar organisations, for example through benchmarking.

70 Intelligence about **operational performance** needs to:

- Provide an accurate, timely and balanced picture of current and recent performance – including patient, clinical, regulatory and financial perspectives.
- Focus on the most important measures of performance, and highlight exceptions.
- Be appropriately standardised in order to take account of known factors that affect outcomes, such as the age and deprivation profile of patients and communities served.
- Integrate informal sources of intelligence from staff and patients.
- Include consideration of assessments from key regulators including comparator information.
- Enable comparisons with the performance of similar organisations.
- Include key workforce indicators, including capacity and capability to deliver future strategy, culture and information on equality and diversity.

71 It is most helpful for boards to receive performance information in a clear, easily digestible format, using graphic overviews, trend analysis and brief commentary. Data can also be presented in the form of dashboards or scorecards, where performance on key measures is presented against nationally or locally established benchmarks. High quality board papers are not purely descriptive – they include analyses that will actively direct the board members' attention to the key issues, implications and consequences.

Focus on Quality

72 Quality is the organising principle of the NHS and needs to be at the heart of everything the board does.

73 While significant progress has been made in shaping and sharpening the finance and activity information generally available to boards, progress has been slower in relation to information that will allow boards to scrutinise the 'quality' of services. Quality accounts should become at least as important as financial statements for boards. Quality comprises three dimensions:

- Clinical effectiveness or patient outcomes.
- Patient safety.
- Quality of the patient experience.

74 As with other organisational priorities, boards should receive this information in an easily digested summary. The closer the data is to 'real time' the greater its value.

Intelligence on the external local environment

75 Intelligence on the local environment should be as important to boards as performance information. It includes:

- **Stakeholder mapping**: One of the key challenges facing NHS boards is the complex stakeholder and accountability landscape. Boards need to have a clear grasp of the entire system within which they operate. This includes an understanding of who are the key local stakeholders, their agendas, priorities and perspectives. For Foundation Trust boards, this includes developing a good understanding of governor and member perspectives.
- **Competitor analysis**: In an increasingly competitive market, the boards of NHS provider organisations need to keep abreast of their competitors (other NHS organisations, independent providers and the voluntary sector), including an understanding of their relative strengths and weaknesses.
- **Market analysis**: Likewise it is important for boards of provider organisations to build their understanding of the local market and the place that the organization wishes to occupy within it. For boards of commissioning organisations, the challenge is to deliver quality and value for money by enabling the development of a vibrant market of providers. Provider and market intelligence will be critical for effective board strategic decision-making. This 'market-making' function of commissioners becomes increasingly complex in the context of policy drives towards patient choice and 'personalisation' in health services.
- **Health need and demography including diversity and equality issues**: These aspects are particularly important for commissioning boards. It includes intelligence to assist boards to understand the local population, its demographic and health profile, particularly health status, healthcare needs, behaviours and aspirations; and the key equality gaps experienced by different groups within the community, both in relation to each other and compared to similar groups in other localities. This aspect of intelligence should be based on shared analysis and monitoring with local government.

> *"In the end, no amount of data, however clear, will make the decisions."*
>
> PCT chair

76 Board members have a key role to play in actively shaping and designing the sort of intelligence they wish to receive.

77 The research evidence supports the view that the provision of too much or too little information can be a significant risk to effective board functioning, so the key is to strike a balance between providing sufficient and meaningful information without overloading board members.

78 A final, and important, thought on intelligence: there is an increasing recognition that paperbased intelligence can only take the board so far. Appropriate interaction between the board and key stakeholders underpins the development of strategy, gives 'texture' to ensuring accountability and shapes a culture of openness and dialogue within the organisation. This brings us to the third key building block: engagement.

Engagement

79 The effective board gives priority to engaging with key stakeholders and opinion formers within and beyond the organisation. Engaging effectively is an important way that a board and organisation demonstrates its openness and transparency and ultimately its accountability. There are also some circumstances where there is a legal obligation to involve the public[16]. Engagement informs and supports the board in formulating strategy, shaping culture, and even aspects of ensuring accountability. The range of internal and external stakeholders with which boards engage includes:

- Patients and the public.
- Members and governors (for Foundation Trusts).
- Clinicians and staff.
- Partners in delivery (e.g. local authorities, third and independent sector partners).
- Key institutional stakeholders (ranging from other NHS organisation to regulators).

80 Engagement with staff, patients, the public and stakeholders is not new, and has long been a priority of senior leaders in NHS organisations. Boards as a whole generally receive and consider the results of these processes in the form of reports and papers.

81 Recent research has however begun to identify the role that direct interaction between the board and clinicians, patients and the public can play in effective governance.

Patient and public engagement

82 A wide range of guidance is available for boards on patient and public engagement; it is referenced in the compendium. There are three main aspects for boards to consider:

- **Empowering people**: Patients and the public want to be able to influence both their own healthcare and the organisations that provide this care.
- **Putting patient experience centre stage**: Organisations need to ensure the routine, systematic collection and analysis of feedback from people who use services (including realtime patient feedback and an understanding of the perspectives of minority and hard to reach groups). Crucially, boards need to demonstrate that this feedback, alongside intelligence on effectiveness and patient safety, actively informs board priority setting, resource allocation and decision-making.
- **Accountability to local communities**: The organisation, and therefore the board, has a statutory 'duty to involve'[16]. In addition, the organisation exercises its local accountability through overview and scrutiny arrangements led by local government.

Members and governors (for Foundation Trusts)

83 Boards of Foundation Trusts need to recognise that the autonomy and freedoms granted to them rest on the twin pillars of robust independent regulation and effective accountability to patients and the public delivered through membership and governors.

84 Governors of Foundation Trusts are at the heart of ensuring that the organisation remains accountable in this way. If governors are to exercise this aspect of their role effectively, they require regular and meaningful engagement with the board. Governors need to be supported to engage with the members and the wider public so that they can contribute these wider perspectives and expectations in their discussions with Directors.

Staff including clinicians

85 Engagement with clinicians and staff is an important means by which the organisation's leaders shape organisational culture. It can help boards drive culture change, for example in encouraging staff to feed into the risk management system or engage in quality improvement.

86 A recent review[17] of how best to engage staff suggests that use of established approaches, such as surveys seeking staff opinion, are deficient in this area as they leave engagement as an 'add-on'. Ideally, boards should aim to achieve 'transformational engagement', where clinicians and staff are integral to developing and delivering organisational strategy. Boards can project a

'human face of leadership' through direct engagement including holding 'Question Time' style events and participating in web-chats. Clinicians might be engaged to lead improvement and innovation work as 'change agents'; to provide input and leadership on quality committees; and as a key source of 'wisdom' in an engaging approach to governance.

Key institutional stakeholders

87   Boards are advised to develop a coherent strategy for engagement with key institutional stakeholders. These include commissioners, NHS providers, local government, universities and further education, the voluntary sector, independent sector and of course regulators.

88   This stakeholder engagement is most often led by the chair and chief executive. While this is sound, it must form part of a systematic and agreed approach that allows other directors to be engaged in a targeted way.

89   A number of boards choose to hold board-to-board meetings with key institutional stakeholders. Properly focused, this can be an important part of building understanding of, and relationships with, stakeholders.

3 SYSTEM GOVERNANCE – THE BOARD'S ROLE

The guidance so far has focused on the board's role in ensuring good governance within its own NHS organisation. This chapter considers the NHS board's role in the wider health system.

90   NHS boards exist within a crowded organizational landscape that includes a range of public, private and community organisations all serving broadly the same citizens. To deliver their core purpose of building public and stakeholder confidence in health and healthcare, NHS boards need to see beyond the boundaries of their individual organisations. This delicate balance involves operating within a 'community of governance' while simultaneously respecting divergent interests in a vibrant market.

91   In a financially constrained environment this becomes particularly pertinent, as boards consider options for strategic partnerships, joint management arrangements, outsourcing, major service reconfigurations, and potential mergers. But whatever the economic environment, the need to develop an effective community of governance is important because:

- Patients and users travel across organizational boundaries to receive services.
- Approaches to health improvement and prevention, as well as tackling health inequalities can only be addressed by taking a whole health economy perspective.
- NHS organisations and other public bodies have a legal duty to co-operate on improving local health outcomes.

92   Boards need to consider their ways of working in the wider system in two main dimensions:

- The requirement for them to operate constructively in the health and social care system.
- The effective governance of established and formalised partnerships.

Operating constructively in the health and social care system

93   The health and social care system in England relies on a complex interplay between collaboration and competition. Boards need to reach finely balanced judgments about how they engage with this complexity.

94   The public interest is best served when all actors in the system reach agreement about:

- Local health need.
- A shared vision for health and healthcare including health outcomes.
- The 'rules of engagement' – how players within the system will work together, including the development of a culture of cooperative transparency.
- Mutual understanding of, and respect for, individual organisational interests and constraints.

95   This shared understanding and agreement can only be reached through regular and ongoing processes of formal and informal dialogue and relationship building. This role is primarily undertaken by the chair and chief executive. Both chair and chief executive play an important role in shaping the climate for inter-organisational engagement and in keeping lines of communication open – especially at times when negotiations may have strained relationships lower down in their organisations. A regular cycle of whole 'board to board' processes has proved valuable in many health economies. The joint production of an annual health system development plan could also be valuable.

Effective governance of formal partnerships

96   A summary of research on inter-organisational working proposes that a partnership might be analysed on two dimensions: its breadth – the range of groups it encompasses; and its depth – ranging from information sharing, through coordinating activities, up to a formal merger of partners.[18]

97   Whatever the form or extent of the partnership, effective governance of these partnerships requires attention to the same three roles that have been described above, as the role of the board. Namely:

- Formulating strategy.
- Ensuring accountability.
- Shaping culture.

Formulating strategy

98   Partnership governance arrangements need to give attention to the three elements of formulating strategy described in section two: the process of developing strategy; the hallmarks of an effective strategy and the approach to strategic decision making.

99   Research on the governance of partnerships identifies the following additional points:

- **Partnership agreements**: It is important to set out and agree a clear purpose for the partnership, which can be formalised through the creation of a partnership agreement. A report on partnerships in public services found that the absence of a partnership agreement can lead to increased difficulties, such as reduced achievement of objectives and even breakdown of the partnership.
- **Care pathway perspective**: for partnerships involved in commissioning or providing care across organisational boundaries, it is important that the strategy takes a clear patient or care pathway perspective.
- **Transparency and openness of strategic decision making**: this is important both to build trust, and also to support shared risk taking. It reduces dominance by any single voice.
- **Clarity of outcomes and performance indicators**: developing a shared agreement on performance measures for the partnership which takes account of the performance expectations of all the constituent partners is key. The aim is to provide assurance that the partnership is operating effectively in terms of its costs and benefits. For many partnerships impact or outcome measures may be long term in nature, in which case identifying appropriate interim measures is important as part of the strategy development process.

Ensuring accountability

100   Ensuring accountability is a particularly key role for the governance of partnerships. The two elements described under roles of the board are highly relevant, namely: holding the partnership to account for the delivery of strategy, and seeking assurance that the systems of control are robust and reliable.

101   Key points for partnership governance include:

- **Develop a performance reporting framework** that captures the various targets of all partners that relate to the partnership. The intelligence provided on performance of the partnership is made available to all involved.

- **Monitor progress on outcomes and performance indicators**. It is important to recognise the challenges in monitoring performance of partnerships, but persevere constructively to find ways of overcoming the challenges.
- **Agree approach to shared quality assurance**: for those partnerships involving commissioning or provision of care, ensure a focus on all three elements of quality: effectiveness; safety and experience.
- **Agree approach to shared risk-taking and risk management**: for major partnerships, consider the development of a partnership assurance framework, to serve a similar purpose to the board assurance framework (paragraph 32).
- **Clarify accountability**: staff working in partnerships have to contend with multiple accountabilities: to the partnership, and to the constituent organisations. It is important to establish where the ultimate responsibility and liability rests.

Shaping culture

102 Shaping culture for a partnership arrangement is more challenging than for a single organisation, as the constituent parts of the partnership will come with very different and distinctive cultures of their own, with different ways of conducting business.

103 Lessons drawn from research in this field emphasise the importance of:

- An open culture that is receptive to engagement.
- A commitment to building trust.
- Transparency and openness in decision making, in reporting and in information sharing.
- A commitment to learning and understanding the different cultures and ways of working of partner organisations.
- A recognition that partnership requires give and take from all sides.

104 The building blocks which underpin and support the delivery of the core board roles are as relevant to the governance of partnerships as they are to the role of the board of a single NHS organisation.

4 IMPROVING BOARD EFFECTIVENESS

This chapter sets out the approaches to improving board effectiveness.

105 This chapter sets out five important clusters of activity that enable boards to improve their effectiveness, namely:

- Building capacity and capability.
- Enabling corporate accountability and good social processes.
- Embedding board disciplines.
- Delegating appropriately.
- Exercising judgment.

106 Further guidance and good practice in this area, and suggested additional reading are provided in the online compendium.

Building capacity and capability

107 This involves activity in the four areas shown in Figure 4.

Board composition, knowledge and skills

108 NHS boards should not be so large as to be unwieldy, but must be large enough to provide the balance of skills and experience that is appropriate for the organisation. The composition of the board should achieve a balance between continuity and renewal. Non-executive Directors (NEDs) serve a maximum of 10 years in the same NHS post to ensure this balance. Within this period, any second reappointment must be through open competition.

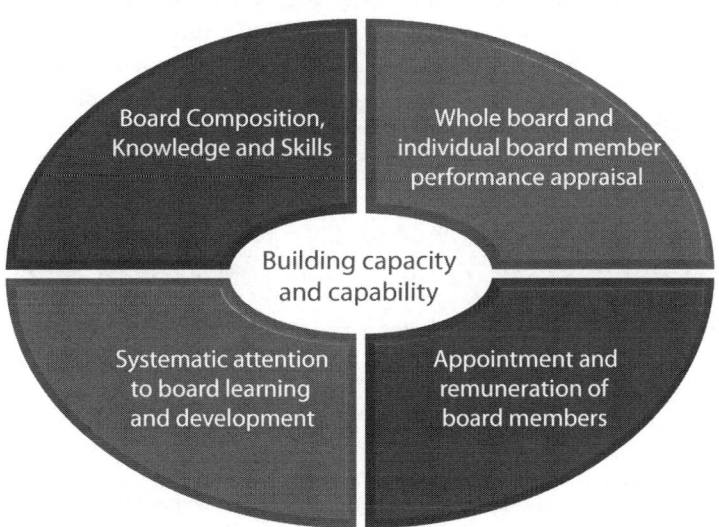

FIGURE 4 Areas of board capacity and capability building

109 In most NHS organisations, governance is the responsibility of a unitary board, with at least half the board, excluding the chair, made up of independent NEDs.

110 The time commitment required of non-executive directors continues to be a focus of debate. Nonexecutive directors should be encouraged to look at their time requirements over an annual cycle. There will be a number of situations where more time is required than on average. This includes the first year after appointment, and when the organisation is considering major strategic changes or significant changes to its status. See also paragraph 160.

111 All directors must be appropriately qualified to discharge their roles effectively, including setting strategy, monitoring and managing performance and driving continuous quality improvement. However, over time the strategic challenges facing boards give rise to the need for specific skills, and this requirement must be kept under review in a systematic way. In order to ensure an effective balance of knowledge, skills and backgrounds boards should undertake regular skills audits of current board members.

112 Guidance suggests that organisations are best served by boards drawn from a wide diversity of backgrounds and sectors. This includes the expectation that board composition reflects the diverse communities they serve.

Whole board and individual board member performance appraisal

113 It is important that the whole board creates opportunities to reflect on its own performance and effectiveness. This should include a formal and rigorous annual evaluation of its own performance and that of its committees. Some boards choose to supplement self-assessment periodically with views obtained from a range of internal and external stakeholders who do not sit on the board but nonetheless experience its impact. This could include leading clinicians, senior managers who are not board members and external partners and stakeholders including patient groups and partner organisations both within and outside of the NHS.

114 A range of approaches to whole board effectiveness review is outlined in the online compendium.

115 It is important for boards to develop a framework of knowledge, skills and competencies that fit their organisational requirements and context and that can serve as the basis for whole board and board member appraisal.

116 Alongside whole board performance evaluation, board members should undergo an annual appraisal of their individual contribution and performance. This appraisal should focus on the director's contribution as a member of the corporate board; in the case of executive directors this is distinct from their functional leadership role. The appraisal of the chief executive by the chair is particularly important because the effective performance management of the chief executive is critical to the success of the organisation and sets the benchmark for other senior NHS managers. Responsibilities for carrying out these appraisals are set out in the table below':

Role	Is appraised by
Chair (non Foundation Trusts)	SHA chair, or the Department of Health for SHA and Arms Length Body chairs
Chair (in Foundation Trusts)	Senior independent director, drawing on the views and perspectives of fellow directors, governors and partners
Chief executive	Chair
NEDs	Chair
EDs	Chief executive with input from the chair on their contribution as a member of the board

117 A growing number of NHS boards are choosing to support the development of individual board members by undertaking a '360 degree review'. This offers board members feedback on their approach, performance and contribution from a wide range of colleagues with whom they have regular contact. This can be very helpful, though experience shows that it requires time and commitment from all board members. It must also be undertaken in a manner that respects and protects confidentiality and trust within the board. The whole process – especially individual feedback needs to be handled independently and professionally. 360 degree review approaches are intended to support individual development rather than to inform re-appointment.

118 All appraisal processes should culminate in a personal development plan, the delivery of which is actively supported by the organisation.

Systematic attention to board learning and development

119 Effective boards use the performance appraisal processes outlined above as the basis for focused board development action plans. The plan should include:

- **A structured process for induction of new board members**. This is an opportunity to attend to the board members' understanding of local and – especially if they are new to the NHS – national context.
- **Individual board member opportunities to refresh and update skills and knowledge**. Conferences and similar events are likely to be very helpful. Organisations should ensure that board members are aware of development opportunities and that new policy and contextual knowledge is systematically shared with board members, including through informal briefings between board meetings.
- **Opportunities for the board to learn together**. Board development should not be limited to externally provided development events and conferences. These are valuable events, especially for the transmission of knowledge and information, but carving out time for the whole board to learn together is valuable. This is particularly true when exploring the applicability of new or innovative ways of working in the board, or when developing new skills and capabilities.

120 Foundation Trust boards should give particular attention to supporting the development of governors. Careful and comprehensive induction is critical. Foundation Trusts have a responsibility to ensure that governors have the skills and capability to deliver their core statutory functions[19] (appointment and removal of chair and NEDs, appointment of auditors, scrutiny of organisational performance, and informing and consenting to annual plan). Governors also need to be supported to build their skills and capacity to engage with their 'constituencies' in order to deliver their role.

121 Support for chairs, chief executives and directors in challenging roles needs particular attention. It should be clear to board members during the appointment process, if the posts are

deemed challenging. Experienced directors should be appointed to these roles, and additional development support clearly agreed and put in place at an early stage.

Appointment and remuneration of board members

122 Formal, rigorous and transparent procedures for both the appointment and the remuneration of directors must be in place. This should include effective processes for checking whether the prospective executive director is appointable.

123 The appointments process must ensure that all appointments are made on merit and against objective criteria. Appointments panels for executives should always include an independent external assessor. Responsibilities for these appointments are summarised in the following table:

Role	In FTs is appointed by	In other organisations is appointed by
Chair	Governors, at a general meeting, informed by the nominations committee and/or governors working group, after taking account of advice of board of directors	Appointments Commission
Chief executive	Committee of the chair and NEDs, approved by the governors	Committee of the chair and NEDs with an independent external assessor, approved by the board
NEDs	Governors, at a general meeting, informed by the nominations committee and/or governors working group, after taking account of advice of board of directors	Appointments Commission
EDs	Committee of the chair, chief executive and NEDs	Committee of the chair, chief executive and NEDs with an independent external assessor

124 Likewise, the responsibilities for setting remuneration are shown in the following table:

Role	In FTs remuneration is decided by	In other organisations remuneration is decided by
Chair	Governors' at a general meeting, informed by the Nominations Committee or a governors working group	Secretary of State
Chief executive	Remuneration committee of at least three independent non-executive directors	Remuneration Committee of at least three non-executive directors
NEDs	Governors' at a general meeting, informed by the Nominations Committee or a governors working group	Secretary of State
EDs	Remuneration Committee of at least three independent non-executive directors	Remuneration Committee of at least three non-executive directors

125 The Remuneration Committee has delegated responsibility for setting not only remuneration for the chief executive and all executive directors, but also including pension rights and compensation payments. This committee also recommends and monitors the level and structure of remuneration for senior management.

126 Remuneration committees are expected to consult with external professionals to market test remuneration levels at least every three years or, where appropriate, apply government guidance on pay awards.

Enabling corporate accountability and good social processes

127 In unitary NHS boards, all directors are collectively and corporately accountable for organizational performance.

128 A key strength of unitary boards is the opportunity provided for the exchange of views between executives and NEDs, drawing on and pooling their experience and capabilities.

129 Boards are 'social systems'. The most effective boards invest time and energy in the development of mature relationships and ways of working.

130 Some techniques and practices that support and hinder the effectiveness of these social systems are summarised in the following table.

Ways of working that support good social processes	Ways of working that obstruct good social processes
Building a crystal clear understanding of the roles of the board and individual board members	Board members behaving in a way that suggests a 'master-servant' relationship between non-executive and executive
Actively working to develop and protect a climate of trust and candour	Executive Directors only contributing in their functional leadership area rather than actively participating across the breadth of the board agenda
Building cohesion by taking steps to know and understand each other's backgrounds, skills and perspectives	Demonstrating an unwillingness to consider points of view that are different from individual directors' starting positions
Encouraging all board members to offer constructive challenges	Challenge primarily coming from non-executive directors, rather than all directors feeling empowered to challenge one another in board meetings
Sharing corporate responsibility and collective decision-making	Challenging in a way that is unnecessarily antagonistic and not appropriately balanced with appreciation, encouragement and support
Ensuring that neither chair nor chief executive power and dominance act to stifle appropriate participation in board debate	Working in ways that don't demonstrate overall confidence in the executive and that feed individual anxiety and insecurity about capability

Embedding board disciplines

131 Competent, systematic board disciplines form the bedrock of good board functioning. These disciplines include:

- Giving thoughtful attention to board agenda planning and management: The chair is central in this process and needs to be vigilant in ensuring that board agendas maintain a complex range of 'balances' between:
- strategy and performance management.
- activity, finance and quality.
- organisational priorities and the demands of regulators.
- information sharing (presentation) by executives and whole board discussion.
- Chairs face the challenge of attending to the full breadth of the board's role while ensuring that board meetings do not descend into a gruelling test of board member endurance.

> International research demonstrates the value of placing quality and safety as a standing item on the board agenda.
>
> Placing quality at the top of the agenda can increase the attention given to the subject across the organisation.
>
> Dedicating significant board time to quality (at least 20%) is associated with improved quality outcomes.

- **Board and committee year planners and annual programmes of work**: the board and its committees should be supported by an annual plan that sets out a coherent overall programme for formal board meetings, board seminars and away-days and committee meetings. It needs to take account of the organisational and system-wide planning cycle including key 'watershed events' such as contract negotiations, budget setting, regulatory returns and so on. It is good practice for the work of every committee of the board to be shaped by an annual plan.
- **Board papers**: The effectiveness of the board is predicated on the timely availability of board papers. Core disciplines for board papers include:
  - Timeliness: papers provided ideally a week ahead of meetings
  - Cover sheets: including, for each paper, the name of the author, a brief summary of the issue, the organisational forums where the paper has been considered, the strategic objective or regulatory requirement to which it relates, and an explicit indication of what is required of the board
  - Executive summaries: Succinct executive summaries that direct the readers' attention to the most important aspects.
- **Action logs**: Boards and committees can be helped to keep track of actions agreed by maintaining and monitoring a log. The log should show all actions agreed by the board, and for each action the 'ownership,' due dates, and status.
- **Declaration of interests and resolution of conflicts**[20]: Probity requires that the board maintains an up to date register of board members' interests. Board agendas should include an opportunity for board members to declare conflicts of interest that may relate to specific agenda items so that these can be managed appropriately.
- **Transparency and openness**: There is an important obligation on public services to ensure that they operate in an open and transparent manner. For many NHS organisations this is partially achieved by holding formal board meetings in public and the publication of papers[20]. The default position ought to be that business is conducted in the public board meeting. However, when a compelling case can be made for an item to be considered in private (for example a matter that involves individual confidentiality or commercial sensitivity), there is provision for attending to it in private. Some boards follow the principles in The Freedom of Information Act[21] for which items are considered in private.

132 Foundation Trust boards are not obliged to hold board meetings in public although some choose to do so. Foundation trusts remain a part of the public service, and thus retain the obligation to ensure openness and transparency to the public. Foundation Trust governors are required to meet in public.

133 Public board meetings alone are not a guarantee of transparency, and boards need to ensure that there is a wide range of ways for the public to access information about the way in which public resources are deployed. These include clear, informative, jargon-free annual reports, regular updating of an easily navigable website, the availability of key information in a range of appropriate languages and in forms that are accessible to those with disabilities.

Delegating appropriately

134 The formal powers of an NHS organization are vested in the board but the NHS Code of Accountability[22] allows the board to delegate some of its business to board committees and to the executive. The board approach to delegation should be set out in:

- Standing orders which specify how the organisation conducts its business.
- Standing financial instructions which detail the financial responsibilities, policies and procedures adopted.

- The scheme of reservation and delegation. This sets out which responsibilities and accountabilities remain at board level and which have been delegated to committees and to the executive, together with the appropriate reporting arrangements that ensure the board has oversight.

135 Approaches and schemes of delegation must be subject to regular board review to ensure that the distribution of functions and accountabilities is accurately and appropriately described, and remains appropriate despite changes in the organisation.

136 A range of approaches to the configuration of board committees and options is set out in the compendium. The following table lists some tests that a board should take into account when considering its committee structure.

Boards may wish to apply the following tests before establishing a new committee:
Are the proposed functions of the committee really board functions or are they executive functions?
Is a standing committee really required – or can the task be undertaken by a short life group?
Are there good reasons why the proposed functions cannot be carried out by the whole board?
Is the committee being established because of one major incident or issue – is it a proportionate response?
Does the creation of the committee reduce clarity of role or create lack of alignment between other committees of the board and the board itself?

Exercising judgment

137 This section recognises that at the heart of good governance is healthy debate about a spectrum of dilemmas that are not amenable to uniform guidance. Resolution of these dilemmas requires good judgment and acumen on the part of the board.

138 Some of the dilemmas that present themselves to boards are set out in the remainder of this section. They are illustrative, not an exhaustive list. The optimal board responses to these issues cannot sensibly be mandated in guidance. Rather, boards are encouraged to set aside the necessary time to debate and explore these issues as part of their developmental journey.

Who is governance for?

139 This dilemma identifies the complex question of who governance is for. It asks how the effective board might balance its responsibility to protect and safeguard the interests of the organization with a duty to take a wider system and community perspective looking at 'the greater good'. Some of the issues to explore include:

- The core purpose of governance in the NHS is to build public and stakeholder confidence. But NHS boards and particularly the boards of Foundation Trusts – also have a duty to act in the best interests of the organisation. How do boards respond if they believe that the public interest is best served by service and whole system changes that are uncomfortable for individual institutions?
- To what extent does the board role need to extend beyond the boundaries of the organisation or even the local health economy to reflect a 'system governance' approach?

Board effectiveness when things get tough

140 Good governance is not judged by 'nothing going wrong'. Even in the best boards and organisations bad things happen and board effectiveness is demonstrated by the appropriateness of the response when there is difficulty. Some of the questions to explore here include:

- How does the board build resilience and capability to respond?
- What are the good foundations that are likely to allow boards to work effectively in good and bad times?

- How do chairs make the best judgments about supporting the chief executive and executive team when there are major organisational performance issues, or where there is significant external pressure to take particular action?

The place of regulatory assurance in ensuring Accountability

141 Boards and organisations devote a great deal of time and resource to responding to the demands and expectations of regulators. Clearly regulatory assurance must be an important component of overall board assurance processes. Some of the dilemmas for board members include:

- To what extent should board members rely on assessments from key regulators in undertaking their accountability role?
- How do board members avoid being lulled into a false sense of security by regulator assurance that inevitably offers a more partial picture than that which the board requires?

Where is power and authority really vested in the NHS system?

142 Formally, NHS boards are both sovereign and accountable; the reality is inevitably less tidy. The Department of Health at central and regional level, major regulators and NHS boards share accountability, power and authority. And the balance of power ebbs and flows over time and in response to circumstances. In this context:

- How does the NHS board remain self-directed and retain an internal locus of control?
- How do board members retain a sense of their purpose and value in a context that may, at times, feel highly constrained?

Achieving a balance between managing risk and encouraging innovation

143 A systematic approach to the management of risk is one way that boards build public confidence. However, it is also clear that the future sustainability of the NHS and its founding values will require creative and innovative solutions. Some of the questions boards may wish to debate include:

- How do we ensure that risk and innovation aren't seen as mutually exclusive?
- How do boards ensure that individuals and teams within the organisation take full and active responsibility for the management of risk without creating a straightjacket of anxiety that stifles creativity?
- Does your board know about and act on best practice emerging from the literature on encouraging innovation?

Hearing the 'lone voice in the wilderness'

144 Reviews of significant governance failure frequently highlight individuals who raised ongoing concerns that were not heard but later turn out to have been early warning signs of impending difficulties. Some of the issues to explore here may include:

- What options are open to directors if they have concerns about board effectiveness and feel that their concerns are not getting a response?
- How do directors continue to express genuine concerns without becoming the proverbial 'dog with a bone'?
- When is it appropriate to let go of concerns that are not shared by others?

Building board engagement without blurring the boundaries

145 In this guide, board members are encouraged to develop a 'textured' understanding of the staff and patient experience through direct processes of engagement. This approach is seen as

a significant contributor to a board with the knowledge and skills effectively to safeguard quality and patient safety. But this approach also brings challenges and questions such as:

- How do we ensure that this approach allows boards to derive the benefits of wide engagement without the risk of being drawn into operational management?
- How do we ensure that the insight gained by individual board members is systematically and actively used in the board process.
- How do we ensure that the engagement by board members does not feel like 'scrutiny' and create unhelpful anxiety among staff?

Enabling effective financial stewardship

146 The whole board is charged with ensuring that there is effective financial stewardship. This means that all board members share accountability for the financial health of the organisation. But board agendas are often crowded and proper financial stewardship and scrutiny takes time. In exploring their options boards may wish to consider:

- Is there a role for a Finance Committee of the board as well as the Audit Committee?
- Does the existence of a Finance Committee tempt board members to abdicate – 'I don't need to be concerned because the finance committee has looked at this?'

What is the board's role in effective clinical engagement?

147 This dilemma explores the approach that boards need to take to clinical engagement as distinct from that of the executive leadership. Boards need to give thought to:

- How to make the best use of clinical advice? How to engage but remain strategic?
- How to ensure that boards make the best use of the scarce resource of clinical leaders' time?

How does the board play a role in developing executive leaders fit for the future?

148 A challenge facing boards is the need to develop leaders that have the knowledge, skills and experience to operate in an increasingly challenging environment. But individual organisations may not have the scale to tackle this challenge. Boards may wish to explore:

- Where is the locus for effective talent management/ succession planning – is it at board or regional level?
- How might boards and organisations within a system collaborate to tackle this challenge?

Meeting in Public

149 Many boards will conduct formal, decision making meetings in public. While board members may be wholly committed to the transparency and public accountability that this offers, they are aware of the respects in which public board meetings can begin to feel a little like 'theatre'. The dilemmas for boards include:

- The balance of what goes onto the public versus private board agenda.
- The need to ensure that boards are able to reflect freely on a wide spectrum of strategic options without fuelling unnecessary public anxiety and 'setting hares running.'

Avoiding 'the curse of recentness'

150 The NHS has never been short of new ideas and while this renewal and innovation is a real strength, the latest big idea can also exercise a form of tyranny over board and organisational agendas.

- How do boards ensure that they recognize and respond to valuable new ideas while simultaneously ensuring that longer-standing ideas and programmes are given the time and attention they need?

5 ROLES OF BOARD MEMBERS

The distinct roles of members of NHS boards are outlined in this section.

> "It is sometimes said that the board needs to be on the bridge of the ship and not in the engine room. I think it is sometimes important to go into the engine room – because how else will you know how it works? The important thing is to remember that its not your job to play with the instruments!"
>
> NHS chair

151 All board members share corporate responsibility for formulating strategy, ensuring baccountability and shaping culture. They also share responsibility for ensuring that the board operates as effectively as possible.

152 The chair and chief executive have complementary roles in board leadership. These are set out in more detail at the end of this section, but it is helpful to identify the essence of these two roles, which are:

- The chair leads the board and ensures the effectiveness of the board.
- For Foundation Trusts, the chair also chairs the council of governors.
- The chief executive leads the executive and the organisation.

153 However there are also distinct roles for different members of the board, and indeed there are distinct roles depending on the type of NHS organisation. The compendium sets these out in more detail.

154 These distinct roles are set out in the table below, showing how they are aligned to the role of the board. The following abbreviations are used:

- CE: chief executive
- NED: non-executive director
- ED: executive director
- FT: Foundation Trust.

Roles of board members

155 While all board members share corporate responsibilities, their distinctive roles are set out in the following table.

Chair	Chief executive	Non-executive director	Executive director
Formulate Strategy			
Ensures board develops vision, strategies and clear objectives to deliver organisational purpose	Leads strategy development process	Brings independence, external skills and perspectives, and challenge to strategy development	Takes lead role in developing strategic proposals – drawing on professional and clinical expertise (where relevant)
Ensure Accountability			
Holds CE to account for delivery of strategy Ensures board committees that support accountability are properly constituted	Leads the organisation in the delivery of strategy Establishes effective performance management arrangements and controls Acts as Accountable Officer	Holds the executive to account for the delivery of strategy Offers purposeful, constructive scrutiny and challenge Chairs or participates as member of key committees that support accountability	Leads implementation of strategy within functional areas

Shape Culture

Provides visible leadership in developing a positive culture for the organisation, and ensures that this is reflected and modelled in their own and in the board's behaviour and decision making Board culture: Leads and supports a constructive dynamic within the board, enabling contributions from all directors	Provides visible leadership in developing a positive culture for the organisation, and ensures that this is reflected in their own and the executive's behaviour and decision making	Actively supports and promotes a positive culture for the organisation and reflects this in their own behaviour Provides a safe point of access to the board for whistle-blowers	Actively supports and promotes a positive culture for the organisation and reflects this in their own behaviour

Context

Ensures all board members are well briefed on external context	Ensures all board members are well briefed on external context		

Intelligence

Ensures requirements for accurate, timely and clear information to board/ directors (and governors for FTs) are clear to executive	Ensures provision of accurate, timely and clear information to board/ directors (and governors for FTs)	Satisfies themselves of the integrity of financial and quality intelligence	Takes principal responsibility for providing accurate, timely and clear information to the board

Engagement

Plays key role as an ambassador, and in building strong partnerships with: • Patients and public • Members and governors (FT) • Clinicians and Staff • Key institutional stakeholders • Regulators	Plays key leadership role in effective communication and building strong partnerships with: • Patients and public • Member and governors (FT) • Clinicians and Staff • Key institutional stakeholders • Regulators	Ensures board acts in best interests of the public Senior independent director is available to members and governors if there are unresolved concerns (FTs)	Leads on engagement with specific internal or external stakeholder groups

Board members' roles in building capacity and capability

156 The table above described roles of board members that are related to the role of the board as a whole. Some members have, in addition, specific responsibilities to support board effectiveness. These specific responsibilities relate in particular to building the capacity and capability of the board. They are summarised in the table below, and explained below.

Chair	Chief executive	Non-executive director
Ensures that the board has the right balance and diversity of skills, knowledge and perspective, both NED and ED	Ensures that the executive team has the right balance and diversity of skills, knowledge and perspectives	
For FTs, supports the Nomination committee to undertake its role of appointing NEDs effectively		
With NEDs, appoints and removes the CE		NEDs including the chair, appoint and remove the chief executive
With the Remuneration Committee, determines appropriate levels of remuneration of EDs		For members of the Remuneration Committee: same as for chair
Has a prime role in appointing, and where necessary removing, executive directors, and in succession planning	With the chair, has a prime role in appointing and where necessary removing executive directors, and in succession planning	As for chair, but a particular responsibility for members of the Remuneration Committee: supports the chair

Ensures that directors (and governors) have a full induction and continually update their skills, knowledge and familiarity with the organisation	With the chair, ensures that development programmes are in place for board members (and governors for FTs)	
Arranges regular evaluation of performance of the board, and its committees and the governors (for FTs) Conducts regular performance reviews of the NEDs, the CE and executive directors in relation to their board contribution. Acts on the results of these evaluations, including supporting personal development planning	Uses the (board) performance evaluations as the basis for determining individual and collective professional development programmes for executive directors relevant to their duties as board members	For FTs: senior independent director (SID) and NEDs meet annually without the chair present to review the chair's performance The SID takes soundings from governors

Chair and chief executive roles and relationship

157 Clarity of role and an effective working relationship between chair and chief executive are crucial to the effectiveness of the board.

158 In essence the chair leads the board and nonexecutive directors, and the chief executive leads the executive and the organisation. In Foundation Trusts, the chair also chairs the council of governors.

159 The table below shows a number of helpful tips and cautionary pointers for chairs and chief executives to support the development of their relationship.[23]

Tips for maintaining a good relationship

- Being honest and open
- Communicating well
- Agreeing clearly defined working styles and roles
- Establishing trust
- Building a personal relationship
- Developing shared values
- Promoting a 'no surprises' culture

Pointers for chairs and chief executives

Chair should NOT ...	Chief executives should NOT ...
Be too operational, interfere with details of management	Be too controlling or autocratic towards the chair
Exceed part time hours	Get too involved in NED role – e.g. no consultation on shaping board agendas
Take specific strategic decisions alone	Break the fundamental rule of 'no surprises'
Adopt bullying, macho 'hire and fire' culture	Be too entrenched in the organisation

Non-executive directors' time commitment

160 The expected time commitment for non-executive directors on NHS boards is often a hotly debated topic. This guidance does not specify the time expected of non-executive directors, but does set out some principles that may help:

- Chairs, in their board leadership role, have a key responsibility to plan and manage the time commitment required of non-executive directors in line with their role on the board in relation to strategy, accountability and culture.
- Some tasks that non-executive directors are asked to do can be undertaken by other, appropriately selected and trained lay people (for example chairing appeals panels or exceptional treatment panels).
- Experience has shown that the higher the time commitment expected of non-executive directors, the less likely boards are to attract and retain candidates with a diverse background (such as people who are younger, of black and minority ethnic origin, women).
- There is a balance to be struck between developing a good understanding of the organisation and how it is functioning in its health economy, and getting too involved in operational functions. It is important for nonexecutive directors to maintain the ability for objectivity and independent scrutiny.
- Newly appointed non-executive directors may find that they need and want to spend more time initially as they learn about the organisation, its people and its context.
- In times of significant organisational or service change, more time may be required of nonexecutive directors for a limited period.

Role of the company secretary

161 The role of company secretary is well established in Foundation Trusts, and is becoming increasingly prominent in other NHS organisations.

162 The company secretary:

- Is accountable to the chair.
- Ensures good information flows within the board and its committees between senior management and non-executive directors.
- Facilitates induction and assists with professional development[24].
- Is responsible for advising the board through the chair on all governance matters, including ensuring that the organisation complies with the relevant legislation and regulations (and in Foundation Trusts the terms of authorisation).
- Is responsible to the board for ensuring compliance with board procedures, and should be accessible to all directors.

163 For Foundation Trusts, the company secretary has additional responsibilities to support the council of governors.

APPENDIX: Perspectives on governance

> "The function of governance is to ensure that an organisation (or partnership) fulfils its overall purpose, achieves its intended outcomes for citizens and service users, and operates in an effective, efficient and ethical manner.'"

> "Ensuring the organisation is doing the right things, in the right way, for the right people in a timely, inclusive, open, honest and accountable manner."

164 There are a wide range of different models of governance, drawn from research, guidance and long standing practise.

165 It is understood that board members will bring past experience and favoured models into their current board role. It is important that, in their developmental processes, boards surface and debate the models that board members carry with them. This guide has not sought to settle on a particular definition of good governance. A sound understanding of governance derives from assimilating and blending this range of perspectives. A helpful overall definition of governance can be found in the Good Governance Standard[25]:

166 Another definition, from the Audit Commission[26], builds on this approach and further develops a strong values basis to effective governance.

167 The **'agency'** model[27] has the 'principal-agent' relationship at its centre. In this approach, the focus is on efforts by those in governance roles to ensure that others within the organization act appropriately on their behalf. The model therefore emphasises monitoring and control systems including performance measures, incentives and sanctions.

168 A rather different view is presented in the **stakeholder** model. It identifies a multiplicity of competing and co-operating interests within organisations. The key aim of governance is to engage with, balance and integrate stakeholder interests ensuring that stakeholders are involved, supportive and are at least 'minimally content'.

169 The **stewardship** model also sees the need to engage with a range of interests but gives priority to the strong link between public bodies and civil society. The key role of those who govern is to create a framework of shared values and then to engage with key stakeholders and a suitably skilled and autonomous workforce, all of whom benefit from helping the organisation to achieve its goals.

170 The **policy governance**[28] model sharply distinguishes between the role of 'owners' (in the public service context, the local public) and 'operators' (those who deliver the service). In this model boards act as 'owner representatives' who set objectives but fully delegate the running of the organisation to operators via the chief executive as the main point of contact. A framework of policies limits the freedom of the management, ensuring that the effectiveness of an activity is not prioritised over its being ethical or prudent.

171 Recently a new approach has emerged from the experience of not-for-profit boards in the United States and is called Governance as Leadership[29] or **generative governance**. It describes three modes in which the board should be effective: fiduciary; strategic and generative. The main contribution of this tri-modal model is to emphasise the role of 'generative thinking' in producing a sense of what knowledge, information and data mean. This requires an active process of dialogue and engagement between the board, staff and service users.

172 Each of these perspectives highlights particular and important elements of the board role. Thus, for example, while good governance clearly flows from a framework of rigorous controls, staff commitment to operating these controls with the necessary consistency may well derive from shared values around patient safety or equality of access. Likewise clearly distinguishing the respective roles of board and management may not necessarily be incompatible with creating opportunities for the board to develop the deep understanding of patient and staff experience that is described within the generative governance model.

References

1 Taking it on Trust. Audit Commission. 2009.
2 Walker D. A review of corporate governance in UK banks and other financial industry entities. London. 2009.
3 Jha AK, Epstein AM. Boards and Governance in U.S. Hospitals and the Relationship to Quality of Care. Health Affairs. November 2009.
4 Section 18 of the Health Act 1999. Later repealed and replaced by Section 45 of the Health and Social Care (Community Health Standards) Act 2003.
5 Schedule 5, para 2(1) of the NHS Act 2006.
6 Corporate governance and the financial crisis. Organisation for Economic Co-operation and Development. Paris. OECD. 2009.

7   Note: Some NHS bodies, notably Primary Care Trusts, are also statutorily required to have a Professional Executive Committee. Primary Care Trust (executive Committee and Standing Financial Instructions) Directions 2007, National Health Service Act 2006.
8   There are interesting lessons on the need for risk committees emerging from the banking crises of 2008. See Walker D. A review of corporate governance in UK banks and other financial industry entities. London. 2009.
9   Baker GR, Denis J-L, Pomey M-P, MacIntosh-Murray A. Effective governance for quality and patient safety in Canadian Healthcare organizations: a report to the Canadian Health Services Research Foundation and the Canadian Patient Safety Institute. Ottawa: 2009.
10 Literature review for The Healthy NHS Board, February 2009.
11 The Intelligent Board. Dr Foster Intelligence. 2006.
12 The Intelligent Commissioning Board. London. Dr Foster Intelligence. 2006.
13 The Intelligent Board 2009: commissioning to reduce inequalities. Dr Foster Intelligence. 2009.
14 The Intelligent Mental Health Board. Dr Foster Intelligence. 2007.
15 The Intelligent Ambulance Board, Dr Foster Intelligence, 2006.
16 See Section 242 of the NHS Act 2006 as amended.
17 MacLeod D, Clarke N. Engaging for success: enhancing performance through employee engagement. London: Crown. 2009.
18 Glasby J, Peck E. We have to stop meeting like this: the governance of inter-agency partnerships. London: Care Services Improvement Partnership. Integrated Care Network. 2006.
19 Your Statutory Duties. A reference guide for NHS Foundation Trust Governors, Monitor, October 2009.
20 Sonnenfeld, Professor Jeffrey. What Makes Great Boards Great. Harvard Business Review 2002.
21 The Freedom of Information Act 2000.
22 Code of Conduct. Code of Accountability in the NHS. Department of Health. July 2004.
23 Leading Together: Co-action and counteraction in Chair-Chief Executive relationships. NHS Institute August 2009.
24 Role of Company Secretary. Institute of Chartered Secretaries and Administrators. http://www.icsa.org.uk.
25 Good Governance Standard for Public Services. Independent Commission on Good Governance in Public Services. January 2005.
26 Audit Commission website. http://www.audit-commission.gov.uk/aboutus/strategic objectives/governanceaccountability/Pages/Default.aspx. Visited December 2009.
27 Denis J-L, Champagne F, Pomey M-P, Préval J, Tré G. Toward a framework for the analysis of governance in healthcare organizations and systems. Ottawa: Canadian Council on Health Services Accreditation. 2005.
28 Carver J. Carver's Policy Governance(r) Model in Nonprofit Organizations. Gouvernance: Revue Internationale. 2001. 2(1)
29 Chait R, Ryan W, Taylor B. Governance as leadership: Reframing the work of nonprofit boards: Wiley. 2005.

APPENDIX 4

FRC Guidance on Board Effectiveness

March 2011

1. THE ROLE OF THE BOARD AND DIRECTORS

An effective board

1.1. The board's role is to provide entrepreneurial leadership of the company within a framework of prudent and effective controls which enables risk to be assessed and managed.

1.2. An effective board develops and promotes its collective vision of the company's purpose, its culture, its values and the behaviours it wishes to promote in conducting its business. In particular it:

- provides direction for management;
- demonstrates ethical leadership, displaying – and promoting throughout the company – behaviours consistent with the culture and values it has defined for the organisation;
- creates a performance culture that drives value creation without exposing the company to excessive risk of value destruction;
- makes well-informed and high-quality decisions based on a clear line of sight into the business;
- creates the right framework for helping directors meet their statutory duties under the Companies Act 2006, and/or other relevant statutory and regulatory regimes;
- is accountable, particularly to those that provide the company's capital; and
- thinks carefully about its governance arrangements and embraces evaluation of their effectiveness.

1.3. An effective board should not necessarily be a comfortable place. Challenge, as well as teamwork, is an essential feature. Diversity in board composition is an important driver of a board's effectiveness – creating a breadth of perspective among directors, and breaking down a tendency towards 'group think'.

The role of the chairman

1.4. Good boards are created by good chairmen. The chairman creates the conditions for overall board and individual director effectiveness.

1.5. The chairman should demonstrate the highest standards of integrity and probity, and set clear expectations concerning the company's culture, values and behaviours, and the style and tone of board discussions.

1.6. The chairman, with the help of the executive directors and the company secretary, sets the agenda for the board's deliberations.

1.7. The chairman's role includes:

- demonstrating ethical leadership;
- setting a board agenda which is primarily focused on strategy, performance, value creation and accountability, and ensuring that issues relevant to these areas are reserved for board decision;
- ensuring a timely flow of high-quality supporting information;

- making certain that the board determines the nature, and extent, of the significant risks the company is willing to embrace in the implementation of its strategy, and that there are no 'no go' areas which prevent directors from operating effective oversight in this area;
- regularly considering succession planning and the composition of the board;
- making certain that the board has effective decision-making processes and applies sufficient challenge to major proposals;
- ensuring the board's committees are properly structured with appropriate terms of reference;
- encouraging all board members to engage in board and committee meetings by drawing on their skills, experience, knowledge and, where appropriate, independence;
- fostering relationships founded on mutual respect and open communication – both in and outside the boardroom – between the non-executive directors and the executive team;
- developing productive working relationships with all executive directors, and the CEO in particular, providing support and advice while respecting executive responsibility;
- consulting the senior independent director on board matters in accordance with the code;
- taking the lead on issues of director development, including through induction programmes for new directors and regular reviews with all directors;
- acting on the results of board evaluation;
- being aware of, and responding to, his or her own development needs, including people and other skills, especially when taking on the role for the first time; and
- ensuring effective communication with shareholders and other stakeholders and, in particular, that all directors are made aware of the views of those who provide the company's capital.

1.8. The chairman of each board committee fulfils an important leadership role similar to that of the chairman of the board, particularly in creating the conditions for overall committee and individual director effectiveness.

The role of the senior independent director

1.9. In normal times the senior independent director should act as a sounding board for the chairman, providing support for the chairman in the delivery of his or her objectives, and leading the evaluation of the chairman on behalf of the other directors, as set out in the code. The senior independent director might also take responsibility for an orderly succession process for the chairman.

1.10. When the board is undergoing a period of stress, however, the senior independent director's role becomes critically important. He or she is expected to work with the chairman and other directors, and/or shareholders, to resolve significant issues. Boards should ensure they have a clear understanding of when the senior independent director might intervene in order to maintain board and company stability. Examples might include where:
- there is a dispute between the chairman and CEO;
- shareholders or non-executive directors have expressed concerns that are not being addressed by the chairman or CEO;
- the strategy being followed by the chairman and CEO is not supported by the entire board;
- the relationship between the chairman and CEO is particularly close, and decisions are being made without the approval of the full board; or
- succession planning is being ignored.

1.11. These issues should be considered when defining the role of the senior independent director, which should be set out in writing.

The role of executive directors

1.12. Executive directors have the same duties as other members of a unitary board. These duties extend to the whole of the business, and not just that part of it covered by their individual executive roles. Nor should executive directors see themselves only as members of the CEO's executive team when engaged in board business. Taking the wider view can help achieve the advantage of a unitary system: greater knowledge, involvement and commitment at the point of decision. The chairman should make certain that executives are aware of their wider responsibilities when joining the board, and ensure they receive appropriate induction, and regular training, to enable them to fulfil the role. Executive directors are also likely to be able to broaden their understanding of their board responsibilities if they take up a non-executive director position on another board.

1.13. The CEO is the most senior executive director on the board with responsibility for proposing strategy to the board, and for delivering the strategy as agreed. The CEO's relationship with the chairman is a key relationship that can help the board be more effective. The code states that the differing responsibilities of the chairman and the CEO should be set out in writing and agreed by the board. Particular attention should be paid to areas of potential overlap.

1.14. The CEO has, with the support of the executive team, primary responsibility for setting an example to the company's employees, and communicating to them the expectations of the board in relation to the company's culture, values and behaviours. The CEO is responsible for supporting the chairman to make certain that appropriate standards of governance permeate through all parts of the organisation. The CEO will make certain that the board is made aware, when appropriate, of the views of employees on issues of relevance to the business.

1.15. The CEO will ensure the board knows the executive directors' views on business issues in order to improve the standard of discussion in the boardroom and, prior to final decision on an issue, explain in a balanced way any divergence of view in the executive team.

1.16. The CFO has a particular responsibility to deliver high-quality information to the board on the financial position of the company.

1.17. Executive directors have the most intimate knowledge of the company and its capabilities when developing and presenting proposals, and when exercising judgement, particularly on matters of strategy. They should appreciate that constructive challenge from non-executive directors is an essential aspect of good governance, and should encourage their non-executive colleagues to test their proposals in the light of the non-executives' wider experience outside the company. The chairman and the CEO should ensure that this process is properly followed.

The role of non-executive directors

1.18. A non-executive director should, on appointment, devote time to a comprehensive, formal and tailored induction which should extend beyond the boardroom. Initiatives such as partnering a non-executive director with an executive board member may speed up the process of him or her acquiring an understanding of the main areas of business activity, especially areas involving significant risk. The director should expect to visit, and talk with, senior and middle managers in these areas.

1.19. Non-executive directors should devote time to developing and refreshing their knowledge and skills, including those of communication, to ensure that they continue to make a positive contribution to the board. Being well-informed about the company, and having a strong command of the issues relevant to the business, will generate the respect of the other directors.

1.20. Non-executive directors need to make sufficient time available to discharge their responsibilities effectively. The letter of appointment should state the minimum time that the non-executive director will be required to spend on the company's business, and seek the individual's confirmation that he or she can devote that amount of time to the role, consistent with other commitments. The letter should also indicate the possibility of additional time commitment when the company is undergoing a period of particularly increased activity, such as an acquisition or takeover, or as a result of some major difficulty with one or more of its operations.

1.21. Non-executive directors have a responsibility to uphold high standards of integrity and probity. They should support the chairman and executive directors in instilling the appropriate culture, values and behaviours in the boardroom and beyond.

1.22. Non-executive directors should insist on receiving high-quality information sufficiently in advance so that there can be thorough consideration of the issues prior to, and informed debate and challenge at, board meetings. High-quality information is that which is appropriate for making decisions on the issue at hand – it should be accurate, clear, comprehensive, up-to-date and timely; contain a summary of the contents of any paper; and inform the director of what is expected of him or her on that issue.

1.23. Non-executive directors should take into account the views of shareholders and other stakeholders, because these views may provide different perspectives on the company and its performance.

2. BOARD SUPPORT AND THE ROLE OF THE COMPANY SECRETARY

2.1. The requirement for a company secretary of a public company is specified in section 271 of the Companies Act 2006. The obligations and responsibilities of the company secretary outlined in the Act, and also in the code, necessitate him or her playing a leading role in the good governance of the company by supporting the chairman and helping the board and its committees to function efficiently.

2.2. The company secretary should report to the chairman on all board governance matters. This does not preclude the company secretary also reporting to the CEO in relation to his or her other executive management responsibilities. The appointment and removal of the company secretary should be a matter for the board as a whole, and the remuneration of the company secretary might be determined by the remuneration committee.

2.3. The company secretary should ensure the presentation of high-quality information to the board and its committees. The company secretary can also add value by fulfilling, or procuring the fulfilment of, other requirements of the code on behalf of the chairman, in particular director induction and development. This should be in a manner that is appropriate to the particular director, and which has the objective of enhancing that director's effectiveness in the board or board committees, consistent with the results of the board's evaluation processes. The chairman and the company secretary should periodically review whether the board and the company's other governance processes, for example board and committee evaluation, are fit for purpose, and consider any improvements or initiatives that could strengthen the governance of the company.

2.4. The company secretary's effectiveness can be enhanced by his or her ability to build relationships of mutual trust with the chairman, the senior independent director and the non-executive directors, while maintaining the confidence of executive director colleagues.

3. DECISION MAKING

3.1. Well-informed and high-quality decision making is a critical requirement for a board to be effective and does not happen by accident. Flawed decisions can be made with the best of intentions, with competent individuals believing passionately that they are making a sound judgment, when they are not. Many of the factors which lead to poor decision making are predictable and preventable. Boards can minimise the risk of poor decisions by investing time in the design of their decision-making policies and processes, including the contribution of committees.

3.2. Good decision-making capability can be facilitated by:

- high-quality board documentation;
- obtaining expert opinions when necessary;

- allowing time for debate and challenge, especially for complex, contentious or business-critical issues;
- achieving timely closure; and
- providing clarity on the actions required, and timescales and responsibilities.

3.3. Boards should be aware of factors which can limit effective decision making, such as:

- a dominant personality or group of directors on the board, which can inhibit contribution from other directors;
- insufficient attention to risk, and treating risk as a compliance issue rather than as part of the decision-making process – especially cases where the level of risk involved in a project could endanger the stability and sustainability of the business itself;
- failure to recognise the value implications of running the business on the basis of self-interest and other poor ethical standards;
- a reluctance to involve non-executive directors, or of matters being brought to the board for sign-off rather than debate;
- complacent or intransigent attitudes;
- a weak organisational culture; or
- inadequate information or analysis.

3.4. Most complex decisions depend on judgment, but the judgment of even the most well intentioned and experienced leaders can, in certain circumstances, be distorted. Some factors known to distort judgment in decision making are conflicts of interest, emotional attachments, and inappropriate reliance on previous experience and previous decisions. For significant decisions, therefore, a board may wish to consider extra steps, for example:

- describing in board papers the process that has been used to arrive at and challenge the proposal prior to presenting it to the board, thereby allowing directors not involved in the project to assess the appropriateness of the process as a precursor to assessing the merits of the project itself; or
- where appropriate, putting in place additional safeguards to reduce the risk of distorted judgements by, for example, commissioning an independent report, seeking advice from an expert, introducing a devil's advocate to provide challenge, establishing a sole purpose sub-committee, or convening additional meetings. Some chairmen favour separate discussions for important decisions; for example, concept, proposal for discussion, proposal for decision. This gives executive directors more opportunity to put the case at the earlier stages, and all directors the opportunity to share concerns or challenge assumptions well in advance of the point of decision.

3.5. Boards can benefit from reviewing past decisions, particularly ones with poor outcomes. A review should not focus just on the merits of the decision itself but also on the decision-making process.

4. BOARD COMPOSITION AND SUCCESSION PLANNING

4.1. Appointing directors who are able to make a positive contribution is one of the key elements of board effectiveness. Directors will be more likely to make good decisions and maximise the opportunities for the company's success in the longer term if the right skill-sets are present in the boardroom. This includes the appropriate range and balance of skills, experience, knowledge and independence. Non-executive directors should possess critical skills of value to the board and relevant to the challenges facing the company.

4.2. The nomination committee, usually led by the chairman, should be responsible for board recruitment. The process should be continuous and proactive, and should take into account the company's agreed strategic priorities. The aim should be to secure a boardroom which achieves the right balance between challenge and teamwork, and fresh input and thinking, while maintaining a cohesive board.

4.3. It is important to consider a diversity of personal attributes among board candidates, including: intellect, critical assessment and judgement, courage, openness, honesty and tact; and the ability to listen, forge relationships and develop trust. Diversity of psychological type, background and gender is important to ensure that a board is not composed solely of like-minded individuals. A board requires directors who have the intellectual capability to suggest change to a proposed strategy, and to promulgate alternatives.

4.4. Given the importance of committees in many companies' decision-making structures, it will be important to recruit non-executives with the necessary technical skills and knowledge relating to the committees' subject matter, as well as the potential to assume the role of committee chairman.

4.5. The chairman's vision for achieving the optimal board composition will help the nomination committee review the skills required, identify the gaps, develop transparent appointment criteria and inform succession planning. The nomination committee should periodically assess whether the desired outcome has been achieved, and propose changes to the process as necessary.

4.6. Executive directors may be recruited from external sources, but companies should also develop internal talent and capability. Initiatives might include middle management development programmes, facilitating engagement from time to time with non-executive directors, and partnering and mentoring schemes.

4.7. Good board appointments do not depend only on the nomination committee. A prospective director should carry out sufficient due diligence to understand the company, appreciate the time commitment involved, and assess the likelihood that he or she will be able to make a positive contribution.

5. EVALUATING THE PERFORMANCE OF THE BOARD AND DIRECTORS

5.1. Boards continually need to monitor and improve their performance. This can be achieved through board evaluation, which provides a powerful and valuable feedback mechanism for improving board effectiveness, maximising strengths and highlighting areas for further development. The evaluation process should aim to be objective and rigorous.

5.2. Like induction and board development, evaluation should be bespoke in its formulation and delivery. The chairman has overall responsibility for the process, and should select an appropriate approach and act on its outcome. The senior independent director should lead the process which evaluates the performance of the chairman. Chairs of board committees should also be responsible for the evaluation of their committees.

5.3. The outcome of a board evaluation should be shared with the whole board and fed back, as appropriate, into the board's work on composition, the design of induction and development programmes, and other relevant areas. It may be useful for a company to have a review loop to consider how effective the board evaluation process has been.

5.4. The code recommends that FTSE350 companies have externally-facilitated board evaluations at least every three years. External facilitation can add value by introducing a fresh perspective and new ways of thinking. It may also be useful in particular circumstances, such as when there has been a change of chairman, there is a known problem around the board table requiring tactful handling, or there is an external perception that the board is, or has been, ineffective.

5.5. Whether facilitated externally or internally, evaluations should explore how effective the board is as a unit, as well as the effectiveness of the contributions made by individual directors. Some areas which may be considered, although they are neither prescriptive nor exhaustive, include:

- the mix of skills, experience, knowledge and diversity on the board, in the context of the challenges facing the company;
- clarity of, and leadership given to, the purpose, direction and values of the company;
- succession and development plans;
- how the board works together as a unit, and the tone set by the chairman and the CEO;

- key board relationships, particularly chairman/CEO, chairman/senior independent director, chairman/company secretary and executive/non-executive;
- effectiveness of individual non-executive and executive directors;
- clarity of the senior independent director's role;
- effectiveness of board committees, and how they are connected with the main board;
- quality of the general information provided on the company and its performance;
- quality of papers and presentations to the board;
- quality of discussions around individual proposals;
- process the chairman uses to ensure sufficient debate for major decisions or contentious issues;
- effectiveness of the secretariat;
- clarity of the decision processes and authorities;
- processes for identifying and reviewing risks; and
- how the board communicates with, and listens and responds to, shareholders and other stakeholders.

6. AUDIT, RISK AND REMUNERATION

6.1. While the board may make use of committees to assist its consideration of audit, risk and remuneration, it retains responsibility for, and makes the final decisions on, all of these areas. The chairman should ensure that sufficient time is allowed at the board for discussion of these issues. All directors should familiarise themselves with the associated provisions of the UK Corporate Governance Code and its related guidance, and any relevant regulatory requirements.

6.2. Sufficient time should be allowed after committee meetings for them to report to the board on the nature and content of discussion, on recommendations, and on actions to be taken. The minutes of committee meetings should be circulated to all board members, unless it would be inappropriate to do so, and to the company secretary (if he or she is not secretary to the committee). The remit of each committee, and the processes of interaction between committees and between each committee and the board, should be reviewed regularly.

7. RELATIONS WITH SHAREHOLDERS

7.1. Communication of a company's governance presents an opportunity for the company to improve the quality of the dialogue with its shareholders and other stakeholders, generating greater levels of trust and confidence.

7.2. The Annual Report and Accounts is an important means of communicating with shareholders. It can also be used to provide well thought-out disclosures on the company's governance arrangements and the board evaluation exercise. Thinking about such disclosures can prompt the board to reflect on the quality of its governance, and what actions it might take to improve its structures, processes and systems.

7.3. The code emphasises the importance of continual communication with major shareholders, and of the AGM, as two aspects of a company's wider communications strategy. The chairman has a key role to play in representing the company to its principal audiences, and is encouraged to report personally about board leadership and effectiveness in the corporate governance statement in the annual report.

APPENDIX 5
FRC Guidance on Audit Committees

December 2010

1. Introduction

1.1. This guidance is designed to assist company boards in making suitable arrangements for their audit committees, and to assist directors serving on audit committees in carrying out their role. While boards are not required to follow this guidance, it is intended to assist them when implementing the relevant provisions of the UK Corporate Governance Code.

1.2. The paragraphs in bold are taken from the UK Corporate Governance Code (Section C3). Listed companies that do not comply with those provisions should include an explanation as to why they have not complied in the statement required by the Listing Rules.

1.3. Best practice requires that every board should consider in detail what arrangements for its audit committee are best suited for its particular circumstances. Audit committee arrangements need to be proportionate to the task, and will vary according to the size, complexity and risk profile of the company.

1.4. While all directors have a duty to act in the interests of the company the audit committee has a particular role, acting independently from the executive, to ensure that the interests of shareholders are properly protected in relation to financial reporting and internal control.

1.5. Nothing in the guidance should be interpreted as a departure from the principle of the unitary board. All directors remain equally responsible for the company's affairs as a matter of law. The audit committee, like other committees to which particular responsibilities are delegated (such as the remuneration committee), remains a committee of the board. Any disagreement within the board, including disagreement between the audit committee's members and the rest of the board, should be resolved at board level.

1.6. The code provides that a separate section of the annual report should describe the work of the committee. This deliberately puts the spotlight on the audit committee and gives it an authority that it might otherwise lack. This is not incompatible with the principle of the unitary board.

1.7. The guidance contains recommendations about the conduct of the audit committee's relationship with the board, with the executive management and with internal and external auditors. However, the most important features of this relationship cannot be drafted as guidance or put into a code of practice: a frank, open working relationship and a high level of mutual respect are essential, particularly between the audit committee chairman and the board chairman, the chief executive and the finance director. The audit committee must be prepared to take a robust stand, and all parties must be prepared to make information freely available to the audit committee, to listen to their views and to talk through the issues openly.

1.8 In particular, the management is under an obligation to ensure the audit committee is kept properly informed, and should take the initiative in supplying information rather than waiting to be asked. The board should make it clear to all directors and staff that they must cooperate with the audit committee and provide it with any information it requires. In addition, executive board members will have regard to their duty to provide all directors, including those on the audit committee, with all the information they need to discharge their responsibilities as directors of the company.

1.9. Many of the core functions of audit committees set out in this guidance are expressed in terms of 'oversight', 'assessment' and 'review' of a particular function. It is not the duty of audit committees to carry out functions that properly belong to others, such as the company's management in the preparation of the financial statements or the auditors in the planning or conducting of audits. To do so could undermine the responsibility of management and auditors. Audit committees should, for example, satisfy themselves that there is a proper system and allocation of responsibilities for the day-to-day monitoring of financial controls but they should not seek to do the monitoring themselves.

1.10. However, the high-level oversight function may lead to detailed work. The audit committee must intervene if there are signs that something may be seriously amiss. For example, if the audit committee is uneasy about the explanations of management and auditors about a particular financial reporting policy decision, there may be no alternative but to grapple with the detail and perhaps to seek independent advice.

1.11. Under this guidance, audit committees have wide-ranging, time-consuming and sometimes intensive work to do. Companies need to make the necessary resources available. This includes suitable payment for the members of audit committees themselves. They – and particularly the audit committee chairman – bear a significant responsibility and they need to commit a significant extra amount of time to the job. Companies also need to make provision for induction and training for new audit committee members and continuing training as may be required.

1.12. This guidance applies to all companies to which the code applies – i.e. companies with a Premium Listing of equity shares. For groups, it will usually be necessary for the audit committee of the parent company to review issues that relate to particular subsidiaries or activities carried on by the group. Consequently, the board of a UK-listed parent company should ensure that there is adequate cooperation within the group (and with internal and external auditors of individual companies within the group) to enable the parent company audit committee to discharge its responsibilities effectively.

2. Establishment and role of the audit committee; membership, procedures and resources

Establishment and role

2.1 The board should establish an audit committee of at least three, or in the case of smaller companies two, members.

2.2 The main role and responsibilities of the audit committee should be set out in written terms of reference and should include:

- to monitor the integrity of the financial statements of the company and any formal announcements relating to the company's financial performance, reviewing significant financial reporting judgements contained in them;
- to review the company's internal financial controls and, unless expressly addressed by a separate board risk committee composed of independent directors or by the board itself, the company's internal control and risk management systems;
- to monitor and review the effectiveness of the company's internal audit function;
- to make recommendations to the board, for it to put to the shareholders for their approval in general meeting, in relation to the appointment of the external auditor and to approve the remuneration and terms of engagement of the external auditor;
- to review and monitor the external auditor's independence and objectivity and the effectiveness of the audit process, taking into consideration relevant UK professional and regulatory requirements;

- to develop and implement policy on the engagement of the external auditor to supply non-audit services, taking into account relevant ethical guidance regarding the provision of non-audit services by the external audit firm;

and to report to the board, identifying any matters in respect of which it considers that action or improvement is needed, and making recommendations as to the steps to be taken.

Membership and appointment

2.3 The board should establish an audit committee of at least three, or in the case of smaller companies two, independent non-executive directors. In smaller companies the company chairman may be a member of, but not chair, the committee in addition to the independent non-executive directors, provided he or she was considered independent on appointment as chairman. The board should satisfy itself that at least one member of the audit committee has recent and relevant financial experience.

2.4 Appointments to the audit committee should be made by the board on the recommendation of the nomination committee (where there is one), in consultation with the audit committee chairman.

2.5 Appointments should be for a period of up to three years, extendable by no more than two additional three-year periods, so long as members continue to be independent.

Meetings of the audit committee

2.6 It is for the audit committee chairman, in consultation with the company secretary, to decide the frequency and timing of its meetings. There should be as many meetings as the audit committee's role and responsibilities require. It is recommended there should be not fewer than three meetings during the year, held to coincide with key dates within the financial reporting and audit cycle[1]. However, most audit committee chairmen will wish to call more frequent meetings.

2.7 No one other than the audit committee's chairman and members is entitled to be present at a meeting of the audit committee. It is for the audit committee to decide if non-members should attend for a particular meeting or a particular agenda item. It is to be expected that the external audit lead partner will be invited regularly to attend meetings as well as the finance director. Others may be invited to attend.

2.8 Sufficient time should be allowed to enable the audit committee to undertake as full a discussion as may be required. A sufficient interval should be allowed between audit committee meetings and main board meetings to allow any work arising from the audit committee meeting to be carried out and reported to the board as appropriate.

2.9 The audit committee should, at least annually, meet the external and internal auditors, without management, to discuss matters relating to its remit and any issues arising from the audit.

2.10 Formal meetings of the audit committee are the heart of its work.

However, they will rarely be sufficient. It is expected that the audit committee chairman, and to a lesser extent the other members, will wish to keep in touch on a continuing basis with the key people involved in the company's governance, including the board chairman, the chief executive, the finance director, the external audit lead partner and the head of internal audit.

Resources

2.11 The audit committee should be provided with sufficient resources to undertake its duties.

2.12 The audit committee should have access to the services of the company secretariat on all audit committee matters including: assisting the chairman in planning the audit committee's work, drawing up meeting agendas, maintenance of minutes, drafting of material about its activities for the annual report, collection and distribution of information and provision of any necessary practical support.

2.13 The company secretary should ensure that the audit committee receives information and papers in a timely manner to enable full and proper consideration to be given to the issues.

2.14 The board should make funds available to the audit committee to enable it to take independent legal, accounting or other advice when the audit committee reasonably believes it necessary to do so.

Remuneration

2.15 In addition to the remuneration paid to all non-executive directors, each company should consider the further remuneration that should be paid to members of the audit committee to recompense them for the additional responsibilities of membership. Consideration should be given to the time members are required to give to audit committee business, the skills they bring to bear and the onerous duties they take on, as well as the value of their work to the company. The level of remuneration paid to the members of the audit committee should take into account the level of fees paid to other members of the board. The chairman's responsibilities and time demands will generally be heavier than the other members of the audit committee and this should be reflected in his or her remuneration.

Skills, experience and training

2.16 It is desirable that the committee member whom the board considers to have recent and relevant financial experience should have a professional qualification from one of the professional accountancy bodies. The need for a degree of financial literacy among the other members will vary according to the nature of the company, but experience of corporate financial matters will normally be required. The availability of appropriate financial expertise will be particularly important where the company's activities involve specialised financial activities.

2.17 The company should provide an induction programme for new audit committee members. This should cover the role of the audit committee, including its terms of reference and expected time commitment by members; and an overview of the company's business, identifying the main business and financial dynamics and risks. It could also include meeting some of the company staff.

2.18 Training should also be provided to members of the audit committee on an ongoing and timely basis and should include an understanding of the principles of and developments in financial reporting and related company law. In appropriate cases, it may also include, for example, understanding financial statements, applicable accounting standards and recommended practice; the regulatory framework for the company's business; the role of internal and external auditing and risk management.

2.19 The induction programme and ongoing training may take various forms, including attendance at formal courses and conferences, internal company talks and seminars, and briefings by external advisers.

3. Relationship with the board

3.1 The role of the audit committee is for the board to decide and to the extent that the audit committee undertakes tasks on behalf of the board, the results should be reported to, and considered by, the board. In doing so it should identify any matters in respect of which it considers that action or improvement is needed, and make recommendations as to the steps to be taken.

3.2 The terms of reference should be tailored to the particular circumstances of the company.

3.3 The audit committee should review annually its terms of reference and its own effectiveness and recommend any necessary changes to the board.

3.4 The board should review the audit committee's effectiveness annually.

3.5 Where there is disagreement between the audit committee and the board, adequate time should be made available for discussion of the issue with a view to resolving the disagreement. Where any such disagreements cannot be resolved, the audit committee should have the right to report the issue to the shareholders as part of the report on its activities in the annual report.

4. Role and responsibilities

Financial reporting

4.1 The audit committee should review the significant financial reporting issues and judgements made in connection with the preparation of the company's financial statements, interim reports, preliminary announcements and related formal statements.

4.2 It is management's, not the audit committee's, responsibility to prepare complete and accurate financial statements and disclosures in accordance with financial reporting standards and applicable rules and regulations. However the audit committee should consider significant accounting policies, any changes to them and any significant estimates and judgements. The management should inform the audit committee of the methods used to account for significant or unusual transactions where the accounting treatment is open to different approaches. Taking into account the external auditor's view, the audit committee should consider whether the company has adopted appropriate accounting policies and, where necessary, made appropriate estimates and judgements. The audit committee should review the clarity and completeness of disclosures in the financial statements and consider whether the disclosures made are set properly in context.

4.3 Where, following its review, the audit committee is not satisfied with any aspect of the proposed financial reporting by the company, it shall report its views to the board.

4.4 The audit committee should review related information presented with the financial statements, including the operating and financial review, and corporate governance statements relating to the audit and to risk management. Similarly, where board approval is required for other statements containing financial information (for example, summary financial statements, significant financial returns to regulators and release of price sensitive information), whenever practicable (without being inconsistent with any requirement for prompt reporting under the Listing Rules) the audit committee should review such statements first.

Internal controls and risk management systems

4.5 The audit committee should review the company's internal financial controls (that is, the systems established to identify, assess, manage and monitor financial risks); and unless expressly addressed by a separate board risk committee comprised of independent directors or by the board itself, the company's internal control and risk management systems.

4.6 The company's management is responsible for the identification, assessment, management and monitoring of risk, for developing, operating and monitoring the system of internal control and for providing assurance to the board that it has done so. Except where the board or a risk committee is expressly responsible for reviewing the effectiveness of the internal control and risk management systems, the audit committee should receive reports from management on the effectiveness of the systems they have established and the conclusions of any testing carried out by internal and external auditors.

4.7 Except to the extent that this is expressly dealt with by the board or risk committee, the audit committee should review and approve the statements included in the annual report in relation to internal control and the management of risk.

4.8 If the external auditor is being considered to undertake aspects of the internal audit function, the audit committee should consider the effect this may have on the effectiveness of the company's overall arrangements for internal control and investor perceptions in this regard. Investor perceptions are likely to be influenced by:

- the rationale set out in the annual report for the work being performed by the external auditor;
- the nature and extent of the work performed by the external auditor;
- how the independence and objectivity of the external auditor and internal audit function have been safeguarded; and
- whether, in the absence of internal audit work, the audit committee is wholly reliant on the views of the external auditor about the effectiveness of its system of controls relating to core activities and significant locations.

Whistleblowing

4.9 The audit committee should review arrangements by which staff of the company may, in confidence, raise concerns about possible improprieties in matters of financial reporting or other matters. The audit committee's objective should be to ensure that arrangements are in place for the proportionate and independent investigation of such matters and for appropriate follow-up action.

The internal audit process

4.10 The audit committee should monitor and review the effectiveness of the company's internal audit function. Where there is no internal audit function, the audit committee should consider annually whether there is a need for an internal audit function and make a recommendation to the board, and the reasons for the absence of such a function should be explained in the relevant section of the annual report.

4.11 The need for an internal audit function will vary depending on company specific factors including the scale, diversity and complexity of the company's activities and the number of employees, as well as cost/benefit considerations. Senior management and the board may desire objective assurance and advice on risk and control. An adequately resourced internal audit function (or its equivalent where, for example, a third party is contracted to perform some or all of the work concerned) may provide such assurance and advice. There may be other functions within the company that also provide assurance and advice covering specialist areas such as health and safety, regulatory and legal compliance and environmental issues.

4.12 When undertaking its assessment of the need for an internal audit function, the audit committee should also consider whether there are any trends or current factors relevant to the company's activities, markets or other aspects of its external environment, that have increased, or are expected to increase, the risks faced by the company. Such an increase in risk may also arise from internal factors such as organisational restructuring or from changes in reporting processes or underlying information systems. Other matters to be taken into account may include adverse trends evident from the monitoring of internal control systems or an increased incidence of unexpected occurrences.

4.13 In the absence of an internal audit function, management needs to apply other monitoring processes in order to assure itself, the audit committee and the board that the system of internal control is functioning as intended. In these circumstances, the audit committee will need to assess whether such processes provide sufficient and objective assurance.

4.14 The audit committee should review and approve the internal audit function's remit, having regard to the complementary roles of the internal and external audit functions. The audit committee should ensure that the function has the necessary resources and access to information to enable it to fulfil its mandate, and is equipped to perform in accordance with appropriate professional standards for internal auditors[2].

4.15 The audit committee should approve the appointment or termination of appointment of the head of internal audit.

4.16 In its review of the work of the internal audit function, the audit committee should, inter alia:

- ensure that the internal auditor has direct access to the board chairman and to the audit committee and is accountable to the audit committee;
- review and assess the annual internal audit work plan;
- receive a report on the results of the internal auditors' work on a periodic basis;
- review and monitor management's responsiveness to the internal auditor's findings and recommendations;
- meet with the head of internal audit at least once a year without the presence of management; and
- monitor and assess the role and effectiveness of the internal audit function in the overall context of the company's risk management system.

The external audit process

4.17 The audit committee is the body responsible for overseeing the company's relations with the external auditor.

Appointment

4.18 The audit committee should have primary responsibility for making a recommendation on the appointment, reappointment and removal of the external auditors. If the board does not accept the audit committee's recommendation, it should include in the annual report, and in any papers recommending appointment or reappointment, a statement from the audit committee explaining its recommendation and should set out reasons why the board has taken a different position.

4.19 The audit committee's recommendation to the board should be based on the assessments referred to below. If the audit committee recommends considering the selection of possible new appointees as external auditors, it should oversee the selection process.

4.20 The audit committee should assess annually the qualification, expertise and resources, and independence (see paragraph 4.27 below) of the external auditors and the effectiveness of the audit process. The assessment should cover all aspects of the audit service provided by the audit firm, and include obtaining a report on the audit firm's own internal quality control procedures and consideration of audit firms' annual transparency reports, where available. It might also be appropriate for the audit committee to consider whether there might be any benefit in using firms from more than one audit network[3].

4.21 If the external auditor resigns, the audit committee should investigate the issues giving rise to such resignation and consider whether any action is required.

4.22 The audit committee should consider the need to include the risk of the withdrawal of their auditor from the market in their risk evaluation and planning.

4.23 The audit committee section of the annual report should explain to shareholders how it reached its recommendation to the board on the appointment, reappointment or removal of the external auditors. This explanation should normally include supporting information on tendering frequency, the tenure of the incumbent auditor, and any contractual obligations that acted to restrict the audit committee's choice of external auditors.

Terms and Remuneration

4.24 The audit committee should approve the terms of engagement and the remuneration to be paid to the external auditor in respect of audit services provided.

4.25 The audit committee should review and agree the engagement letter issued by the external auditor at the start of each audit, ensuring that it has been updated to reflect changes in circumstances arising since the previous year. The scope of the external audit should be reviewed by the audit committee with the auditor. If the audit committee is not satisfied as to its adequacy it should arrange for additional work to be undertaken.

4.26 The audit committee should satisfy itself that the level of fee payable in respect of the audit services provided is appropriate and that an effective audit can be conducted for such a fee.

Independence, including the provision of non-audit services

4.27 The audit committee should assess the independence and objectivity of the external auditor annually, taking into consideration relevant UK law, regulation and professional requirements. This assessment should involve a consideration of all relationships between the company and the audit firm (including the provision of non-audit services) and any safeguards established by the external auditor. The audit committee should consider whether, taken as a whole and having regard to the views, as appropriate, of the external auditor, management and internal audit, those relationships appear to impair the auditor's independence and objectivity.

4.28 The audit committee should seek reassurance that the auditors and their staff have no financial, business, employment or family and other personal relationship with the company which could adversely affect the auditor's independence and objectivity, taking account of relevant Ethical Standards. The audit committee should seek from the audit firm, on an annual basis, information about policies and processes for maintaining independence and monitoring compliance with relevant requirements, including current requirements regarding the rotation of audit partners and staff.

4.29 The audit committee should develop and recommend to the board the company's policy in relation to the provision of non-audit services by the auditor, and keep the policy under review. The audit committee's objective should be to ensure that the provision of such services does not impair the external auditor's independence or objectivity. In this context, the audit committee should consider:

- whether the skills and experience of the audit firm make it the most suitable supplier of the non-audit service;
- whether there are safeguards in place to eliminate or reduce to an acceptable level any threat to objectivity and independence in the conduct of the audit resulting from the provision of such services by the external auditor;
- the nature of the non-audit services;
- the fees incurred, or to be incurred, for non-audit services both for individual services and in aggregate, relative to the audit fee; and
- the criteria which govern the compensation of the individuals performing the audit.

4.30 The audit committee should set and apply a formal policy specifying the types of non-audit service (if any):

- for which the use of the external auditor is pre-approved (i.e. approval has been given in advance as a matter of policy, rather than the specific approval of an engagement being sought before it is contracted);
- for which specific approval from the audit committee is required before they are contracted; and
- from which the external auditor is excluded.

4.31 Pre-approval of the use of the external auditor may be appropriate where the threats to auditor independence are considered low, for example if the engagement is:

- routine in nature and the fee is not significant in the context of the audit fee; or
- for an audit related service.[4]

4.32 The non-audit services that fall within the second category in paragraph 4.30 above are likely to be those which, because of their size or nature or because of special terms and conditions (for example, contingent fee arrangements), are thought to give rise to threats to the auditor's independence. As a consequence, careful consideration will be needed when determining whether it is in the interests of the company that they should be purchased from the audit firm (rather than another supplier) and, if so, whether any safeguards to be put in place by the audit firm are likely to be effective.

4.33 In determining the policy, the audit committee should take into account the possible threats to auditor objectivity and independence[5] and APB Ethical Standards for Auditors regarding the provision of non-audit services by the external audit firm.

4.34 The audit committee should agree with the board the company's policy for the employment of former employees of the external auditor, taking into account the APB Ethical Standards for Auditors paying particular attention to the policy regarding former employees of the audit firm who were part of the audit team and moved directly to the company. The audit committee should monitor application of the policy, including the number of former employees of the external auditor currently employed in senior positions in the company, and consider whether in the light of this there has been any impairment, or appearance of impairment, of the auditor's independence and objectivity in respect of the audit.

4.35 The audit committee should monitor the external audit firm's compliance with APB Ethical Standards for Auditors relating to the rotation of audit partners, the level of fees that the company pays in proportion to the overall fee income of the firm, or relevant part of it[6], and other related regulatory requirements.

4.36 A degree of flexibility over the timing of rotation of the audit engagement partner is possible where the audit committee decides that it is necessary to safeguard the quality of the audit. In such circumstances, the audit engagement partner may continue in this position for an additional period of up to two years, so that no longer than seven years in total is spent in this position. The audit committee should disclose this fact and the reasons for it to the shareholders as early as practicable.

4.37 The annual report should explain to shareholders how, if the auditor provides non-audit services, auditor objectivity and independence is safeguarded.

4.38 The explanation should:

- describe the work of the committee in discharging its responsibilities;
- set out the audit committee's policy on the engagement of the external auditor to supply non-audit services in sufficient detail to describe each of the elements in paragraph 4.30, or cross-refer to where this information can be found on the company's website;
- set out, or cross refer to, the fees paid to the auditor for audit services, audit related services and other non-audit services[7]; and
- if the auditor provides non-audit services, other than audit related services, explain for each significant engagement, or category of engagements, what the services are, why the audit committee concluded that it was in the interests of the company to purchase them from the external auditor (rather than another supplier) and how auditor objectivity and independence has been safeguarded.

Annual audit cycle

4.39 At the start of each annual audit cycle, the audit committee should ensure that appropriate plans are in place for the audit.

4.40 The audit committee should consider whether the auditor's overall work plan, including planned levels of materiality, and proposed resources to execute the audit plan appears consistent with the scope of the audit engagement, having regard also to the seniority, expertise and experience of the audit team.

4.41 The audit committee should review, with the external auditors, the findings of their work. In the course of its review, the audit committee should:

- discuss with the external auditor major issues that arose during the course of the audit and have subsequently been resolved and those issues that have been left unresolved;
- review key accounting and audit judgements; and
- review levels of errors identified during the audit, obtaining explanations from management and, where necessary, the external auditors as to why certain errors might remain unadjusted.

4.42 The audit committee should also review the audit representation letters before signature by management and give particular consideration to matters where representation has been requested that relate to non-standard issues[8]. The audit committee should consider whether the information provided is complete and appropriate based on its own knowledge.

4.43 As part of the ongoing monitoring process, the audit committee should review the management letter (or equivalent). The audit committee should review and monitor management's responsiveness to the external auditor's findings and recommendations.

4.44 At the end of the annual audit cycle, the audit committee should assess the effectiveness of the audit process. In the course of doing so, the audit committee should:

- review whether the auditor has met the agreed audit plan and understand the reasons for any changes, including changes in perceived audit risks and the work undertaken by the external auditors to address those risks;
- consider the robustness and perceptiveness of the auditors in their handling of the key accounting and audit judgements identified and in responding to questions from the audit committees, and in their commentary where appropriate on the systems of internal control;
- obtain feedback about the conduct of the audit from key people involved, e.g. the finance director and the head of internal audit; and
- review and monitor the content of the external auditor's management letter, in order to assess whether it is based on a good understanding of the company's business and establish whether recommendations have been acted upon and, if not, the reasons why they have not been acted upon.

5. Communication with shareholders

5.1 The terms of reference of the audit committee, including its role and the authority delegated to it by the board, should be made available. A separate section in the annual report should describe the work of the committee in discharging those responsibilities.

5.2 The audit committee section should include, inter alia:

- a summary of the role of the audit committee;
- the names and qualifications of all members of the audit committee during the period;
- the number of audit committee meetings;
- a report on the way the audit committee has discharged its responsibilities; and
- the explanations provided for in paragraphs 4.23 and 4.37 above.

5.3 The chairman of the audit committee should be present at the AGM to answer questions, through the chairman of the board, on the report on the audit committee's activities and matters within the scope of the audit committee's responsibilities.

Notes:

1 For example, when the audit plans (internal and external) are available for review and when interim statements, preliminary announcements and the full annual report are near completion.

2 Further guidance can be found in the Chartered Institute of Internal Auditors' Code of Ethics and the International Standards for the Professional Practice of Internal Auditing.

3 Guidance on the considerations relevant to the use of firms from more than one audit network can be found in the Appendix.

4 Audit related services are those non-audit services specified as such in APB Ethical Standards for Auditors as including:

- reporting required by law or regulation to be provided by the auditor;
- reviews of interim financial information;
- reporting on regulatory returns;
- reporting to a regulator on client assets:
- reporting on government grants;
- reporting on internal financial controls when required by law or regulation; and
- extended work that is authorised by those charged with governance on financial information and/or financial controls performed where this work is integrated with the audit work and is performed on the same principal terms and conditions.

5 APB Ethical Standards for Auditors explain that threats to auditor objectivity and independence may arise from:

- Self-interest threats which arise when the auditor has financial or other interests which might cause it to be reluctant to take actions that would be adverse to the interests of the audit firm or any individual in a position to influence the conduct and outcome of the audit;
- Self-review threats which arise when the results of a non-audit service performed by the auditor or others within the firm are reflected in the amounts included or disclosed in the financial statements of the audited entity;
- Management threats which arise where partners and employees of the audit firm make judgments or take decisions on behalf of the management of the audited entity;
- Advocacy threats which arise when the audit firm undertakes work that involves acting as an advocate for an audited entity and supporting a position taken by management in an adversarial context;
- Familiarity threats which arise when the auditor is predisposed to accept or is insufficiently questioning of the audited entity's point of view; and
- Intimidation threats which arise when the auditor's conduct is influenced by fear or threats.

6 Where the audit firm's profits are not shared on a firm-wide basis, the relevant part of the firm is that by reference to which the audit engagement partner's profit share is calculated.

7 The statutory requirement for disclosure in the financial statements is contained in the Companies (Disclosure of Auditor Remuneration and Liability Limitation Agreements) Regulations 2008. A template for the provision of this information by the auditors to the audit committee is set out in Appendix A to Ethical Standard 1 issued by the Auditing Practices Board.

8 Further guidance can be found in the Auditing Practices Board's International Standard on Auditing (UK and Ireland) 580: 'Management Representations'.

Appendix

Revised guidance on use of firms from more than one network

Introduction

This guidance was produced in response to a recommendation made by the Markets Participants Group (MPG) that advised the FRC on the Choice in the Audit Market project.

The MPG recommended that: 'The FRC should provide independent guidance for audit committees and other market participants on considerations relevant to the use of firms from more than one network.'

The MPG intended that the guidance would provide audit committees of growing companies using non-Big Four firms with relevant factors they may wish to consider when their activities expand geographically beyond the perceived capacity of their existing firm.

More generally, it was expected that the guidance could also help audit committees to select auditors for individual components of the group financial statements based on how best to achieve audit quality for that particular component and for the group as a whole.

To assist users to compare different group audit arrangements, the guidance includes a description of considerations relevant to the use of firms from one audit network as well as those relevant to the use of firms from more than one network.

Drivers of audit quality for group audits

Under UK auditing standards, the group auditor has sole responsibility for the audit opinion on the group accounts, the group auditor cannot limit its responsibility by referring to the work of another firm.

For the group auditor's work to be effective there are key quality drivers that need to be in place, including:

- a well structured and efficient methodology;
- arrangements to safeguard auditor integrity, objective and independence;
- arrangements to ensure partners and staff understand their client's business and staff performing detailed 'on-site' audit work have sufficient experience;
- effective, understood and applied quality control procedures;
- effective communication between the group auditor and the parent company's audit committee covering the key risks identified and judgements made in reaching the group audit opinion.

Achieving each of these drivers on a group audit presents some challenges to the auditor where there are international components. The extent of this challenge will vary by group depending on factors that may include the:

- extent to which the group has international operations and subsidiary undertakings;
- countries and regions in which the group has international components;
- extent to which the components of the group transact with each other;
- diversity of the groups operations including the industries in which it operates;
- extent to which the finance function of the firm is centralised;
- extent to which the components require local statutory audits.

Use of firms from a single network

It is common practice to appoint one firm to audit the parent group and the consolidated group accounts. This firm then uses other firms from within its international network to carry out audit work on components that are needed for group audit purposes. It is common for the same firms to carry out statutory audits of subsidiaries where these are needed.

The 'single network' arrangement is common because firms from a single network may have:

- common audit methodology that is generally seen as well-structured, efficient and effective;
- effective inter-office communication arrangements;
- partners and staff in network firms internationally that understand the group's business and have staff available to perform detailed 'on-site' audit work with that experience;
- common quality control policies and monitoring arrangements across the network that are effective, understood and applied.

In assessing the use of firms from a single network, audit committees may wish to consider:

- Do each of the network's member firms that will be involved in the group audit have partners and staff that understand the group's business?
- Will each of the network's member firms select a staff with sufficient experience to perform detailed 'on-site' audit work?
- In considering the findings of each of the other firms from within its network, will the group auditor review the degree to which the firm has followed the network's common audit methodology and associated procedures?
- What quality checks and inspections are carried out by the network organisation on its member firms?
- What information is available to the group auditor on the results of these quality inspections and on any follow-up actions?

Use of firms from more than one network

In some circumstances it may be appropriate to use a firm from more than one network to achieve a high quality and cost-effective audit. The group would still appoint a single firm to audit the parent company and the group's consolidated financial statements. However, the group would agree with the group auditor that for some components the audit work that is needed for group audit purposes will be carried out by one or more firms from other networks.

However, where consideration is given to using firms from more than one network, groups should be mindful that the firm appointed to audit the parent company and group's consolidated financial statements must be able to demonstrate that they can satisfy the principal auditor requirements as set out in International Standards on Auditing (UK and Ireland) 600.

It is likely that the same firms will be used to carry out audits of subsidiaries where these are needed for local statutory purposes.

Groups for which this arrangement may be useful include:

- groups that consider their current auditor delivers high quality audits but have growing or new subsidiaries in locations not well served by their current auditor's network;
- groups wishing to give subsidiaries the option of which audit firm to use for local audits;
- groups wishing to have the flexibility to select the firms in each country with the most suitable capabilities to carry out audit work on the relevant subsidiary.

In assessing the use of firms from more than one network, audit committees may wish to consider:

- How will the group auditor assess the independence and professional competence of the firms from other networks?
- How the group auditor will ensure that they are familiar with the methodology of the other firms, in order to enable them to evaluate the audit evidence obtained?
- The arrangements the group auditor will make with different networks to ensure that they communicate effectively with each other.
- The overall costs and benefits associated with using firms from more than one network.
- What costs will be attached to the group auditor assessing firms from other networks evaluating audit evidence obtained by them and addressing any issues?

Use of joint auditors

This is a special case of use of firms from more than one audit network. The group appoints two firms who are expected to reach a single group audit opinion for which they are jointly responsible. Audit work that is needed for group audit purposes would normally be carried out by firms from the joint auditors' networks.

The groups may find this arrangement useful if they:

- have completed a merger and wish to maintain audit experience and knowledge by keeping the auditors involved in each of the merged entities;
- wish to have the benefits of an audit opinion from two firms;
- wish to reduce the scope for close relationships to build up with the auditor or for the auditor to become complacent;
- wish to facilitate the rotation of audit firms by maintaining audit knowledge and experience;
- wish to have a safeguard against the withdrawal from the market of their auditor.

In assessing the uses of joint auditors, audit committees may wish to consider:

- how effectively will the two joint auditors coordinate their work and cooperate with each other in reviewing findings?
- how effectively will the joint auditors ensure that all key issues are addressed?
- how effectively will the joint auditors conclude on highly judgemental matters?
- balancing the benefits of a joint opinion with the underlying costs.

APPENDIX 6

Guidance on internal control (The Turnbull Guidance)

October 2005

One – Introduction

The importance of internal control and risk management

1. A company's system of internal control has a key role in the management of risks that are significant to the fulfilment of its business objectives. A sound system of internal control contributes to safeguarding the shareholders' investment and the company's assets.

2. Internal control (as referred to in paragraph 19) facilitates the effectiveness and efficiency of operations, helps ensure the reliability of internal and external reporting and assists compliance with laws and regulations.

3. Effective financial controls, including the maintenance of proper accounting records, are an important element of internal control. They help ensure that the company is not unnecessarily exposed to avoidable financial risks and that financial information used within the business and for publication is reliable. They also contribute to the safeguarding of assets, including the prevention and detection of fraud.

4. A company's objectives, its internal organisation and the environment in which it operates are continually evolving and, as a result, the risks it faces are continually changing. A sound system of internal control therefore depends on a thorough and regular evaluation of the nature and extent of the risks to which the company is exposed. Since profits are, in part, the reward for successful risk-taking in business, the purpose of internal control is to help manage and control risk appropriately rather than to eliminate it.

Objectives of the guidance

5. This guidance is intended to:
   - reflect sound business practice whereby internal control is embedded in the business processes by which a company pursues its objectives;
   - remain relevant over time in the continually evolving business environment; and
   - enable each company to apply it in a manner which takes account of its particular circumstances.

   The guidance requires directors to exercise judgement in reviewing how the company has implemented the requirements of the Combined Code relating to internal control and reporting to shareholders thereon.

6. The guidance is based on the adoption by a company's board of a risk-based approach to establishing a sound system of internal control and reviewing its effectiveness. This should be incorporated by the company within its normal management and governance processes. It should not be treated as a separate exercise undertaken to meet regulatory requirements.

Internal control requirements of the Combined Code

7 Principle C.2 of the Code states that 'The board should maintain a sound system of internal control to safeguard shareholders' investment and the company's assets'.

8 Provision C.2.1 states that 'The directors should, at least annually, conduct a review of the effectiveness of the group's system of internal control and should report to shareholders that they have done so. The review should cover all material controls, including financial, operational and compliance controls and risk management systems'.

9 Paragraph 9.8.6 of the UK Listing Authority's Listing Rules states that in the case of a listed company incorporated in the United Kingdom, the following items must be included in its annual report and accounts:

- a statement of how the listed company has applied the principles set out in Section 1 of the Combined Code, in a manner that would enable shareholders to evaluate how the principles have been applied;
- a statement as to whether the listed company has:
    - complied throughout the accounting period with all relevant provisions set out in Section 1 of the Combined Code; or
    - not complied throughout the accounting period with all relevant provisions set out in Section 1 of the Combined Code and if so, setting out:
        (i) those provisions, if any, it has not complied with;
        (ii) in the case of provisions whose requirements are of a continuing nature, the period within which, if any, it did not comply with some or all of those provisions; and
        (iii) the company's reasons for non-compliance.

10 The Preamble to the code makes it clear that there is no prescribed form or content for the statement setting out how the various principles in the code have been applied. The intention is that companies should have a free hand to explain their governance policies in the light of the principles, including any special circumstances which have led to them adopting a particular approach.

11 The guidance in this document applies for accounting periods beginning on or after 1 January 2006, and should be followed by boards of listed companies in:

- assessing how the company has applied Code Principle C.2;
- implementing the requirements of Code Provision C.2.1; and
- reporting on these matters to shareholders in the annual report and accounts.

12 For the purposes of this guidance, internal controls considered by the board should include all types of controls including those of an operational and compliance nature, as well as internal financial controls.

Groups of companies

13 Throughout this guidance, where reference is made to 'company' it should be taken, where applicable, as referring to the group of which the reporting company is the parent company. For groups of companies, the review of effectiveness of internal control and the report to the shareholders should be from the perspective of the group as a whole.

The Appendix

14 The Appendix to this document contains questions which boards may wish to consider in applying this guidance.

Two – Maintaining a sound system of internal control

Responsibilities

15 The board of directors is responsible for the company's system of internal control. It should set appropriate policies on internal control and seek regular assurance that will enable it to satisfy itself that the system is functioning effectively. The board must further ensure that the system of internal control is effective in managing those risks in the manner which it has approved.

16 In determining its policies with regard to internal control, and thereby assessing what constitutes a sound system of internal control in the particular circumstances of the company, the board's deliberations should include consideration of the following factors:

- the nature and extent of the risks facing the company;
- the extent and categories of risk which it regards as acceptable for the company to bear;
- the likelihood of the risks concerned materialising;
- the company's ability to reduce the incidence and impact on the business of risks that do materialise; and
- the costs of operating particular controls relative to the benefit thereby obtained in managing the related risks.

17 It is the role of management to implement board policies on risk and control. In fulfilling its responsibilities management should identify and evaluate the risks faced by the company for consideration by the board and design, operate and monitor a suitable system of internal control which implements the policies adopted by the board.

18 All employees have some responsibility for internal control as part of their accountability for achieving objectives. They, collectively, should have the necessary knowledge, skills, information, and authority to establish, operate and monitor the system of internal control. This will require an understanding of the company, its objectives, the industries and markets in which it operates, and the risks it faces.

Elements of a sound system of internal control

19 An internal control system encompasses the policies, processes, tasks, behaviours and other aspects of a company that, taken together:

- facilitate its effective and efficient operation by enabling it to respond appropriately to significant business, operational, financial, compliance and other risks to achieving the company's objectives. This includes the safeguarding of assets from inappropriate use or from loss and fraud and ensuring that liabilities are identified and managed;
- help ensure the quality of internal and external reporting. This requires the maintenance of proper records and processes that generate a flow of timely, relevant and reliable information from within and outside the organisation;
- help ensure compliance with applicable laws and regulations, and also with internal policies with respect to the conduct of business.

20 A company's system of internal control will reflect its control environment which encompasses its organisational structure. The system will include:

- control activities;
- information and communications processes; and
- processes for monitoring the continuing effectiveness of the system of internal control.

21 The system of internal control should:

- be embedded in the operations of the company and form part of its culture;
- be capable of responding quickly to evolving risks to the business arising from factors within the company and to changes in the business environment; and

- include procedures for reporting immediately to appropriate levels of management any significant control failings or weaknesses that are identified together with details of corrective action being undertaken.

22 A sound system of internal control reduces, but cannot eliminate, the possibility of poor judgement in decision-making; human error; control processes being deliberately circumvented by employees and others; management overriding controls; and the occurrence of unforeseeable circumstances.

23 A sound system of internal control therefore provides reasonable, but not absolute, assurance that a company will not be hindered in achieving its business objectives, or in the orderly and legitimate conduct of its business, by circumstances which may reasonably be foreseen. A system of internal control cannot, however, provide protection with certainty against a company failing to meet its business objectives or all material errors, losses, fraud, or breaches of laws or regulations.

8 *Internal Control: Revised Guidance for Directors on the Combined Code (October 2005)*

Three – Reviewing the effectiveness of internal control Responsibilities

24 Reviewing the effectiveness of internal control is an essential part of the board's responsibilities. The board will need to form its own view on effectiveness based on the information and assurances provided to it, exercising the standard of care generally applicable to directors in the exercise of their duties. Management is accountable to the board for monitoring the system of internal control and for providing assurance to the board that it has done so.

25 The role of board committees in the review process, including that of the audit committee, is for the board to decide and will depend upon factors such as the size and composition of the board; the scale, diversity and complexity of the company's operations; and the nature of the significant risks that the company faces. To the extent that designated board committees carry out, on behalf of the board, tasks that are attributed in this guidance document to the board, the results of the relevant committees' work should be reported to, and considered by, the board. The board takes responsibility for the disclosures on internal control in the annual report and accounts.

The process for reviewing effectiveness

26 Effective monitoring on a continuous basis is an essential component of a sound system of internal control. The board cannot, however, rely solely on the embedded monitoring processes within the company to discharge its responsibilities. It should regularly receive and review reports on internal control. In addition, the board should undertake an annual assessment for the purposes of making its public statement on internal control to ensure that it has considered all significant aspects of internal control for the company for the year under review and up to the date of approval of the annual report and accounts.

27 The board should define the process to be adopted for its review of the effectiveness of internal control. This should encompass both the scope and frequency of the reports it receives and reviews during the year, and also the process for its annual assessment, such that it will be provided with sound, appropriately documented, support for its statement on internal control in the company's annual report and accounts.

28 The reports from management to the board should, in relation to the areas covered by them, provide a balanced assessment of the significant risks and the effectiveness of the system of internal control in managing those risks. Any significant control failings or weaknesses identified should be discussed in the reports, including the impact that they have had, or may have, on the company and the actions being taken to rectify them. It is essential that

there be openness of communication by management with the board on matters relating to risk and control.

29 When reviewing reports during the year, the board should:
- consider what are the significant risks and assess how they have been identified, evaluated and managed;
- assess the effectiveness of the related system of internal control in managing the significant risks, having regard in particular to any significant failings or weaknesses in internal control that have been reported;
- consider whether necessary actions are being taken promptly to remedy any significant failings or weaknesses; and
- consider whether the findings indicate a need for more extensive monitoring of the system of internal control.

30 Additionally, the board should undertake an annual assessment for the purpose of making its public statement on internal control. The assessment should consider issues dealt with in reports reviewed by it during the year together with any additional information necessary to ensure that the board has taken account of all significant aspects of internal control for the company for the year under review and up to the date of approval of the annual report and accounts.

31 The board's annual assessment should, in particular, consider:
- the changes since the last annual assessment in the nature and extent of significant risks, and the company's ability to respond to changes in its business and the external environment;
- the scope and quality of management's ongoing monitoring of risks and of the system of internal control, and, where applicable, the work of its internal audit function and other providers of assurance;

10 Internal Control: Revised Guidance for Directors on the Combined Code (October 2005)
- the extent and frequency of the communication of the results of the monitoring to the board (or board committee(s)) which enables it to build up a cumulative assessment of the state of control in the company and the effectiveness with which risk is being managed;
- the incidence of significant control failings or weaknesses that have been identified at any time during the period and the extent to which they have resulted in unforeseen outcomes or contingencies that have had, could have had, or may in the future have, a material impact on the company's financial performance or condition; and
- the effectiveness of the company's public reporting processes.

32 Should the board become aware at any time of a significant failing or weakness in internal control, it should determine how the failing or weakness arose and reassess the effectiveness of management's ongoing processes for designing, operating and monitoring the system of internal control.

Four – The board's statement on internal control

33 The annual report and accounts should include such meaningful, high-level information as the board considers necessary to assist shareholders' understanding of the main features of the company's risk management processes and system of internal control, and should not give a misleading impression.

34 In its narrative statement of how the company has applied Code Principle C.2, the board should, as a minimum, disclose that there is an ongoing process for identifying, evaluating and managing the significant risks faced by the company, that it has been in place for the year under review and up to the date of approval of the annual report and accounts, that it is regularly reviewed by the board and accords with the guidance in this document.

35 The disclosures relating to the application of Principle C.2 should include an acknowledgement by the board that it is responsible for the company's system of internal control and for reviewing its effectiveness. It should also explain that such a system is designed to manage rather than eliminate the risk of failure to achieve business objectives, and can only provide reasonable and not absolute assurance against material misstatement or loss.

36 In relation to Code Provision C.2.1, the board should summarise the process it (where applicable, through its committees) has applied in reviewing the effectiveness of the system of internal control and confirm that necessary actions have been or are being taken to remedy any significant failings or weaknesses identified from that review. It should also disclose the process it has applied to deal with material internal control aspects of any significant problems disclosed in the annual report and accounts.

37 Where a board cannot make one or more of the disclosures in paragraphs 34 and 36, it should state this fact and provide an explanation. The Listing Rules require the board to disclose if it has failed to conduct a review of the effectiveness of the company's system of internal control.

38 Where material joint ventures and associates have not been dealt with as part of the group for the purposes of applying this guidance, this should be disclosed.

Five – Appendix

Assessing the effectiveness of the company's risk and control processes

Some questions which the board may wish to consider and discuss with management when regularly reviewing reports on internal control and when carrying out its annual assessment are set out below. The questions are not intended to be exhaustive and will need to be tailored to the particular circumstances of the company.

This Appendix should be read in conjunction with the guidance set out in this document.

Risk assessment

- Does the company have clear objectives and have they been communicated so as to provide effective direction to employees on risk assessment and control issues? For example, do objectives and related plans include measurable performance targets and indicators?
- Are the significant internal and external operational, financial, compliance and other risks identified and assessed on an ongoing basis? These are likely to include the principal risks identified in the Operating and Financial Review.
- Is there a clear understanding by management and others within the company of what risks are acceptable to the board?

Control environment and control activities

- Does the board have clear strategies for dealing with the significant risks that have been identified? Is there a policy on how to manage these risks?
- Do the company's culture, code of conduct, human resource policies and performance reward systems support the business objectives and risk management and internal control system?
- Does senior management demonstrate, through its actions as well as it policies, the necessary commitment to competence, integrity and fostering a climate of trust within the company?
- Are authority, responsibility and accountability defined clearly such that decisions are made and actions taken by the appropriate people? Are the decisions and actions of different parts of the company appropriately co-ordinated?
- Does the company communicate to its employees what is expected of them and the scope of their freedom to act? This may apply to areas such as customer relations; service levels

for both internal and outsourced activities; health, safety and environmental protection; security of tangible and intangible assets; business continuity issues; expenditure matters; accounting; and financial and other reporting.
- Do people in the company (and in its providers of outsourced services) have the knowledge, skills and tools to support the achievement of the company's objectives and to manage effectively risks to their achievement?
- How are processes/controls adjusted to reflect new or changing risks, or operational deficiencies?

Information and communication

- Do management and the board receive timely, relevant and reliable reports on progress against business objectives and the related risks that provide them with the information, from inside and outside the company, needed for decision-making and management review purposes? This could include performance reports and indicators of change, together with qualitative information such as on customer satisfaction, employee attitudes etc.
- Are information needs and related information systems reassessed as objectives and related risks change or as reporting deficiencies are identified?
- Are periodic reporting procedures, including half-yearly and annual reporting, effective in communicating a balanced and understandable account of the company's position and prospects?
- Are there established channels of communication for individuals to report suspected breaches of law or regulations or other improprieties?

Monitoring

- Are there ongoing processes embedded within the company's overall business operations, and addressed by senior management, which monitor the effective application of the policies, processes and activities related to internal control and risk management? (Such processes may include control self-assessment, confirmation by personnel of compliance with policies and codes of conduct, internal audit reviews or other management reviews).
- Do these processes monitor the company's ability to re-evaluate risks and adjust controls effectively in response to changes in its objectives, its business, and its external environment?
- Are there effective follow-up procedures to ensure that appropriate change or action occurs in response to changes in risk and control assessments?
- Is there appropriate communication to the board (or board committees) on the effectiveness of the ongoing monitoring processes on risk and control matters? This should include reporting any significant failings or weaknesses on a timely basis.
- Are there specific arrangements for management monitoring and reporting to the board on risk and control matters of particular importance? These could include, for example, actual or suspected fraud and other illegal or irregular acts, or matters that could adversely affect the company's reputation or financial position.

Glossary

accountability The requirement for a person in a position of responsibility to justify, explain or account for the exercise of his/her authority and his/her performance or actions. Accountability is to the person or persons from whom the authority is derived.

accountable officer The primary authority for providing financial management and accountability for NHS property and services.

agency theory Theory based on the separation of ownership from control in a large organisation and the conflict of interests between the individuals who direct the organisation and the people who own it. In a company, the directors act as agents for the shareholders, and the conflict of interests between them should be controlled.

'apply or explain' rule Similar to the 'comply or explain' rule. Companies should apply the principles of a code or explain why they have not done so.

audit committee Committee of the board, consisting entirely of independent non-executive directors, with responsibility (among other things) for monitoring the reliability of the financial statements, the quality of the external audit and the organisation's relationship with its external auditors.

audit firm rotation Changing the firm of external auditors on a regular basis, say every seven years. Not common in practice.

audit partner rotation Changing the lead partner (and possibly other partners) involved with an organisation's audit on a regular basis, typically every five or seven years.

audit report Report for stakeholders produced by the external auditors on completion of the annual audit, and included in the organisation's published annual report and accounts. The report gives the opinion of the auditors on whether the financial statements present a true and fair view of the organisation's financial performance and position.

balance of power A situation in which power is shared out more or less evenly between a number of different individuals or groups, so that no single individual or group is in a position to dominate.

board committee A committee established by the board of directors, with delegated responsibility for a particular aspect of the board's affairs. For example, audit committee, remuneration/ compensation committee and nominations committee.

board/council of governors (to be known as a Council of Governors in accordance with the Health and Social Care Act 2012) A council of governors is a several member group that oversees or manages the running of an institution. In the context of an NHS foundation trust it is an elected body of members who hold the board of directors to account.

board succession The replacement of a senior director (typically the chairman or CEO) when he or she retires or resigns.

bounded rationality The idea that in decision-making, rationality of individuals is limited by the information they have, the cognitive limitations of their minds, and the finite amount of time they have to make a decision.

box-ticking approach An approach to compliance based on following all the specific rules or provisions in a code, and not considering the principles that should be applied and circumstances where the principles are best applied by not following the detailed provisions.

Bribery Act UK Act (2010) making it a criminal offence to give or receive bribes, to bribe a foreign public official for business benefit or to fail to prevent the payment of bribes by employees or agents.

business ethics Standards of business behaviour, sometimes set out by companies in a code of corporate ethics.

business risk The risk from unexpected events or developments in a business or in the business environment, which are outside the control of management. In the NHS, business risks are to patient safety and financial security.

business risk management The management of business risks within a strategy based on risk appetite and risk tolerance. The board is responsible for business risk strategy and management is responsible for implementing the strategy within a business risk management system. The board is also responsible for monitoring the effectiveness of the business risk management system, at least annually according to the UK Corporate Governance Code.

Cadbury Code A code of corporate governance, published by the Cadbury Committee in the UK in 1992 (and since superseded).

Care Quality Commission (CQC) The safety and quality regulator for all health services, which is also responsible for the regulation of adult social care services.

chairman Leader of the board of directors. Often referred to as the 'company chairman' in companies and 'chair' in public bodies and voluntary organisations.

chief executive officer The executive director who is head of the executive management team in an organisation.

clinical commissioning groups (CCGs) Groups of GPs and other health professionals responsible under the Health and Social Care Act 2012 for commissioning most healthcare, and replacing PCTs.

Combined Code The UK code on corporate governance for listed companies from 1998 to 2010. It was revised in 2010 and re-named the UK Corporate Governance Code.

comply or explain rule Requirement (e.g. in the UK, a requirement of the Listing Rules) for a company to comply with a voluntary code of corporate governance (in the UK, the UK Corporate Governance Code) or explain any non-compliance.

connected person A person with whom a director has an enduring and direct relationship, such as a family member, including a spouse, civil partner, children and step children (and equivalent relationships arising through civil partnerships) and companies in which the director has an interest of 20% or more.

corporate governance The system by which a company is directed, so as to achieve its overall objectives. It is concerned with relationships, structures, processes, information flows, controls, decision-making and accountability at the highest level in a company.

Davies Review A government-sponsored report (published February 2011) recommending greater diversity on the boards of companies and in particular a greater proportion of women on the boards of FTSE350 companies.

directors' report The 'report' in the annual report and accounts of a company or organisation. A report by the board of directors to the stakeholders, contained in the annual report and accounts and containing a variety of reports and information disclosures, such as the business review and remuneration report.

Disclosure and Transparency Rules In the UK, rules on disclosures that listed companies are required to comply with. The rules (like the Listing Rules) are issued and enforced by the UK financial markets regulator.

downside risk A risk that actual events will turn out worse than expected. Downside risk can be measure in terms of the amount by which profits could be worse than expected. The expected outcome is the forecast or budget expectation.

duty of skill and care A duty owed by a director to the company or organisation. In the UK, this has been a common law duty, but became a statutory duty under the provisions of the Companies Act 2006. A question can be raised, however, about what level of skill and care should be expected from a director.

elective care Planned specialist medical care

enlightened shareholder approach Approach to corporate governance based on the view that the objective of a company's directors should be to meet the needs of shareholders, while also showing concern for other major stakeholders. Also called an inclusive approach to governance.

emergency preparedness Emergency preparedness is a plan of what to do if a disaster that is unconnected with the organisation's business and outside the control of management occurs.

EU Directive An instruction, devised by the European Commission and approved by the European Council and European Parliament. The contents of a Directive must be introduced into national law or regulations by all members states of the EU. Some Directives, such as the Shareholder Rights Directive, deal wholly or partly with corporate governance issues.

European Commission The managing and administrative body of the EU.

executive director A director who also has executive responsibilities in the management structure. Usually a full-time employee with a contract of employment.

external audit Statutory annual audit of an organisation by independent external auditors.

fairness Impartiality, a lack of bias. In a corporate governance context, the quality of fairness refers to things that are done or decided in a reasonable manner, and with sense of justice, avoiding bias.

fiduciary duty A duty of a trustee. The directors of a company or organisation are given their powers in trust, and have fiduciary duties towards the company or organisation.

financial risk A risk of a failure or error, deliberate (fraud) or otherwise, in the systems or procedures for recording financial transactions and reporting financial performance and position, or the risk of a failure to safeguard financial assets such as cash and accounts receivable.

fixed pay The elements in a remuneration package that are a fixed amount each year, such as basic salary.

going concern statement A requirement of some corporate governance codes, such as the UK Corporate Governance Code. A statement by the board of directors that in their view the organisation will remain as a going concern for the next financial year.

Greenbury Report Report in the UK in 1995 by the Greenbury Committee, focusing mainly on corporate governance issues related to directors' remuneration.

Hampel Committee Committee set up in the UK to continue the review of corporate governance practices in the UK, following the Cadbury and Greenbury Committee Reports. The Hampel Committee suggested that the recommendations of all three committees should be integrated into a single code of corporate governance, which was published in 1998 as the Combined Code.

health service governance The system, practices and procedures by which power is shared and exercised by the board of directors (and the council of governors in foundation trusts) and how the holders of that power are held accountable for ensuring that the individual parts of the NHS achieve their objectives and are in line with public sector values such as VFM and providing universal and free healthcare benefits to all those in need.

Higgs Report The 2003 UK government commissioned review into the role and effectiveness of non-executive directors.

induction Process of introducing a newly-appointed director into his or her role, by providing appropriate information, site visits, meetings with management and (where necessary) training.

insider dealing Dealing in the shares of a company by an 'insider' (such as a company director or professional adviser) on the basis of knowledge of price-sensitive information that has not yet been made available to the public. A criminal activity.

institutional investor An organisation or institution that invests funds of clients, savers or depositors. The main institutional investors in the UK are pension funds, insurance/life assurance companies, investment trust companies and mutual organisations such as unit trusts.

internal audit Investigations and checks carried out by internal auditors of an organisation. Internal audit is a function rather than a specific activity. However, work programme of the internal audit team might reduce the amount of work the external auditors need to carry out in their annual audit, provided the internal and external auditors collaborate properly.

internal control A procedure or arrangement that is implemented to prevent an internal control risk, reduce the potential impact of such a risk, or detect a failure of internal control when it occurs (and initiate remedial action).

internal control risk A risk of failure in a system or procedure due to causes that are within the control of management. They can be categorised as financial risks, operational risk and compliance risks.

internal control system A system of internal controls within an organisation. The system should have a suitable control environment, and should provide for the identification and assessment of internal control risks, the design and implementation of internal controls, communication and information and monitoring. In the UK, the board of directors of a listed company has responsibility for the system of internal control.

International Corporate Governance Network (ICGN) A voluntary association of institutional investors that has the objective of raising standards of corporate governance globally, to meet the requirements and expectations of global investors.

King Code Also called the King Report and King III (because it is the third version of the Code/Report, issued in 2009). The corporate governance code for listed companies in South Africa.

lead governor The lead governor's role is to facilitate direct communication between Monitor and the NHS foundation trust's board of governors in a limited number of circumstances and in particular where it may not be appropriate to communicate through the normal channels.

majority shareholder A shareholder holding a majority of the equity shares in a company and so having a controlling interest in the company. A majority shareholder has the voting power to remove directors from the board, and so can control the board.

management board A board of executive managers, chaired by the CEO, within a two-tier board structure. The chairman of the management board reports to the chairman of the supervisory board. The management board has responsibility for the operational performance of the business.

minority shareholders Shareholders holding a fairly small proportion of the total equity shares in a company who could be at risk of having their interests ignored in favour of a controlling shareholder or group of large shareholders.

model articles of association Under UK company law, a company may adopt standard articles of association (company constitution) and amend these as necessary to meet the requirements and particular circumstances of the individual company. In practice, the articles of association of most UK companies formed under the Companies Act 1985 are based on the Table A Articles. Different model articles apply to companies formed under the Companies Act 2006.

Model Code A code of conduct for directors of listed companies, stating when they should (in normal circumstances) avoid buying or selling shares in their company.

modified audit report Audit report in which the auditors express some reservations about the financial statements of the organisation, because of insufficient information to reach an opinion or disagreement with the figures in the statements.

money laundering The process of transferring or using money obtained from criminal activity, so as to make it seem to have come from legitimate (non-criminal) sources. Companies are often used as a cover for money laundering.

Monitor The regulator of Foundation Trusts. Under the Health and Social Care Act its role will be extended to become the sector regulator for health making it responsible for licensing providers of NHS-funded services.

mutual society A mutual, mutual organisation, or mutual society is an organisation (which is often, but not always, a company or business) based on the principle of mutuality. A mutual is therefore owned by, and run for the benefit of, its members – it has no external shareholders to pay in the form of dividends, and as such does not usually seek to maximise and make large profits or capital gains.

Myners Report A UK report into the role and responsibilities of institutional investors.

nomination committee A committee of the board of directors (or council of governors in foundation trusts), with responsibility for identifying potential new members for the board of directors. Suitable candidates are recommended to the main board (or to the council of governors), which then makes a decision about their appointment.

non-audit work Work done by a firm of auditors for a client organisation, other than work on the annual audit, such as consultancy services and tax advice. In the context of corporate governance, the independence of the auditors might be questionable when they earn high fees for non-audit work.

non-executive director (NED) A director who is not an employee of the company and who does not have any responsibilities for executive management in the company.

OECD Principles of Corporate Governance General principles of corporate governance issued by the Organisation for European Cooperation and Development, which all countries are encouraged to adopt.

operational risk Risk of an error, deliberate or otherwise, in operating systems or procedures within an organisation; the risk of failure in equipment or system design; the risk of failures due to weak organisational structure; or risks due to human error including inefficient management. Includes health and safety risks, environmental risks.

policy governance theory Policy governance theory is an integrated set of concepts and principles that describes the job of any governing board. It outlines the manner in which boards can be successful in their servant-leadership role, as well as in their all-important relationship with management.

postcode lottery A situation where local budgets and decision-making can lead to different levels of public services in different places especially with regard to health and social services, e.g. access to cancer drugs en.wikipedia.org/wiki/Postcode_lottery – cite_note-1#cite_note-1 or quality of education.

premium listing One of two categories of listing for companies in the UK. Companies with a premium listing are required to meet the highest standards of regulation and corporate governance.

primary care The first point of healthcare such as GPs, dentists, pharmacists and optometrists.

primary care trust (PCT) The key organisation responsible for ensuring a comprehensive range of health services for the local population, either directly or commissioned (purchased) from a range of different organisations. Due to be replaced by GP Commissioning clusters in 2013.

public benefit corporation A public benefit corporation is usually a corporation created by the government that performs a specific function for the benefit of the public, such as a hospital or public library.

Quality Account A Quality Account is a report about the quality of services provided by an NHS healthcare service. The report is published annually by each NHS healthcare provider, including the independent sector and made available to the public.

quality governance The combination of structures and processes at and below board level to lead on trust-wide quality performance including:

- ensuring required standards are achieved
- investigating and taking action on sub-standard performance
- planning and driving continuous improvement

- identifying, sharing and ensuring delivery of best-practice
- identifying and managing risks to quality of care.

related party transaction A transaction by a company with a 'related party' such as a major shareholder, a director, a company in which a director has a major interest or a member of a director's family.

remuneration committee A committee of the board of directors (or council of governors in foundation trusts), with responsibility for deciding remuneration policy for top executives and the individual remuneration packages of certain senior executives, for example, all the executive directors (or non-executive directors in foundation trusts).

reputation risk Risk to the reputation of a company or other organisation in the mind of the public (including customers and suppliers) when a particular matter becomes public knowledge

responsibility Having power and authority over something. A person in a position of responsibility should be held accountable for the exercise of that authority.

risk appetite The amount and type of business risk that the board of directors would like their organisation to have exposure to. Identifying risk appetite should be a part of strategic planning.

risk assessment An assessment of risks faced by an organisation, Typically risks are assessed according to how probably or how frequent an adverse outcome is likely to be in the planning period and the potential size of the losses if an adverse outcome occurs. The greatest risks are those with a high probability of an adverse outcome combined with the likelihood of a large loss if this were to happen.

risk capacity The maximum risk exposures that the organisation can accept without threatening its financial stability.

risk committee A committee of the board that an organisation may establish, with the responsibility of monitoring the risk management system within the organisation, instead of the audit committee. A risk committee may be established when the audit committee has too many other responsibilities to handle.

risk management A function of the administration of the NHS body directed toward identification, evaluation, and correction of potential risks that could lead to injury to patients, staff members, or visitors and result in loss or damage.

risk management committee A committee of senior executive managers and risk managers, whose responsibility is to implement the risk management strategy of the board.

risk tolerance The amount of business risk that the board is willing to let their organisation be exposed to. Alternatively, the amount of risk that the organisation is able to accept without serious threat to its stability.

safe harbour provisions Provisions in the UK Companies Act whereby directors are not liable for incorrect or misleading statements (or omissions) in a report to shareholders, unless they knew the statements or omissions to be incorrect or misleading. These provisions reduced concern about directors' liability for the information provided by their company in its business review.

Sarbanes-Oxley Act Legislation, largely on corporate governance issues, introduced in the USA in 2002 following a series of corporate scandals such as Enron and WorldCom.

secondary care Acute healthcare, either elective or emergency

secret profit A profit that is not revealed. In the context of corporate governance, a director should not make a secret profit for his/her personal benefit and at the expense of the company or organisation.

senior independent director A non-executive director who is the nominal head of all the non-executive directors on the board. The SID may act as a channel of communication between the NEDs and the chairman, or (in some situations) between major stakeholders and the board.

severance payment Payment to a director (or other employee) on being required to resign (or otherwise leave the company).

shareholder value approach Approach to corporate governance based on the view that the objective of its directors should be to maximise benefits for shareholders.

share options Rights given to an individual giving him (or her) the right but not the obligation to buy new shares in the company at a fixed price (the exercise price), not earlier than a specified date and not later than a specified date in the future (typically not earlier than three years after the options are granted and not later than ten years respectively).

Smith Report A report concerned with the independence of auditors in the wake of the collapse of Arthur Andersen and the Enron scandal in the US in 2002. It raised the important point that an auditor himself should look at whether a company's corporate governance structure provides safeguards to preserve his own independence.

stakeholder A stakeholder group is an identifiable group of individuals or organisations with a vested interest. Stakeholder groups in a company include the shareholders, the directors, senior executive management and other employees, customers, suppliers. In the NHS stakeholders will also include patients, employees, the regulators, the general public and the government.

stakeholder approach Approach to governance based on the view that the organisation should aim to satisfy the needs of all stakeholders. Also called a pluralist approach.

stakeholder theory The view that the purpose of corporate governance should be to satisfy, as far as possible, the objectives of all key stakeholders.

Statement on Internal Control The SIC is a mandatory disclosure for all central government entities that comply with the FReM. All public bodies (including NHS organisations) must provide assurance that they are appropriately managing and controlling the resources for which they are responsible. This has now been replaced by the AGS.

statutory duties Duties imposed by statute law.

stewardship theory Stewardship theory emphasises the role of top management acting as stewards, integrating their goals as part of the organisation. The stewardship theory suggests that stewards are satisfied and motivated when organisational success is attained.

strategic health authority Before the Health and Social Care Act 2012, SHAs were the regional headquarters of the NHS, overseeing the performance and management of the healthcare system in its area.

strategic risk the risks of taking decisions on strategy that will result in exposures to excessive business risk and so could lead to losses or even business collapse.

stress testing Testing the ability of a business to withstand the effects of extreme adverse events or developments in the business environment.

succession planning Planning for the eventual replacement of a senior member of the board (chairman, CEO and possibly finance director) by his or her successor.

supervisory board A board of non-executive directors, found in an organisation with a two-tier board structure. The supervisory board reserves some responsibilities to itself. These include oversight of the management board.

sustainability Conducting business operations in a way that can be continued into the foreseeable future, without using natural resources at such a rate or creating such environmental damage that the continuation of the business will eventually become impossible.

sustainability report Report on the economic, social and environmental performance of a company or organisation.

total shareholder returns The total returns in a period earned by the company's shareholders, consisting normally of the dividends received and the gain (or minus the fall) in the share price during the period. The returns might be expressed as a percentage of the share value, e.g. the share price at the start of the period.

transaction cost theory A theory about organisations that includes the view that management are opportunistic and may take opportunities that arise to pursue their personal interests.

transparency Openness. Being clear about historical performance and future intentions, and not trying to hide information.

Turnbull Guidance Initially a report of the Turnbull Committee in the UK, giving listed companies guidance on how the directors should carry out their responsibility for the internal control system, as required by the UK corporate governance code. Now the responsibility of the FRC.

two-tier board Board structure in which the responsibilities are divided between a supervisory board of non-executive directors led by the chairman, and a management board of executives led by the CEO.

UK Corporate Governance Code The code of corporate governance issued by the FRC in the UK, which is applied to UK listed companies. Formerly (until 2010) called the Combined Code.

UK Listing Rules Rules that apply to all listed companies in the UK. They include the 'comply or explain' rule on compliance with the UK Corporate Governance Code.

ultra vires In corporate law, ultra vires describes acts attempted by a corporation that are beyond the scope of powers granted by the corporation's objects clause, articles of incorporation or in a clause in its Bylaws, in the laws authorizing a corporation's formation, or similar founding documents.

unitary board Board structure in which decisions are taken by a single group of executive and non-executive directors, led by the company chairman.

upside risk A risk that actual events will turn out better than expected and will provide unexpected profits. Some risks, such as the risk of a change in foreign exchange rates, or a change in interest rates, or a change in consumer buying patterns could be 'two-way' with both upside and downside potential.

variable pay The elements in a remuneration package that vary each year according to the individual's performance, such as annual bonuses, and the grant of shares or share options

voluntary code of governance A code of governance that is not enforced by law or regulation. However, as in the UK and South Africa, listed companies may be encouraged to adopt a voluntary code by means of a 'comply or explain' or 'apply or explain' regulation.

Walker Report A report published in the UK in 2009 about corporate governance in banks and other financial services organisations, following the banking crisis of 2007–2008.

whistleblowing The disclosure by a person, usually an employee in a government agency or private enterprise, to the public or to those in authority, of mismanagement, corruption, illegality, or some other wrongdoing.

window dressing of accounts Applying accounting policies that are just within the limits of permissible accounting practice, but which have the effect of making the company's performance or financial position seem better than it would if more conservative accounting policies were used. For example, accounting policies might be used that recognise income at an early stage in a transaction process, or defer the recognition of expenses.

Women on Boards Report A report highlighting the poor representation of women on boards, relative to their male counterparts, and raised questions about whether board recruitment is in practice based on skills, experience and performance. This report presents practical recommendations to address this imbalance.

wrongful trading Wrongful trading occurs when a company continues to trade when the directors are aware that the company had gone into (or would soon go into) insolvent liquidation.

Directory

Further reading, codes of practice and guidance

A First Class Service: Quality in the new NHS, Department of Health, 1998.
Audit Code for NHS Foundation Trusts, Monitor, 2011.
Board Governance Assurance Framework, Department of Health, 2011.
Carver, J. Boards that Make a Difference: a new design for leadership in nonprofit and public organisations, Jossey-Bass, 2006.
Chait, R., Ryan, W. and Taylor, B. Governance as leadership: Reframing the work of nonprofit boards, Wiley, 2005.
Code and Report on Governance for South Africa (King III), Institute of Directors South Africa, 2009. *See* www.iodsa.co.za
Code of Ethics for Professional Accountants, IFAC, 2006.
Code of Governance for Foundation Trusts, Monitor, 2010. *See* Appendix 2.
Corporate Governance Policy and Voting Guidelines, NAPF, 2011.
Davies Review into Women on Boards, BIS, 2011.
Director–Governor Interaction in NHS Foundation Trusts: a best practice guide for boards of directors, Monitor, 2012
Dr Foster Intelligent Board series
  See http://drfosterintelligence.co.uk/thought-leadership/intelligent-board
Effective Boards in the NHS, NHS Confederation, 2005
Equity and Excellence: liberating the NHS, Department of Health White Paper, 2010.
The Foundations of Good Governance: a compendium of best practice, Foundation Trust Network, 2011.
Good Governance: a code for the voluntary sector, NCVO, 2010.
  See www.ncvo-vol.org.uk/codeofgovernance
Government Financial Reporting Manual (FReM), HM Treasury, annual.
Guidance on Audit Committees, FRC, 2010. *See* Appendix 5.
Guidance on Board Effectiveness, FRC, 2011. *See* Appendix 4.
Guidance on Internal Control (The Turnbull Guidance), FRC, 2005. *See* Appendix 6.
The Handbook to the NHS Constitution for England, DH, 2012
The Healthy NHS Board: principles for good governance, NHS Leadership Council, 2010
  See Appendix 3.
High Quality Care for All (Darzi Report), Department of Health, 2008.
Hutton Review of Fair Pay in the Public Sector, HM Treasury, 2011.
ICGN Global Corporate Governance Principles, ICGN, 2009.
ICSA Mapping the Gap, ICSA, July 2011
The Integrated Governance Handbook, Department of Health, 2006
New Voices, New Accountabilities: a guide to wider governance in foundation trusts, Foundation Trust Network, 2005.
NHS Audit Committee Handbook, HFMA and Department of Health, 2011.
The NHS Emergency Planning Guidance, Department of Health, 2005.
The Nolan Principles of Standards in Public Life, 1995
Plurality, Stewardship and Engagement, The Ownership Commission, 2012.
Quality Governance Framework, Monitor, 2010.
Quality Governance in the NHS: a guide for provider boards, Department of Health, 2011.
Sonnenfeld, J.A. What Makes Boards Great, Harvard Business Review, September 2002.
Taking it on Trust, Audit Commission, 2009
The UK Corporate Governance Code, FRC, 2010. *See* Appendix 1.
Walker Review of Corporate Governance of UK Banking Industry, HM Treasury, 2009.
Your Statutory Duties: a reference guide for NHS Foundation Trust governors, Monitor, 2009.

Useful websites

Association of British Insurers (ABI)
www.abi.org.uk

Audit Commission
www.audit-commission.gov.uk/Pages/default.aspx

Care Quality Commission
www.cqc.org.uk

Chartered Institute of Internal Auditors
www.iia.org.uk

The Chartered Institute of Public Finance and Accountancy
www.cipfa.org.uk

Department for Business, Innovation and Skills (BIS)
www.bis.gov.uk

Department of Health
www.dh.gov.uk

European Corporate Governance Institute
www.ecgi.org/codes/all_codes.php.

Financial Reporting Council (FRC)
www.frc.org.uk

Foundation Trust Governors Association
www.ftga.org.uk

Foundation Trust Network
www.foundationtrustnetwork.org

HM Treasury
www.hm-treasury.gov.uk

The Institute of Chartered Secretaries and Administrators (ICSA)
www.icsaglobal.com

International Corporate Governance Network (ICGN)
www.icgn.org

The International Federation of Accountants (IFAC)
www.ifac.org

National Association of Pension Funds (NAPF)
www.napf.co.uk

Monitor
www.monitor-nhsft.gov.uk

NHS Confederation
www.nhsconfed.org

OECD
www.oecd.org

The Ownership Commission
www.ownershipcomm.org

Index

References to Figures or Tables will be in *italics*.

access to healthcare, NHS Constitution 28
accountability 19, 72, 116, 282, 314, 315, 316
  audit committee/auditors 283–4
  boards of directors 313–17
  definition 368
  Foundation Trusts 100–1
  and Health and Social Care (HSC) Act 2012 37–9
  local 35–6
  NHS Appointment Commission, Code of Conduct and Accountability 96, 138–9, 180
  quality assurance and clinical governance 314–15
  quality corporate governance 8–9
  reporting 217–18
  risk management 282, 315–16
  UK Code 217, 275, 282–4
  see also transparency
accountable officer 368
accounts
  misleading 10–11
  window dressing 10, 57, 217, 375
adverse opinion, audit reports 223
agency theory 71–3, 75, 368
Agenda for Change 13, 115, 189
Annual General Meeting (AGM), constructive use 286
annual governance statement (AGS) 14, 90, 262–5, 374
annual report and accounts, duties of PCT company secretary 60
'apply or explain' rule 84, 368
appointment and removal, company secretary 57–8
Appointments Commission (NHS) 163, 172, 180, 201
appointments to board 162–5, 279
  FT Code of Governance (2010) 297–9
  in NHS 163–4
area health authorities (AHAs) 42
Arthur Andersen 11, 12, 17
articles of association, model 128–9, 371
Association of British Insurers (ABI) 16, 78, 205–7
Association of Chartered Certified Accountants (ACCA) 227
Audit Code for Foundation Trusts 235
Audit Commission Act 1998 221
Audit Commission Code of Audit Practice 2010 222
Audit Committee Handbook, NHS 231, 232
audit committees 231–7, 262, 353
  annual audit cycle 236–7, 356
  appointment and removal 234–5, 350
  composition 232–3
  definition 368
  establishment and role 349–50
  financial reporting 234, 352
  firms from more than one network 357–60
  FRC review 237, 348–60
  FT Code of Governance (2010) 305–6
  independence of members 354–6
  meetings 233, 350
  non-audit services, provision 235–6
  remuneration of members 233, 351, 354
  resources 350–1
  role and responsibilities 231–2, 260, 352–6
  shareholder relations 357–8
  UK Code 283–4
  whistleblowing 353
audit firm/partner rotation 230, 368
audit reports 223–4
  definition 368
  modified 223, 372
  opinions 223
  unmodified 224
auditing
  annual audit cycle 236–7, 356
  auditors *see* auditors
  committees *see* audit committees
  external audit, role and responsibilities 223–31
  group audits 358–9
  key issues 10–12
  non-audit work 228–9, 372
  relationship between internal and external 220–2
  reporting *see* audit reports
  review of audits by FRC 237
  UK Code 55
  see also external audit; internal audit
Auditing Practices Board 253
auditors
  appointment and removal 109–10, 234–5
  Foundation Trust boards of governors 109–10
  FT Code of Governance (2010) 305–6
  independence of external 227–8
  joint 360
  liability to third parties 226
  objectivity and independence of internal 266–7
  UK Code 283–4
autonomy 95

balance of power 368
banks, role of non-executive directors in 148–9, 375
Barking, Havering and Redbridge University Hospital NHS Trust 91
base pay and bonuses 206–7
beneficence 95
Board Assurance Framework (BAF) 60, 103, 157, 177
  annual governance statement (AGS) 264–5
board committees 129, 178, 316–17, 368
  non-executive directors (NEDs) 151, 153
board of directors 123–56
  accountability, ensuring 313–17
  appointments to 162–5, 279, 297–9
  behaviour 159–62
  composition 53–4, 145–6, 162–3, 278–9, 345–6
  culture 317–19

decision-making 125, 344–5
effectiveness, improving 326–34
  board disciplines, embedding 330–1
  capacity and capability building 326–30, 335
  corporate accountability and good social processes, enabling 330
  delegation 331–2
  judgement, exercising 332–4
  role of board and directors 341–4
engagement 323–4
evaluation of performance 346–7
FT Code of Governance (2010) 292–4, 294–6
governance responsibilities 123–5
individual members, evaluation 178
information, development and relationships 54
intelligence 320–2
leadership role 276
male dominated 164–5
matters reserved for 139–40
meetings 59, 158
National Health Service (NHS) 311–24
performance evaluation 175–80
procedures 53–4
refreshing membership 171–2
roles and responsibilities 312–24
roles of board members 335–8
shareholder relations 347
size 145, 162–3
and stakeholders 77–8
strategy formulation 312–13
succession 368
support 344–5
two-tier 126–8
UK Code 123–4
unitary 7, 126, 375
see also boardroom practice; directors; non-executive directors (NEDs)
board of governors, Foundation Trusts (NHS) 99, 106–11
  auditors, appointment and removal 109–10
  chief executives, approval of appointment 109
  as Councils 113–14
  forward planning 110
  FT Code of Governance (2010) 296–7, 299–300
  future role of governors 110–11
  lead governor 107, 371
  non-executive directors (NEDs), appointment or removal 108
  re-election of governors 110, 299–300
  remuneration of a chair or non-executive director (NED) 108
  statutory duties 107–10
boardroom practice 157–86
  agenda 158
  appointments to board 162–5
  board behaviour 159–62
  board meetings, frequency 158
  conflicts of interest, avoiding 134–5, 180–2
  definition of good quality 157–8
  guidance on behaviour 162
  Hospitality Policy see Hospitality Policy
  ICSA report 160–1
  induction and training of directors 172–5
  information 158–9
  Mapping the Gap (ICSA research project) 97, 161
  performance evaluation of board 175–80
  quality 157–9
  refreshing board membership 171–2
  succession planning 166, 170–1, 345–6, 374
  support 159
  terms of engagement 170
  see also board of directors
borrowing powers of directors 136
bounded rationality 74, 368
Bower, Cynthia 270
box-ticking approach 22, 84, 368
bribery
  Bribery Act 2010 see Bribery Act 2010
  prevention, guiding principles 184
  reporting of acts 269
Bribery Act 2010 50, 368
  Hospitality Policy 183–4
  statutory duties of directors 135
  and whistleblowing 272
Bristol Royal Infirmary, children's heart surgery at (1984–1995) 68, 147
business continuity management 268–9
business environment risks 246
business ethics 95, 369
  code 96
business reporting, accountability 282
business review 238–9
business risk management 369
business risks
  categories 246–7
  corporate governance and risk management 14
  definition 369
  and internal control risks 246–7
  relevance for health service governance 243–4

Cadbury, takeover by Kraft 5
Cadbury Code/Report 1992 15, 92, 244, 369
Caparo Industries plc v Dickman (1990) 226
Care Quality Commission (CQC) 33, 86, 369
Care Trusts 42
Carver, John 75
CEO see chief executive officer (CEO)
chairman
  chief executive officer compared 142–3
  commitments 144–5
  consultation with regarding executive remuneration 199
  definition of role 369
  evaluation 178–9
  Foundation Trusts (NHS)
    appointment and removal 108
    dual role 116–17
    FT Code of Governance (2010) 294
  independence 141–2
  leadership 277
  remuneration 108
  role 140–1, 142, 341–2
Chait, Richard 75
Charity Commission Statement of Recommended Practice 22
Chartered Institute of Internal Auditors 220
chief executive officer (CEO)
  approval of appointment (Foundation Trusts) 109
  chairman compared 142–3
  consultation with regarding executive remuneration 199
  definition of role 77, 369
  FT Code of Governance (2010) 294
  governance and management 7

role 140, *142*, 335, *336–7*
   in United States 51
chief finance officer (CFO), in United States 51
chief risk officer (CRO) 249
Civil Contingencies Act 2004 268
civil liability of directors 137
Clinical Commissioning Groups (CCGs) 37, 38, 369
Code of Audit Practice, NHS 235
Combined Code on Corporate Governance (1998) 16, 92, 369
   internal control requirements 362
Commission for Healthcare Audit and Inspection (CHAI) 43
Commissioner for Public Appointment, Code of Practice 163
Commissioners 9
Commissioning for Quality Improvement (CQINs) 210
Committee of Sponsoring Organizations of the Treadway Commission (COSO), US 254, 258
Committee on the Financial Aspects of Corporate Governance (Cadbury Report) 15
committees
   board 151, 153, 178
   nomination 165–70
   overview and scrutiny 36
Commonwealth Association for Corporate Governance (CACG) 21
Companies Act 2006 49, 124, 133
   conflicts of interest, avoiding 134–5
   error and fraud detection 225–6
company law 49–51
company secretary 53–62
   appointment and removal 57–8
   as conscience of company 57
   and corporate social responsibility 55–7
   general responsibilities 53
   and in-house lawyer 59
   independence of 57–8
   primary care trust, core duties 59–61
   role 117, 335, *336–7*, 338, 344
   specific responsibilities under *UK Code* 53–5
company-stakeholder relations 13
competition risk 246
compliance, 61, 256
compliance error 369
compliance risk 94, 254
'comply or explain' rule 16, 84, 369
compulsory regulation 51–2
conflicts of interest, avoiding
   declaration of interests requirement 181–2
   definition of conflicts of interest 180–1
   direct and indirect financial interests 181
   loyalties, conflict of 181
   non-financial/personal conflicts 181
   statutory duty of directors 134–5
connected person 134, 180, 369
co-operatives, and Foundation Trusts 117–18
corporate governance
   board of directors, responsibilities 123–5
   definitions 1, 6, 369
   disclosure requirements 287–91
   health service governance compared 6
   history 15–18
   international perspective 17

national variations 18
poor quality, consequences 69–70
quality 8–9
and risk management 14
stakeholders specific to 76–7
and UK Listing Regime 50
in United Kingdom 15–17
see also governance; health service governance
Corporate Governance Code *see* UK Corporate Governance Code 2010 (*UK Code*)
corporate sector, board appointments in 164–5
corporate social responsibility (CSR), 15, 55–7
Council for Healthcare Regulatory Excellence 34
Council of Governors *see* board of governors, Foundation Trusts (NHS)
Counter Fraud and Security Management Service (CFSMS) 48
criminal liability of directors 137
Crisp, Sir Nigel 86, 96

Data Protection Act 1998 46
Data Protection Commissioner 44
Davies Review (2011) 16, 164–5, 369
decision-making
   accountability 316
   board of directors 125, 344–5
   delays, non-executive directors 155
   health service governance 97
deferred bonuses 207
Deighan, Michael 86
delegation 133, 331–2
Department of Health (DH) 33, 47, 103, 124
   Model Election Rules 107, 111
dignity 95
directors
   board of *see* board of directors
   borrowing powers 136
   dismissal, and severance payments 202–3
   duties to their organisation 129–33
   executive *see* executive directors
   FT Code of Governance (2010) 292–6
   general powers, private sector 128–9
   indemnity, liability for 138
   induction and training 172–5
   liability of 136–8
   new
      induction of 172–3
      talent pool 168–9
   non-executive *see* non-executive directors (NEDs)
   powers 128–9
      duty to act within 133
   re-appointment 299–300
   remuneration *see* directors' remuneration
   report *see* directors' report
   resignation 300
   risk training 249
   senior independent (SID) 78, 152–3, 342, 374
   statutory duties 133–6
   Trust claims, liability in relation to 137–8
directors' remuneration 13
   compensation for loss of office 202–3
   disclosure of details 203–5
   executive directors 195–6
      ABI guidance 205–7
      component elements 195
      consultants, use of 195

consultation with chairman/CEO 199
EU recommendations 207
FT Code of Governance (2010) 302–3
NAF policy 207
non-executive directors (NEDs) 108, 200–1
report 204–5
reward to performance links, problems 196
severance payments 190, 202–3, 374
see also remuneration
Directors' Remuneration Report Regulations 13
directors' report 14, 369
disclaimer of opinion, audit reports 223
disclosure
   corporate governance arrangements 287–91
   directors' remuneration 203–5
   financial reporting 219
   governance arrangements 238
   internal control weaknesses 264
   UK Code 55, 287–91
   see also UK Disclosure and Transparency Rules (DTR)
district health authorities (DHAs) 42
D'Jan of London, Re [1993] 131, 132
Dorchester Finance Co. Ltd v Stebbing [1989] 131
duties of directors
   common law 130
   delegation 133
   fiduciary 130, 139, 370
   financial reporting 218–19
   skill and care, exercise of 130–2, 370
   statutory *see* statutory duties of directors
   to their organisation 129–33
   wrongful trading 132
'duty to consult' legislation 47–8

effectiveness
   appointments to board 279
   board composition 278–9
   commitments 279–80
   development 280
   evaluation 281
   information and support 280–1
   re-election 281
   UK Code 275, 278–81
elective care 31, 370
emergency preparedness 268–9, 370
enlightened shareholder approach 80–1, 93, 370
Enron 10, 11, 12, 230
Equality Act 2010 168
'Equity and Excellence: Liberating the NHS' (White Paper), 2010 32, 36, 100
ethical codes, implementation 97
ethics
   business ethics 95, 96, 369
   and corporate social responsibility 15
   and governance 94–7
European Commission 49, 207, 370
European Union (EU)
   Directives 17, 49, 370
   executive remuneration guidelines 207
executive directors
   compared to non-executive directors 151–2
   definition of role 77, 342–3, 370
   governance and management 7
   induction of executive manager as 174
   non-executive directors overriding influence of 154–5
   remuneration 195–6
      ABI guidance 205–7
      component elements 195
      consultants, use of 195
      consultation with chairman/CEO 199
      EU recommendations 207
external audit
   appointment and removal of external auditors 234–5
   audit committees 353
   definition 370
   error and fraud detection 225–6
   function and scope 221–2
   key issues 11
   roles and responsibilities 223–31

fairness 8, 370
Fastow, Andrew 11
fiduciary duty of directors 130, 139, 370
financial controls 255–6
financial interests, direct and indirect 181
financial markets and services, legal aspects 49–50
financial reporting 215–17
   accountability 282
   annual planning and monitoring cycle *216*
   audit committees 234, 352
   duties of directors for 218–19
   FT Code of Governance (2010) 304–5
   going concern statement 219, 370
   initiative for greater disclosure 219
   key issues 10–12
   UK Code 282
Financial Reporting Advisory Board (FRAB) 215
Financial Reporting Council (FRC) 16, 148
   audit committees, review 233, 236, 237, 348–60
   chairman 140–1
   Guidance on Board Effectiveness 124, 157, 171
Financial Reporting Manual (FReM) 215
financial risks 14, 246, 254, 370
financial statements 370
financial stewardship 315
fixed pay 195, 370
Foundation Trust Network (FTN) 112–13
Foundation Trusts (NHS) 34–5, 39, 99–119
   accountability 100–1
   authorisation terms 100
   becoming 102–3
   board of governors 106–11
   and co-operatives 117–18
   directors 114
   elections 111–12
   evidence 115–16
   freedoms 100
   future 113–14
   governance challenge 114–18
   governance structures 103–5
   and hybrid organisations 118
   issues 116–17
   membership 105–6
   and mutual organisations 117
   overview 99–101
   and quality reporting 212–14
   regulation 101–3
   two-tier structure 114
   see also FT Code of Governance (2010); governors, Foundation trusts; Monitor (regulator of Foundation Trusts)

FRC *see* Financial Reporting Council (FRC)
Freedom of Information Act 2000 (FOIA) 9, 15, 44, 46
FT Code of Governance (2010) 85, 87–9, 108, 125, 292–308
   accountability 304–6
   audit committees/auditors 305–6
   board of directors 292–4
      appointment to 297–9
      balance and independence 294–6
   chairman and CEO 294
   cooperation with third parties 308
   directors 292–6
      non-executive 149, 150, 151, 171
      remuneration 302–3
      resignation 300
      senior independent 152
   governors *see* governors, Foundation Trusts
   information and professional development 300–1
   internal controls 305
   performance evaluation 175, 176, 301–2
   re-election of governors 110
   reporting 304–5
   risk management 247
   shareholder relations 307–8
   see also Foundation Trusts (NHS); governors, Foundation trusts; Monitor (regulator of Foundation Trusts)

GatNet 173
General Medical Council (GMC) 34
generative governance model 75
German Corporate Governance Code 128
Gibb v Maidstone and Tunbridge Wells NHS Trust 190
gifts, acceptance 183
Global Crossing 10
going concern statement 219, 370
'Good Governance: a code for the voluntary and community sector' 23–4
Good Governance Standard for Public Service 19–21
governance 3–25
   approaches to 79–82
   and boardroom practice *see* boardroom practice
   compulsory regulation, advantages 52
   definition 1, 4–7
   disclosure of arrangements 238
   and ethics 94–7
   of Foundation Trusts *see* Foundation Trusts (NHS)
   generative governance model 75
   importance 7
   and insolvency law 49
   key issues 10–15
   and law *see under* law
   and management 7
   policy governance theory 75, 81–2
   principles-based code 372–3
   in public sector *see* public sector governance
   quality 210–14, 373
   regimes, arguments for and against 21–2
   remuneration as governance issue 187–93
   and risk management 243–5
   and voluntary sector 23–4
   see also corporate governance; health service governance
Governing the NHS (2003) 168

governors, Foundation trusts
   accountability 116
   appointed 106
   capability 116
   chair 106
   FT Code of Governance (2010) 296–7
   future role 110–11, 113
   lead governor 107, 371
   public 106
   re-election of 110, 299–300
   staff 106
   see also board of governors, Foundation Trusts (NHS)
Greenbury Report (1995) 13, 16, 370
Guide to NHS Foundation Trusts (DH) 103

Hampel, Sir Ronald 16
Hampel Committee 16, 370
Handbook to the NHS Constitution 26–7
Health Act 1999 42
Health Act 2009 26, 43, 211
Health and Social Care (HSC) Act 2001 42–3, 48
Health and Social Care (HSC) Act 2003 43
Health and Social Care (HSC) Act 2008 43
Health and Social Care (HSC) Act 2012 31, 36–9, 43, 67
   and Foundation Trusts 102, 105, 114, 116
Health and Social Care (Community Health and Standards) Act 2003 102
Health and Social Care (HSC), Northern Ireland 3
Health and Wellbeing (CCG) 38
Health Authorities Act 1995 42
health service governance
   clinical and quality matters 97–8
   corporate governance compared 6
   decision-making 97
   definition 1, 67, 370
   duties of PCT company secretary 60–1
   Foundation Trusts 103–5
   issues 67–82
   levels of operation 4
   poor quality 67–9, 70
   probity and transparency 98
   and reporting 210–18
   stakeholders specific to 76
   strategy 97
   theoretical frameworks 71–5
   see also corporate governance; governance
health service governance codes 85–92
   case examples 91–2
   FT Code of Governance (2010) 85, 87–9, 292–308
   Healthy NHS Board: principles of good governance (2010) 85, 89–90, 141
   Integrated Governance Handbook (2006) 53, 58, 59, 85, 86–7, 126
   Intelligent Board (2006) 85, 165
   Intelligent Board – Modernising Mental Health Services (2007) 85
   Nolan Principles 18–19, 85
   Taking it on Trust (2009) 85, 90
   see also health service governance
Health Services Act 1980 42
Healthcare Commission 115
healthcare law, UK 42–8
HealthWatch Committees 36
Healthwatch England (CCG) 38

Healthy NHS Board: principles of good governance (2010) 85, 89–90, 141
Heart of England NHS Foundation Trust 35, 247
Higgs Report (2003) 16, 92, 370
honesty 19, 95
Hospitality Policy 182–6
  acceptable hospitality 183
  Bribery Act 2010 183–4
  gifts, acceptance 183
Hutton Review of Fair Pay in public sector (2011) 189, 192–3
hybrid organisations 118

incentives, performance-related 195, 197, 206
independence
  audit committees 354–6
  auditors 235
    external 227–8
    internal 266–7
  chairman 141–2
  company secretary 57–8
  directors 134
  non-executive directors 149–50
Independent Commission for Good Governance in Public Service 19–21
induction
  audit committee members 233
  definition 371
  of new directors 172–3
  and training 172–5, 233
information 14–15
in-house lawyer, and company secretary 59
insider dealing 50, 371
insolvency law 49
Institute of Chartered Accountants in England and Wales (ICAEW) 228, 267
institutional investor 371
integrated approach 79
Integrated Governance Handbook (2006) 53, 58, 59, 85, 86–7, 126
integrity 19
Intelligent Board (2006) 85, 165
Intelligent Board – Modernising Mental Health Services (2007) 85
internal audit 265–7
  audit committees 353
  definition 371
  function and scope 220–1, 265–6
  investigation of internal financial controls 266
  objectivity and independence of internal auditors 266–7
  reliance on work of 222
  review of effectiveness of function 267
internal control risk 246–7, 371
internal control systems 253–74
  case examples 257–8
  definition 371
  elements 253–9
  purpose 255
  review of effectiveness 364–5
  sound, maintaining 363–4
internal controls
  annual governance statement (AGS) 262–5
  assessing effectiveness of risk and control processes 366–7
  audit committees 352
  board statement 365–6

compliance 256
control environment 258
definition 371
emergency preparedness and business continuity 267–8
financial 255–6
FT Code of Governance (2010) 305
groups of companies 362
importance 361–7
investigation of financial controls 266
operational 256
purpose 255
review of effectiveness 261–2
risk categories 254
Turnbull Guidance 92, 255, 260–2, 361–7, 375
UK Code 55, 261, 282
UK corporate governance framework 259–60
and whistleblowing 269–70
see also internal audit; internal control systems
International Corporate Governance Network (ICGN) 18, 371
International Federation of Accountants (IFAC) 227

justice 95

Kay, John 8–9
King Code (King Report and King III, 2009) 17, 81, 93–4, 141, 371
Kraft, takeover of Cadbury 5

law
  company 49–51
  compulsory regulation and voluntary best practice 51–2
  'duty to consult' legislation 47–8
  financial markets and services 49–50
  and governance 41–2
  insolvency 49
  UK healthcare 42–8
  see also specific Acts
lead governor 107, 371
leadership
  board, role of 276
  chairman 277
  division of responsibilities 277
  governance as leadership approach 82
  King Code 93
  Nolan Principles 19
  non-executive directors (NEDs) 277–8
  UK Code 275, 276–8
Leeson, Nick 132
Lehman Brothers 16, 227
Levitt, Arthur 69
liability of directors 136–8
liquidity risk 246
Listing Rules 289
Local Authority Overview and Scrutiny Committees 48
Local Government and Public Involvement in Health Act 2007 43, 47, 48
Local Involvement Network Regulations 2008 48
Local Involvement Networks (Duty of Service Providers to Allow Entry) Regulations 2008 48
Local Involvement Networks (LINks) 35–6, 48, 79
loyalties, conflict of 181

Maidstone and Tunbridge Wells NHS Trust, review into board leadership 90, 91
majority shareholders 371
management, and governance 7
management boards 126, 371
Mapping the Gap (ICSA research project) 97, 161
Marks & Spencer 143
Maxwell Corporation 69
Medicines and Healthcare Products Regulatory Agency 34
meetings
  audit committees 233, 350
  board of directors 59, 158
Mid Staffordshire NHS Foundation Trust, failures in patient care 90
Mid-Staffordshire NHS Foundation Trust Public Inquiry (2010) 68
Mills, Cliff 117
minority shareholders 8, 371
model articles of association 128–9, 371
Model Code 372
Model Publication Scheme for NHS organisations 45–6
modified audit reports 372
money laundering 50, 372
Monitor (regulator of Foundation Trusts) 12, 34, 39, 100, 101, 102, 212, 372
  Compliance Framework 110
  Model Core Constitution 104
  Quality Governance Framework 214
Monitor *Audit Code for NHS Foundation Trusts* 222
Moore, Roger 86
moral hazard 72
Moyes, Bill 144
mutual organisations 117, 372
Myners Report (2002) 15, 155, 372

Nadir, Asil 143
National Association of Pension Funds (NAPF) 16, 78, 207
  Corporate Governance Policy and Voting Guidelines 2011 142
National Audit Office (NAO) 263
National Council of Voluntary Organisations (NCVO) 22
National Health Service Act 1977 42, 43
National Health Service Act 2006 43, 47, 87, 100, 101, 107, 111
National Health Service and Community Care Act 1990 42
National Health Service (NHS) 26–40
  appointments to boards in 163–4
  board of directors 311–24
  Constitution *see* NHS Constitution for England
  creation 3
  definitions 3–4
  history/context 26–7
  principles 27
  stakeholders, relationships with 35–6
  Statement of Accountability 31–4
  values 27–8
National Health Service Reform and Health Care Professions Act 2002 43
National Institute for Health and Clinical Excellence (NICE) 29, 34
National Quality Board 211

NEDs *see* non-executive directors (NEDs)
New York Stock Exchange (NYSE) 17
NHS *see* National Health Service (NHS)
NHS Act 1948 3
NHS Act 1977 34
NHS Appointment Commission, *Code of Conduct and Accountability* 96, 138–9, 180
NHS Blood and Transplant Authority 34
NHS Choices (website) 215
NHS Commissioning Board 38
NHS Constitution for England
  approved treatments, drugs and programmes (NHS Constitution) 29
  background 3–4
  confidentiality 29
  consent 29
  definition of 'RIGHTS' 29–30
  definitions/purpose 26
  informed choice 30
  involvement in one's own healthcare and NHS 30
  quality of care 29
  redress, rights of 30
  renewal 26
  respect 29
  rights and privileges provided by 28–30
  transparency 9
NHS Foundation Trust Code of Governance (2010) *see FT Code of Governance* (2010)
NHS Plan 2000 42
NHS Reorganisation Act 1973 42
NHS trust boards 124–5
NHS Trust Development Agency 38
NHS Trusts (Membership and Procedures) Regulations 1990 42
Nolan Standards in Public Life 9
  Principles 18–19, 85
nomination committees 144, 165–70
  accepting offer of appointment as non-executive director 169–70
  appointment criteria 167
  definition 372
  main duties 166–7
  new directors, talent pool 168–9
  terms of engagement 170
  time commitment 167–8
non-audit work 228–9, 235–6, 372
non-departmental public bodies (NDPBs) 18
non-executive directors (NEDs)
  accepting offer of appointment, by nomination committee 169–70
  appointment or removal 108
  board committees 151, 153
  boards of governors, Foundation Trusts 108
  company-stakeholder relations 13
  compared to executive 151–2
  criteria for judging independence 150
  criticisms 153–5
    decision-making delays 155
    insufficient knowledge 154
    overriding influence of executive directors 154–5
    time constraints 154, 338
  definition of role 77, 372
  duties of PCT company secretary in relation to 61
  FRC Guidance 148
  independence 149–50
  leadership 277–8

Myners Report (2002) 15, 155, 372
  remuneration 108, 200–1
  role 147, 343–4
  serving, independence of 151
  supervisory boards 127
  UK Code 148
  Walker Report on role in banks 148–9
non-malificence 95
Northern Rock bank 16
Nursing and Midwifery Council 34

objectivity 19
OECD Principles of Corporate Governance 17, 71, 93, 372
Office for Public Management (OPM) 19
Office of the Information Commissioner 44
Ombudsman, Parliamentary and Health Service 36
openness *see* transparency
Operating Framework (OF) 215
operational controls 256
operational risks 14, 254, 372
opportunism 74–5
overview and scrutiny committees (OSCs) 36, 42–3, 60

Parliamentary and Health Service Ombudsman 36
Parmalat 10, 69
partnerships, effective governance 325–6
Patients and Public Involvement Forum (PPIF) 48, 60
'Patients' Forums' 43
performance evaluation of board 175–80
  board committees 178
  chairman 178–9
  FT Code of Governance (2010) 301–2
  individual board members 178
  problems with performance reviews 179–80
  requirement for annual evaluation 175–6
  UK Code requirements 176
  using results of review 179
performance reporting 215
performance-related remuneration
  design 196–8
  longer-term incentives 197, 206
  short-term incentives 197
  UK Code 287
personal ethics 95
pluralist (stakeholder) approach 80
policy governance theory 75, 81–2, 372
political scrutiny 9
Polly Peck 143
postcode lottery 372
premium listing 50, 372
primary care 31, 372
primary care trusts (PCTs)
  company secretary, core duties 59–61
  definition 372
  identity 61
  seal 61
  Statement of Accountability (NHS) 31–2
principles-based code of governance 372–3
professional ethics 95
professional regulators 34
public, duty to involve and report to 35
public benefit corporations 87, 99, 373

public opinion 9
public sector governance 18–21
  definition 1
  Good Governance Standard for Public Service 19–21
  Nolan Principles 18–19, 85
  state-owned industries, emerging countries 21

qualified opinion, audit reports 223
Quality Account 373
quality boardroom practice 157–9
quality governance 210–14, 373
  formal partnerships 325–6
  NHS boards 311–24
  operating constructively in health and social care system 324–5
  principles 8–9, 309–40
  system governance 324–6
Quality Governance Framework (Monitor) 214
quality reporting
  and Foundation Trusts 212–14
  FT Code of Governance (2010) 304–5
  and quality governance 210–14

Rank Xerox 10
'Real Involvement: working with people to improve health services' (DH) 47
red top notices 205
regional health authorities (RHAs) 42
Register of Interest 182
registers, statutory 60
regulation
  compulsory 51–2
  duties of PCT company secretary 60
  Foundation Trusts (NHS) 101–3
  regulators 9, 32–4
  regulatory framework 83–98
  voluntary governance frameworks 83–4
related party transactions 136, 373
remuneration 187–208
  audit committee members 233, 351, 354
  base pay and bonuses 206–7
  chairman (Foundation Trusts) 108
  directors *see* directors' remuneration
  failure, rewards for 189–90
  as governance issue 187–93
  guidance 205–7
  Hutton Review (2011) 189, 192–3
  performance-related *see* performance-related remuneration
  public attitudes 189–90
  senior executive 193–4
  UK Code see under UK Corporate Governance Code 2010
remuneration committees 198–200
  consultation with chairman/CEO regarding executive remuneration 199
  definition 373
  and guidance 206
  principle duties 199–200
  UK Code requirements 198–9
reporting 211–40
  accountability 217–18
  annual report and accounts 60
  audit reports *see* audit reports
  business review 238–9
  directors' remuneration 204–5

directors' report 14, 369
financial *see* financial reporting
FT Code of Governance (2010) 304–5
governance arrangements, disclosure 238
and health service governance 210–18
management reports to audit committee 262
performance 215
public, duty to report to 35
quality 210–14
sustainability report 375
transparency 217–18
UK Code 55
see also auditing; *specific reports, such as Myners Report (2002)*
reports, quality 211
reputation risk 21, 246, 373
resignation of directors 300
responsibilities
auditor independence 235
definitions 373
division of 277
quality corporate governance 9
risk management 247–8
risk appetite 244–5, 373
risk assessment 251, 373
risk capacity 244, 373
risk committees 248, 373
risk management
audit committees 352
control and review 251
and corporate governance 14
definition 373
effective systems 250–1
and governance 243–4
importance 361
policies, systems and procedures 249–51
quality governance 315–16
responsibilities for 247–8
UK Code 282
see also internal control systems; internal controls; risks
risk management committees 373
risk officers 249
risk register 251
risk tolerance 244–5, 373
RiskMetrics 18
risks 243–52
business *see* business risks
business environment 246
categories of internal control 254
competition 246
compliance 94, 254
evaluation 250
financial 14, 246, 254, 370
liquidity 246
measures 250
nature of 245
operational 14, 254, 372
reputation 21, 246, 373
strategic 246, 374
upside 245, 375
see also risk appetite; risk management; risk management committees; risk officers; risk register; risk tolerance
Rose, Sir Stuart 143
Royal Bank of Scotland 16
Ryan, William 75

safe harbour provisions 238, 373
Sarbanes-Oxley Act (SOX) 2002, US 17, 49, 51, 374
secondary care 31, 374
secret profits 130, 374
selflessness 18
Sema 56–7
senior executive
remuneration 193–4
replacement 368
senior independent director (SID) 78, 152–3, 342, 374
severance payments 190, 202–3, 374
share options 13, 374
shareholders/shareholder relations
AGM, constructive use 286
audit committees 357–8
board of directors 347
dialogue with shareholders 285–6
enlightened shareholder approach 80–1, 93, 370
FT Code of Governance (2010) 307–8
minority shareholders 8, 371
shareholder value approach 79–80, 374
UK Code 55, 276, 285–6
Sharman Panel of Enquiry 219
Shipman, Harold 68
skill and care, duty of 130–2, 370
Slipman, Sue 118
Sonnenfeld, Jeffrey 160
special health authorities 34
stakeholders 76–9
and board of directors 77–8
company-stakeholder relations 13
definition 5, 374
duties of PCT company secretary in relation to 60
and employees 78
and general public 78–9
governance, approaches to 79–82
influence of other 77–9
and NHS 35–6
and representative bodies 78
specific to corporate governance 76–7
specific to health service governance 76
stakeholder approach 79, 80, 374
stakeholder theory 71, 374
and suppliers 78
standing orders, duties of PCT company secretary 60
Statement of Accountability (NHS) 31–4
Statement of Internal Control (SIC) *see* annual governance statement (AGS)
Board Assurance Framework 264–5
required elements to support 263
weaknesses, disclosure 264
statutory duties of directors
to act within powers 133
and common law duties 130
conflicts of interest, avoiding 134–5
corporate governance 17
to declare interests in proposed transactions 135
definition 374
to exercise independent judgement 134
to exercise reasonable care, skill and diligence 134
NHS Code of Conduct and Accountability 139
non-acceptance of third party benefits 135
organisation outsiders, responsibilities to 135–6
to promote success of organisation 133–4
related party transactions 136

UK Disclosure and Transparency Rules (DTR) for listed companies 136
  see also duties of directors
statutory returns, duties of PCT company secretary 60
stewardship theory 73, 374
Stout, David 188
Strategic Health Authorities (SHAs) 33, 34, 374
strategic risk 246, 374
strategy, health service governance 97
stress testing 251, 374
succession planning 166, 170–1, 345–6, 374
supervisory boards 126, 127, 374
sustainability 93, 374
sustainability report 170, 375

Taking it on Trust (2009) 85, 90
Taylor, Barbara 75
terms of engagement 170
theoretical frameworks, health service governance 71–5
third party benefits, duty of directors not to accept 135
time considerations
  nomination committees 167–8
  non-executive directors 154, 338
total shareholder returns 9, 375
training
  audit committee members 233
  directors 172–5
  and professional development 174–5
  risk 249
transaction cost theory 73–5, 375
transparency
  definition 375
  health service governance 98
  Nolan Principles 19
  quality corporate governance 9
  reporting 217–18
  see also accountability
Tuckey, Andrew 132
Turnbull Guidance on internal control 92, 255, 260–2, 361–7
  definitions/purpose 375
  importance of internal controls 361
  maintaining sound systems 261
  management reports to audit committee 262
  review of effectiveness 261–2
two-tier boards 126–7, 375
  criticisms 127–8
Tyson Report on Recruitment and Development of Non-Executive Directors (2003) 168

UK Corporate Governance Code 2010 (*UK Code*) 92–3, 275–91
  accountability 217, 275, 282–4
  auditing 55
  background 16
  board of directors, responsibilities under 123–4
  chairman 140
  description 375
  disclosure requirements 55, 287–91
  effectiveness 275, 278–81
  going concern statement 219
  internal controls 55, 261, 282
  leadership 275, 276–8
  main principles 275–6
  non-executive directors (NEDs) 148
  performance review 176, 179
  remuneration 54, 284–5
    committee, requirements for 198–9
    design of packages 196–7
    guidance 206
    main principles 276
    non-executive directors (NEDs) 201
    performance-related 197, 287
    severance payments 203
    short-term incentives 197
  reporting 55
  risk training 249
  shareholder relations 55, 276, 285–6
  specific responsibilities derived from 53–5
  whistleblowing 269
UK Disclosure and Transparency Rules (DTR) 50, 136, 288–9, 369
UK Listing Authority Rules 50
UK Listing Rules 50, 375
ultra vires acts 137, 375
unitary boards 7, 126, 375
United States (US)
  business code of ethics 96
  Committee of Sponsoring Organizations of the Treadway Commission 254, 258
  Sarbanes-Oxley Act (SOX) 2002 17, 49, 51, 374
University College London Hospital NHS Foundation Trust 214
upside risk 245, 375

Vandevelde, Luc 143
variable pay 195, 375
Very Senior Managers (VSM) Pay Framework 13, 189, 191
voluntary best practice, and compulsory regulation 51–2
voluntary sector, and governance 23–4
  advantages of voluntary system 52
  voluntary codes of governance 375
  voluntary governance frameworks 83–4

Walker, Sir David 16
Walker Report (2009) 16, 128, 148–9, 159, 249, 375
whistleblowing
  audit committees 353
  best practice 270–1
  and Bribery Act 2010 272
  case example 12
  definition 375
  and Enron 11
  and internal controls 269–70
  internal procedures for allegations 271–2
  procedures 269–72
window dressing of accounts 10, 57, 217, 375
WorldCom 10, 230
wrongful trading 132, 375
Wyman, Peter 230

ASTRONOMICAL SOCIETY OF THE PACIFIC
CONFERENCE SERIES

Volume 450

MOLECULES IN THE ATMOSPHERES OF EXTRASOLAR PLANETS

Proceedings of a conference held at
Observatoire de Paris, Paris, France
19–21 November 2008

Edited by

Jean Philippe Beaulieu
UPMC Univ Paris 06, UMR7095, Institut d'Astrophysique de Paris, F-75014, Paris, France

Stefan Dieters
School Maths and Physics, University Tasmania, Hobart, Tasmania, Australia

Giovanna Tinetti
Department Physics and Astronomy, University College London, London, UK

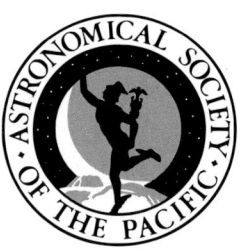

SAN FRANCISCO

ASTRONOMICAL SOCIETY OF THE PACIFIC
390 Ashton Avenue
San Francisco, California, 94112-1722, USA

Phone: 415-337-1100
Fax: 415-337-5205
E-mail: service@astrosociety.org
Web site: www.astrosociety.org
E-books: www.aspbooks.org

First Edition
© 2011 by Astronomical Society of the Pacific
ASP Conference Series
All rights reserved.

No part of the material protected by this copyright notice may be reproduced or utilized in any form or by any means—graphic, electronic, or mechanical, including photocopying, taping, recording, or by any information storage and retrieval system—without written permission from the Astronomical Society of the Pacific.

ISBN: 978-1-58381-782-7
e-book ISBN: 978-1-58381-783-4

Library of Congress (LOC) Cataloging in Publication (CIP) Data:
Main entry under title
Library of Congress Control Number (LCCN): 2011940728

Printed in the United States of America by Sheridan Books, Ann Arbor, Michigan.
This book is printed on acid-free paper.